DISEASE MANAGEMENT
SOURCEBOOK
FOURTH EDITION

Health Reference Series

DISEASE MANAGEMENT
SOURCEBOOK
FOURTH EDITION

Basic Consumer Health Information about Coping with Chronic and Serious Illnesses, Navigating the Medical System, Communicating with Health-Care Providers, Evaluating Health-Care Quality, and Making Informed Decisions, Including Facts about Second Opinions, Hospitalization, Surgery, and Medications

Along with Information about Legal, Financial, and Insurance Issues, a Glossary of Related Terms, and Directories of Additional Resources

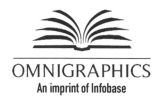

OMNIGRAPHICS
An imprint of Infobase

Bibliographic Note

Because this page cannot legibly accommodate all the copyright notices, the Bibliographic Note portion of the Preface constitutes an extension of the copyright notice.

* * *

OMNIGRAPHICS
An imprint of Infobase
8 The Green
Suite 19225
Dover, DE 19901
www.infobase.com
James Chambers, *Editorial Director*

* * *

Copyright © 2024 Infobase
ISBN 978-0-7808-2130-9
E-ISBN 978-0-7808-2131-6

Library of Congress Cataloging-in-Publication Data

Names: Chambers, James (Editor), editor.

Title: Disease management sourcebook / edited by James Chambers.

Description: Fourth edition. | Dover, DE: Omnigraphics, an imprint of Infobase, [2024] | Series: Health reference series | Includes index. | Summary: "Provides basic consumer health information on chronic diseases and their management, along with facts about health literacy, patient rights and responsibilities, medications, health-care technologies, and legal and financial aspects related to disease management. Includes an index, glossary of related terms, and other resources"-- Provided by publisher.

Identifiers: LCCN 2024007770 (print) | LCCN 2024007771 (ebook) | ISBN 9780780821309 | ISBN 9780780821316 (eISBN)

Subjects: LCSH: Chronic diseases--Treatment. | Consumer education.

Classification: LCC RC108.D58 2024 (print) | LCC RC108 (ebook) | DDC 616/.044--dc23/eng/20240327

LC record available at https://lccn.loc.gov/2024007770
LC ebook record available at https://lccn.loc.gov/2024007771

Electronic or mechanical reproduction, including photography, recording, or any other information storage and retrieval system for the purpose of resale is strictly prohibited without permission in writing from the publisher.

The information in this publication was compiled from the sources cited and from other sources considered reliable. While every possible effort has been made to ensure reliability, the publisher will not assume liability for damages caused by inaccuracies in the data, and makes no warranty, express or implied, on the accuracy of the information contained herein.

This book is printed on acid-free paper meeting the ANSI Z39.48 Standard. The infinity symbol that appears above indicates that the paper in this book meets that standard.

Printed in the United States

Table of Contents

Preface xi

Part 1. Introduction to Diseases
Chapter 1—Understanding Human Diseases 3
Chapter 2—Health and Economic Costs of
                Chronic Diseases 9
Chapter 3—Risk Factors for Preventable
                Chronic Diseases 13
Chapter 4—Family Health History 23
                Section 4.1—What Is Family Health History? 25
                Section 4.2—Family Health History and
                            Chronic Disease 26
Chapter 5—Preventing Chronic Diseases 39
Chapter 6—Common Screening and Diagnostic Tests 41
                Section 6.1—Screening Tests: What You Need
                            to Know 43
                Section 6.2—Screening Tests for Women 45
                Section 6.3—Screening Tests for Men 48
                Section 6.4—Laboratory-Developed Tests 51
                Section 6.5—Home-Use Tests 52
                Section 6.6—Direct-to-Consumer Genetic
                            Testing 55
                Section 6.7—Biomarkers 60
Chapter 7—After Your Diagnosis: Getting Support 67

Part 2. Treatment and Management of Common Diseases
Chapter 8—Respiratory Diseases 73
Chapter 9—Cardiovascular Diseases 81

Chapter 10—Gastrointestinal Diseases 99
Chapter 11—Muscle and Bone Diseases 111
Chapter 12—Urinary System Diseases 123
Chapter 13—Nervous System Diseases 133
Chapter 14—Immune System Diseases 157

Part 3. Working with Health-Care Providers and the Health-Care System
Chapter 15—Choosing Your Doctor 169
Chapter 16—Talking with Your Health-Care Provider
 before Making Decisions...175
   Section 16.1—Why Being Able to Talk with
    Your Doctor Matters............................177
   Section 16.2—How to Prepare for a Doctor's
    Appointment 179
   Section 16.3—Make the Most of Your Time at the
    Doctor's Office......................................183
   Section 16.4—Be More Involved in Your
    Health Care..187
Chapter 17—Making Decisions with Your Doctor 189
Chapter 18—Seeking Out Information 193
Chapter 19—Getting a Second Opinion..197
Chapter 20—Selecting a Complementary and Alternative
 Medicine Practitioner 201
Chapter 21—Health-Care Quality Issues 209
   Section 21.1—Understanding Health-Care
    Quality..211
   Section 21.2—Identifying Quality Laboratory
    Services..218
   Section 21.3—Patient Safety in Ambulatory
    Care..224
Chapter 22—Hospitalization..229
   Section 22.1—Choosing a Hospital 231
   Section 22.2—Medicare and Hospital Expenses.......234
   Section 22.3—Caregivers and Their Role during
    a Hospital Stay......................................238

Chapter 23—Surgery 245
    Section 23.1—What You Need to Know about
                    Surgery 247
    Section 23.2—Anesthesia Basics 249
    Section 23.3—Robotic Interventions........................252
    Section 23.4—Wrong-Site, Wrong-Procedure,
                    and Wrong-Patient Surgery...............257

Part 4. Health Literacy and Making Informed Health Decisions
Chapter 24—Understanding Health Literacy 261
Chapter 25—eHealth Literacy..265
Chapter 26—Health Communication and Technology..................269
Chapter 27—Patient Rights and Responsibilities...........................275
    Section 27.1—Health-Care Rights and
                    Responsibilities...................................277
    Section 27.2—Health Information Privacy
                    Rights...281
    Section 27.3—How to Keep Your Health
                    Information Private and Secure 287
Chapter 28—Personal Health Records and Patient Portals 291
Chapter 29—Making Sense of Internet Health Information 293
Chapter 30—Informed Consent 299
Chapter 31—Preventing Medical Errors 305
Chapter 32—Health-Care Fraud Scams 309
Chapter 33—Medical Identity Theft 313

Part 5. Prescription and Over-the-Counter Medications
Chapter 34—Understanding Medications 319
    Section 34.1—About Medication and
                    Their Categories 321
    Section 34.2—Medicine's Life inside the Body.........327
    Section 34.3—Pharmacogenomics 329
    Section 34.4—As You Age: You and Your
                    Medications 333
Chapter 35—Using Medications Safely 341
Chapter 36—Over-the-Counter Medicines 349

Chapter 37—Buying Prescription Drugs..355
    Section 37.1—Using Your Health Insurance
                           Coverage for Getting Prescription
                           Medications 357
    Section 37.2—Cost May Result in Underuse of
                           Medications 359
    Section 37.3—E-prescribing 361
    Section 37.4—Safely Purchase Prescription
                           Medicine Online 362
    Section 37.5—Truth in Advertising:
                           Advertisements for
                           Prescription Drugs..............................364
    Section 37.6—Imported Drugs Raise Safety
                           Concerns 367
Chapter 38—Generic Drugs..375
Chapter 39—Other Types of Drugs 383
    Section 39.1—Biosimilars 385
    Section 39.2—Precision Medicine 387
Chapter 40—Taking Medicine 393
    Section 40.1—Tips for Taking Medications.............395
    Section 40.2—Know When Antibiotics
                           Work 396
    Section 40.3—Kids Are Not Just Small
                           Adults: Advice on Giving
                           Medicine to Your Child......................399
Chapter 41—Adverse Drug Reactions..403
Chapter 42—Drug Interactions: What You Should Know............407
Chapter 43—Preventing Medication Errors 411
Chapter 44—Unapproved, Counterfeit, and Misused Drugs 417
    Section 44.1—Unapproved Drugs and
                           Counterfeit Drugs...............................419
    Section 44.2—Misuse of Prescription
                           Pain Relievers 424

Part 6. Managing Chronic Disease

Chapter 45—Self-Management of Chronic Illness 429
        Section 45.1—Take Charge of Your Health 431
        Section 45.2—Adopt a Healthy Eating Plan 433
        Section 45.3—Stress and Your Health 438
        Section 45.4—Exercise Can Improve Some Chronic Disease Conditions 442
        Section 45.5—Tips for Dealing with Pain 448
        Section 45.6—The Health Benefits of Having Pets 450
Chapter 46—Caring for Children 453
        Section 46.1—Children's Health 455
        Section 46.2—Developmental and Behavioral Screening Tests 456
        Section 46.3—Vaccines for Children 460
        Section 46.4—Caring for a Seriously Ill Child 473
Chapter 47—Preventing Infection at Home and Work 481
Chapter 48—Chronic Illness and Depression 487
Chapter 49—Technologies in Disease Management 493
        Section 49.1—Rehabilitative and Assistive Technology 495
        Section 49.2—Artificial Pancreas 499
        Section 49.3—Artificial Intelligence 504
        Section 49.4—Biosensors and Biomaterials 507
Chapter 50—Preventive Care Services 511
Chapter 51—Palliative and Hospice Care 515

Part 7. Legal, Financial, and Insurance Aspects of Disease Management

Chapter 52—The Americans with Disabilities Act 523
Chapter 53—The Family and Medical Leave Act 531
Chapter 54—Advance Directives 537
Chapter 55—Legal and Financial Planning for People with Chronic Disease 545

Chapter 56—Health-Care Benefit Laws 551
Chapter 57—Medicaid and Hill-Burton Free and
             Reduced-Cost Health Care 557
             Section 57.1—Medicaid..559
             Section 57.2—Hill-Burton Free and
                          Reduced-Cost Health Care.................562
Chapter 58—Paying for Complementary and Integrative
             Health Approaches..567
Chapter 59—Medicare's Preventive Services 571
Chapter 60—Medicare Coverage of Home Health Care 579
Chapter 61—Health Savings Account: Eligible Plans.....................587
Chapter 62—Medical Discount Plans: Service or Scam? 591
Chapter 63—Low-Cost or Free Health Insurance
             for Children...599
Chapter 64—Things to Know before You Pick a
             Health Insurance Plan 601
Chapter 65—Filing a Claim for Your Health or
             Disability Benefits 609

Part 8. Additional Help and Information
Chapter 66—Glossary of Disease Management Terms 621
Chapter 67—Resources for Information about Disease
             Management 627

Index 637

Preface

ABOUT THIS BOOK

Making informed health-care decisions is vital for everyone, especially those living with chronic illnesses such as cardiovascular disease, diabetes, and cancer. According to the Centers for Disease Control and Prevention (CDC), about 6 in 10 people in the United States have a chronic disease, and 4 in 10 have two or more chronic diseases. Health literacy is crucial for individuals to make informed decisions about their health and well-being. Limited health literacy has been linked to poor health outcomes, including higher rates of morbidity and mortality, which are associated with higher health-care costs.

Disease Management Sourcebook, Fourth Edition addresses these concerns by providing a basic understanding of chronic diseases along with tips for treating and managing them. It also offers guidance on navigating the health-care system, communicating with health-care providers, and finding and evaluating health information. The book covers the importance of health literacy, patient rights and responsibilities, privacy, medical errors, and health-care scams. It includes information about medications—prescription, generic, over-the-counter, and counterfeit drugs. Additionally, it explains assistive technologies available to help people with chronic illnesses and provides tips for dealing with legal, financial, and health-insurance matters. The concluding chapter features a glossary and directories of resources for patients, their families, and caregivers.

HOW TO USE THIS BOOK

This book is divided into parts and chapters. Parts focus on broad areas of interest. Chapters are devoted to single topics within a part.

Part 1: Introduction to Diseases presents presents an overview of chronic diseases in the United States. It includes information about family health history, risk factors for chronic disease, and symptoms that may indicate serious health conditions or medical emergencies. It describes common screening and diagnostic tests and offers tips for finding support after receiving a diagnosis.

Part 2: Treatment and Management of Common Diseases discusses the treatment and management of the most common diseases of the respiratory system, cardiovascular system, musculoskeletal system, urinary system, nervous system, and immune system. It also covers gastrointestinal (GI) diseases and the treatment and management options for some common conditions of the digestive system.

Part 3: Working with Health-Care Providers and the Health-Care System provides information about effective communication in a doctor's office or hospital setting. Topics include making decisions in consultation with the doctor, second opinions, complementary and alternative medicine, and laboratory services. It also includes basic information about choosing a hospital and undergoing surgery, and addresses issues related to health-care quality.

Part 4: Health Literacy and Making Informed Health Decisions discusses the skills essential for making knowledgeable health-care choices. Developments in health information technology are covered, along with insights into eHealth literacy. The part also discusses patients' rights and responsibilities, patient privacy rights, informed consent, medical errors, and health-care fraud.

Part 5: Prescription and Over-the-Counter Medications provides information about what medications do and how to use them safely. It discusses purchasing and using prescription, generic, and over-the-counter (OTC) drugs. It also covers buying prescription drugs online, adverse drug reactions, common drug interactions, counterfeit and misused drugs, and safety concerns with imported drugs.

Part 6: Managing Chronic Disease offers guidelines for self-management practices such as healthy eating plans, physical activity, and relaxation techniques. Along with tips for dealing with pain, stress, and depression, it provides information about infection prevention, assistive technology, and preventive care. The part concludes with options for palliative and hospice care for individuals with chronic diseases.

Part 7: Legal, Financial, and Insurance Aspects of Disease Management includes information about the Americans with Disabilities Act (ADA), the Family and Medical Leave Act (FMLA), and health-care benefit laws. It describes advance directives and explains how to access free or reduced-cost health care. It also includes information on health insurance and provides guidelines for paying for complementary health approaches, preventive services, and home health care. Additionally, it discusses topics such as health savings accounts, medical discount plans, and the insurance claim process.

Part 8: Additional Help and Information includes a glossary of related terms and directories of resources for information about disease management, health insurance, and financial assistance for medical treatments.

BIBLIOGRAPHIC NOTE

This volume contains documents and excerpts from publications issued by the following U.S. government agencies: ADA.gov; Agency for Healthcare Research and Quality (AHRQ); Centers for Disease Control and Prevention (CDC); Centers for Medicare & Medicaid Services (CMS); *Eunice Kennedy Shriver* National Institute of Child Health and Human Development (NICHD); Federal Trade Commission (FTC); Health Resources and Services Administration (HRSA); HealthIT.gov; HIV.gov; MedlinePlus; National Cancer Institute (NCI); National Center for Chronic Disease Prevention and Health Promotion (NCCDPHP); National Center for Complementary and Integrative Health (NCCIH); National Center on Birth Defects and Developmental Disabilities (NCBDDD); National Heart, Lung, and Blood Institute (NHLBI); National Human Genome Research Institute (NHGRI); National Institute of Arthritis and Musculoskeletal and Skin Diseases (NIAMS); National Institute of Biomedical Imaging and Bioengineering (NIBIB); National Institute of Diabetes and Digestive and Kidney Diseases (NIDDK); National Institute of Environmental Health Sciences (NIEHS); National Institute of General Medical Sciences (NIGMS); National Institute of Mental Health (NIMH); National Institute of Neurological Disorders and Stroke (NINDS); National Institute on Aging (NIA); *NIH News in Health*; Office of Disease Prevention and Health Promotion (ODPHP); Surveillance, Epidemiology, and End Results (SEER) Program; U.S. Department of Health and Human Services (HHS); U.S. Department of Labor (DOL); and U.S. Food and Drug Administration (FDA).

ABOUT THE *HEALTH REFERENCE SERIES*

The *Health Reference Series* is designed to provide basic medical information for patients, families, caregivers, and the general public. Each volume provides comprehensive coverage on a particular topic. This is especially important for people who may be dealing with a newly diagnosed disease or a chronic disorder in themselves or in a family member. People looking for preventive guidance, information about disease warning signs, medical statistics, and risk factors for health problems will also find answers to their questions in the *Health Reference Series*. The *Series*, however, is not intended to serve as a tool for diagnosing illness, in prescribing treatments, or as a substitute for the physician-patient relationship. All people concerned about medical symptoms or the possibility of disease are encouraged to seek professional care from an appropriate health-care provider.

A NOTE ABOUT SPELLING AND STYLE

Health Reference Series editors use *Stedman's Medical Dictionary* as an authority for questions related to the spelling of medical terms and *The Chicago Manual of Style* for questions related to grammatical structures, punctuation, and other editorial concerns. Consistent adherence is not always possible, however, because the individual volumes within the *Series* include many documents from a wide variety of different producers, and the editor's primary goal is to present material from each source as accurately as is possible. This sometimes means that information in different chapters or sections may follow other guidelines and alternate spelling authorities. For example, occasionally a copyright holder may require that eponymous terms be shown in possessive forms (Crohn's disease vs. Crohn disease) or that British spelling norms be retained (leukaemia vs. leukemia).

HEALTH REFERENCE SERIES UPDATE POLICY

The inaugural book in the *Health Reference Series* was the first edition of *Cancer Sourcebook* published in 1989. Since then, the *Series* has been enthusiastically received by librarians and in the medical community. In order to maintain the standard of providing high-quality health information for the layperson, the editorial staff felt it was necessary to implement a policy of updating volumes when warranted.

Medical researchers have been making tremendous strides, and it is the purpose of the *Health Reference Series* to stay current with the most recent advances. Each decision to update a volume is made on an individual basis. Some of the considerations include how much new information is available and the feedback we receive from people who use the books. If there is a topic you would like to see added to the update list, or an area of medical concern you feel has not been adequately addressed, please write to: custserv@infobaselearning.com.

Part 1 | Introduction to Diseases

Chapter 1 | Understanding Human Diseases

Diseases are pathological conditions that impair the regular structure or functioning of the body, organs, or systems, identified by signs and symptoms. Human diseases manifest in various forms, causing symptoms that range from slight discomfort to severe sickness. These conditions harm individuals physically, intellectually, and emotionally. Diseases arise from diverse sources, including infectious agents (bacteria, viruses, fungi, and parasites), genetic mutations, environmental influences (diet, exercise, and substance addiction), and underlying disorders.

CLASSIFICATION OF DISEASES
Diseases are classified based on location, organs affected, nature, and causes. Classifications include the following:
- **Topographical**. These are diseases classified based on their location within the body, such as the central nervous system (CNS), cardiovascular system, respiratory system, and so on.
- **Anatomical**. This classification is determined by the specific tissues or organs affected by a particular condition, such as the heart, lungs, liver, kidney, muscles, or joints.
- **Physiological**. These diseases are classified based on improper functioning of the organs, such as diabetes, asthma, glaucoma, and so on.
- **Pathological**. These diseases are categorized based on their nature, such as neoplastic diseases (tumors) and inflammatory diseases.

- **Etiological.** These are diseases classified based on their cause or origin, including infectious diseases, genetic disorders, immune system dysregulation, and metabolic disruptions.
- **Jurisdictional.** These are diseases classified based on legal or administrative borders, mortality locations, and jurisdiction-specific factors.
- **Epidemiological.** These diseases are categorized based on occurrence patterns, distribution, age, socioeconomic status, geography, and risk within a defined population.

CAUSES OF DISEASE TRANSMISSION IN HUMANS

Human disease transmission occurs through various paths, influenced by the type of illness, environmental conditions, human behavior, and vectors (disease-carrying insects). Transmission modes include the following:

- **Direct contact (communicable).** Direct contact with an infected individual is the most common mode of transmission involving physical contact, such as touching, sharing body fluids, or transmitting droplets by coughing or sneezing. Illnesses such as the common cold, influenza, and sexually transmitted infections (STIs) are transferred by direct contact.
- **Indirect contact (noncommunicable).** Pathogens can be transmitted by contact with infected surfaces, such as doorknobs, handrails, countertops, or faucets, where they can remain viable after exposure for a period of time, depending on the pathogen. When individuals are in contact with these contaminated surfaces and subsequently touch their eyes, nose, or mouth, they transfer the germs into their bodies, resulting in infection. Other aspects of transmission include airborne, foodborne, waterborne, environmental, and animal-to-person.
    - **Airborne transmission.** Infections transmitted through respiratory droplets may lead to

tuberculosis (TB), measles, influenza, and coronavirus disease 2019 (COVID-19).
- **Vector transmission.** Infections transmitted through vectors (mosquitoes, fleas, and ticks) may cause malaria, dengue, Zika, plague, and Lyme disease.
- **Food transmission.** Consuming contaminated food can result in illnesses caused by bacteria such as *Salmonella*, *Escherichia coli* (*E. coli*), *Listeria*, and *Campylobacter*.
- **Water transmission.** Contaminated water sources can lead to cholera, typhoid fever, and cryptosporidiosis.
- **Hospital-borne transmission.** Infections acquired within health-care settings include pneumonia, methicillin-resistant *Staphylococcus aureus* (MRSA), sepsis, and urinary tract infections (UTIs).

SIGNS AND SYMPTOMS OF HUMAN DISEASES
Manifestations of human diseases vary based on the disease, intensity, and affected organs. Common indicators include:
- breathing difficulty
- chills
- congestion
- coughing
- diarrhea
- fatigue
- fever
- inflammation
- pain
- sweats
- vomiting

DIAGNOSIS OF HUMAN DISEASES
Diagnosing diseases involves a multistep process:
- **Medical history.** Gathering information on current symptoms, concurrent or preexisting illnesses, family

history, lifestyle, and recent contacts with infected persons or infectious agents.
- **Clinical assessment.** Conducting a comprehensive physical examination, including vital signs, body system assessment, and identification of physical irregularities.
- **Laboratory tests.** Identifying abnormalities such as infections, inflammation, hormonal imbalances, nutritional inadequacies, and chemical compounds through blood tests, urine analysis, or examination of other body fluids.
- **Radiological examinations.** Using imaging modalities such as x-rays, computed tomography (CT) scans, magnetic resonance imaging (MRI), and ultrasound for detailed internal images of bones, organs, and tissues.
- **Sample testing.** Conducting biopsies (taking tissue samples for microscopic analysis) to detect cancer, infectious diseases, autoimmune disorders, or specific organ abnormalities.
- **Psychological assessments.** Evaluating intelligence, emotional issues, personality, and cognitive performance.

PREVENTION OF HUMAN DISEASES

Various strategies can be followed to prevent diseases, including the following:
- **Sanitary behavior.** Practice good hygiene and use protective measures during contact with an infected individual.
- **Medications.** Antibiotic, antiviral, antiparasitic, antifungal, and antiinflammatory drugs can help control symptoms and disease progression.
- **Vaccinations.** Vaccines safely train the body's immune system for specific diseases to enhance its natural defense mechanisms.
- **Lifestyle changes.** Follow a balanced diet, engage in regular physical activity, and limit alcohol consumption

to moderate levels (up to one drink per day for women and up to two drinks per day for men).
- **Exercise.** Maintain a healthy weight, strengthen muscles and bones, and reduce stress through regular physical activity.
- **Therapies.** Complementary and alternative therapies, such as acupuncture, chiropractic care, massage therapy, dietary supplements, yoga, tai chi, and meditation, may help reduce stress and increase fitness to lessen the risk of disease.

Understanding human diseases requires a complete approach involving the classification system, diagnosis, treatment, and prevention. This knowledge empowers individuals and health-care professionals in managing and easing the effects of diseases on society.

References

Burrows, William; and Scarpelli, Dante G. "Disease," Britannica, February 15, 2024. Available online. URL: www.britannica.com/science/disease. Accessed February 28, 2024.

Higuera, Valencia. "How Are Diseases Transmitted?" Healthline, September 23, 2022. Available online. URL: www.healthline.com/health/disease-transmission. Accessed February 28, 2024.

"Infection Prevention and Control," Physiopedia, December 4, 2023. Available online. URL: www.physiopedia.com/Infection_Prevention_and_Control. Accessed February 28, 2024.

Rakel, Robert Edwin. "Diagnosis," Britannica, January 11, 2024. Available online. URL: www.britannica.com/science/diagnosis. Accessed February 28, 2024.

Robbins, Stanley L.; Robbins, Jonathan H.; and Scarpelli, Dante G. "Classification of Diseases," Britannica, August 10, 2023. Available online. URL: www.britannica.

com/science/human-disease/Classifications-of-diseases.
Accessed February 28, 2024.

"Routes of Transmission: Acute and Communicable Disease," Oregon Health Authority, March 11, 2011. Available online. URL: www.oregon.gov/oha/ph/diseasesconditions/communicabledisease/pages/transmission.aspx. Accessed February 28, 2024.

Torrey, Trisha. "Overview of Disease Management," Verywell Health, May 25, 2023. Available online. URL: www.verywellhealth.com/disease-management-2615164. Accessed February 28, 2024.

Chapter 2 | Health and Economic Costs of Chronic Diseases

Chronic diseases are defined broadly as conditions that last one year or more and require ongoing medical attention or limit activities of daily living (ADLs) or both. Chronic diseases such as heart disease, cancer, and diabetes are the leading causes of death and disability in the United States.[1]

Chronic diseases have significant health and economic costs in the United States. Interventions to prevent and manage these diseases have significant health and economic benefits. The following are the economic costs of some common chronic conditions:

- **Heart disease and stroke**. Nothing kills more Americans than heart disease and stroke. More than 877,500 Americans die of heart disease or stroke every year—that is one-third of all deaths. These diseases take an economic toll, as well, costing our health-care system $216 billion per year and causing $147 billion in lost productivity on the job.
- **Cancer**. Each year in the United States, more than 1.7 million people are diagnosed with cancer, and almost 600,000 die from it, making it the second leading cause of death. The cost of cancer care continues to rise and is expected to reach more than $240 billion by 2030.

---

[1] National Center for Chronic Disease Prevention and Health Promotion (NCCDPHP), "About Chronic Diseases," Centers for Disease Control and Prevention (CDC), July 21, 2022. Available online. URL: www.cdc.gov/chronicdisease/about/index.htm. Accessed February 12, 2024.

- **Diabetes.** More than 37 million Americans have diabetes, and another 96 million adults in the United States have a condition called "prediabetes," which puts them at risk for type 2 diabetes. Diabetes can cause serious complications, including heart disease, kidney failure, and blindness. In 2017, the total estimated cost of diagnosed diabetes was $327 billion in medical costs and lost productivity.
- **Obesity.** This disease affects 20 percent of children and 42 percent of adults, putting them at risk of chronic diseases such as type 2 diabetes, heart disease, and some cancers. Over 25 percent of young people aged 17–24 are too heavy to join the U.S. military. Obesity costs the U.S. health-care system nearly $173 billion a year.
- **Arthritis.** This disease affects 58.5 million adults in the United States, which is about one in four adults. It is a leading cause of work disability in the United States, one of the most common chronic conditions, and a common cause of chronic pain. The total cost attributable to arthritis and related conditions was about $303.5 billion in 2013. Of this amount, nearly $140 billion was for medical costs and $164 billion was for indirect costs associated with lost earnings.
- **Alzheimer disease (AD).** AD, a type of dementia, is an irreversible, progressive brain disease that affects about 5.7 million Americans, including 1 in 10 adults aged 65 and older. It is the sixth leading cause of death among all adults and the fifth leading cause for those aged 65 or older. In 2020, the estimated cost of caring for and treating people with AD was $305 billion. By 2050, these costs are projected to be more than $1.1 trillion.
- **Epilepsy.** In the United States, about 3 million adults and 470,000 children and teens younger than the age of 18 have active epilepsy—meaning that they have been diagnosed by a doctor, had a recent seizure, or both. Adults with epilepsy report worse mental

Health and Economic Costs of Chronic Diseases

health, more cognitive impairment, and barriers in social participation compared to adults without epilepsy. In 2016, health-care spending for epilepsy was $8.6 billion in direct costs.
- **Tooth decay.** Cavities (also called "tooth decay") are one of the most common chronic diseases in the United States. One in six children aged 6–11 and one in four adults have untreated cavities. Untreated cavities can cause pain and infections that may lead to problems eating, speaking, and learning. On average, 34 million school hours are lost each year because of unplanned (emergency) dental care, and over $45 billion is lost in productivity due to dental disease.[2]

---

[2] National Center for Chronic Disease Prevention and Health Promotion (NCCDPHP), "Health and Economic Costs of Chronic Diseases," Centers for Disease Control and Prevention (CDC), March 23, 2023. Available online. URL: www.cdc.gov/chronicdisease/about/costs/index.htm. Accessed February 12, 2024.

Chapter 3 | Risk Factors for Preventable Chronic Diseases

Diseases or conditions that usually last for three months or longer and may get worse over time are called "chronic diseases." Chronic diseases tend to occur in older adults and can usually be controlled but not cured. The most common types of chronic diseases are cancer, heart disease, stroke, diabetes, and arthritis.

Many chronic diseases are caused by the following risk behaviors:
- tobacco use and exposure to secondhand smoke
- poor nutrition
- physical inactivity
- excessive alcohol use

TOBACCO USE
Commercial* tobacco use is the leading cause of preventable disease, disability, and death in the United States. Every day in the United States, about 1,600 young people under the age of 18 try their first cigarette, and nearly 200 end up smoking cigarettes daily.

Some groups of people have a higher percentage of tobacco use, secondhand smoke exposure, and related health problems, as well as less access to treatment to help them quit. These disparities can be based on where people live, the kind of job they have, whether they have health insurance, and factors such as race, ethnicity, age, or sexual orientation.

Refers to the use of commercial tobacco and not the sacred and traditional use of tobacco by some American-Indian communities.

Over 16 million people live with at least one disease caused by smoking, and smoking-related illnesses cost the United States more than $600 billion in 2018. Preventing people from starting tobacco use and helping tobacco-users to quit could reduce these costs.

The Centers for Disease Control and Prevention (CDC) and its partners work to reduce tobacco-related diseases and deaths by:
- preventing young people from using tobacco products
- helping people quit using tobacco products
- eliminating exposure to secondhand smoke
- advancing health equity by identifying and eliminating tobacco-related disparities

In the United States:
- 30.8 million adults smoke cigarettes
- 3.08 million middle and high school students use tobacco products
- one in four people who do not smoke is exposed to secondhand smoke
- over $240 billion is spent each year to treat smoking-related diseases

The Harmful Effects of Tobacco Use

Cigarette smoking leads to disease and disability and harms nearly every organ of the body. Smoking causes cancer, heart disease, stroke, lung disease, type 2 diabetes, and other chronic health conditions. The effect also extends beyond the person who smokes. For example, smoking during pregnancy increases the risk of premature birth (being born too early) and sudden infant death syndrome (SIDS).

Secondhand smoke, which affects 58 million Americans who do not smoke, also causes stroke, lung cancer, and heart disease in adults. Children who are exposed to secondhand smoke are at increased risk of SIDS, impaired lung function, acute respiratory infections (ARIs), middle ear disease, and more frequent and severe asthma attacks.

Risk Factors for Preventable Chronic Diseases

CANCER

Cigarette smoking causes several forms of cancer, including about 80–90 percent of lung cancer deaths. People who do not smoke can also develop lung cancer, and those who are exposed to secondhand smoke at home or work have a 20–30 percent higher risk of getting lung cancer than those not exposed. Smoking also causes cancers of the voice box (larynx), mouth and throat, esophagus, bladder, kidney, liver, pancreas, cervix, colon, rectum, and stomach, as well as a type of blood cancer called "acute myeloid leukemia" (AML). It can also interfere with cancer treatment, increasing the risk of recurrence, more serious complications, and death.

HEART DISEASE AND STROKE

Cigarette smoking is a major cause of heart disease and stroke and causes one in every four deaths from heart disease and stroke. People who do not smoke but breathe secondhand smoke at home or work have a 25–30 percent higher risk of heart disease and a 20–30 percent higher risk of stroke. Smoking can damage the body by:
- raising triglycerides (a type of fat in the blood) and lowering high-density lipoprotein (HDL) or "good" cholesterol
- making blood sticky and more likely to clot, which can block blood flow to the heart and brain
- damaging cells that line blood vessels, increasing the buildup of plaque (fat, cholesterol, calcium, and other substances) in blood vessels, and causing blood vessels to thicken and narrow

LUNG DISEASE

Cigarette smoking can cause lung disease by damaging the airways and the small air sacs (alveoli) found in the lungs. It can cause chronic obstructive pulmonary disease (COPD), which includes emphysema and chronic bronchitis. Smoking accounts for as many as 8 in 10 COPD-related deaths. If you have asthma, tobacco smoke can trigger an asthma attack or make an attack worse.

DIABETES

The risk of developing type 2 diabetes is 30–40 percent higher for current smokers than nonsmokers. The more cigarettes a person smokes, the higher their risk of type 2 diabetes. People with diabetes who smoke are more likely than nonsmokers to have trouble managing their blood sugar and to have serious complications, including:
- heart disease and kidney disease
- poor blood flow in the legs and feet that can lead to infections, ulcers, and amputation (surgery to remove a body part, such as toes or feet)
- retinopathy (an eye disease that can cause blindness)
- peripheral neuropathy (nerve damage in the hands, arms, feet, and legs that causes numbness, pain, weakness, and poor coordination)

PREGNANCY COMPLICATIONS

Cigarette smoking during pregnancy increases the risk of pregnancy complications, including premature birth, low birth weight, certain birth defects, and SIDS. Smoking can also make it harder for a woman to get pregnant. In addition, exposure to secondhand smoke is dangerous for infants and increases the risk of SIDS, slowed lung growth, and middle ear disease.

POOR NUTRITION

Good nutrition is essential to keeping current and future generations healthy across their lifespan. A healthy diet helps children grow and develop properly and reduces their risk of chronic diseases. Adults who eat a healthy diet live longer and have a lower risk of obesity, heart disease, type 2 diabetes, and certain cancers. Healthy eating can help people with chronic diseases manage these conditions and avoid complications.

However, when healthy options are not available, people may settle for foods that are higher in calories and lower in nutritional value. People in low-income communities and some racial and ethnic groups often lack access to convenient places that offer affordable, healthier foods.

Risk Factors for Preventable Chronic Diseases

Most people in the United States do not eat a healthy diet and consume too much sodium, saturated fat, and sugar, increasing their risk of chronic diseases. For example, fewer than 1 in 10 adolescents and adults eat enough fruits or vegetables. In addition, 6 in 10 young people aged 2–19 and 5 in 10 adults consume at least one sugary drink on any given day.

The CDC supports breastfeeding and works to improve access to healthier food and drink choices in settings such as early care and education facilities, schools, worksites, and communities.

In the United States:
- three in four infants are not exclusively breast-fed for six months
- 9 in 10 Americans consume too much sodium
- one in six pregnant women has iron levels that are too low
- nearly $173 billion a year is spent on health care for obesity

The Harmful Effects of Poor Nutrition
OVERWEIGHT AND OBESITY

Eating a healthy diet, along with getting enough physical activity and sleep, can help children grow up healthy and prevent overweight and obesity. In the United States, 20 percent of young people aged 2–19 and 42 percent of adults have obesity, which can put them at risk of heart disease, type 2 diabetes, and some cancers.

HEART DISEASE AND STROKE

Two of the leading causes of heart disease and stroke are high blood pressure (HBP) and high blood cholesterol. Consuming too much sodium can increase blood pressure and the risk for heart disease and stroke. The guidelines recommend getting less than 2,300 mg a day, but Americans consume more than 3,400 mg a day on average.

Over 70 percent of the sodium that Americans eat comes from packaged, processed, store-bought, and restaurant foods. Eating foods low in saturated fats and high in fiber and increasing access to low-sodium foods, along with regular physical activity, can help prevent high blood cholesterol and HBP.

TYPE 2 DIABETES

People who are overweight or obese are at increased risk of type 2 diabetes compared to those who are at healthy weight because, over time, their bodies become less able to use the insulin they make. Of U.S. adults, 96 million—more than one in three—have prediabetes, and more than 8 in 10 of them do not know they have it. Although the rate of new cases has decreased in recent years, the number of adults with diagnosed diabetes has nearly doubled in the last two decades as the U.S. population has increased, aged, and become more overweight.

CANCER

An unhealthy diet can increase the risk of some cancers. Consuming unhealthy food and beverages, such as sugar-sweetened beverages and highly processed food, can lead to weight gain, obesity, and other chronic conditions that put people at higher risk of at least 13 types of cancer, including endometrial (uterine) cancer, breast cancer in postmenopausal women, and colorectal cancer. The risk of colorectal cancer is also associated with eating red and processed meat.

PHYSICAL INACTIVITY

Physical activity can improve health now and in the future. People of all ages, races and ethnicities, shapes, sizes, and abilities can benefit from more physical activity as it:
- helps prevent unhealthy weight gain
- reduces the risk of many chronic diseases, such as heart disease, cancer, and type 2 diabetes
- helps reduce feelings of anxiety and improves sleep quality
- improves cognitive ability and reduces the risk of dementia
- improves bone and musculoskeletal health

The CDC aims to help 27 million Americans become more physically active by 2027 through Active People, Healthy Nation

Risk Factors for Preventable Chronic Diseases

(www.cdc.gov/physicalactivity/activepeoplehealthynation), a comprehensive initiative to promote physical activity based on strategies recommended by the Guide to Community Preventive Services.

In the United States:
- about one in two adults does not get enough aerobic physical activity
- 77 percent of high school students do not get enough aerobic physical activity
- $117 billion in annual health-care costs are related to low physical activity

The Harmful Effects of Not Getting Enough Physical Activity
HEART DISEASE
Not getting enough physical activity can lead to heart disease—even for people who have no other risk factors. It can also increase the likelihood of developing other heart disease risk factors, including obesity, HBP, high blood cholesterol, and type 2 diabetes.

TYPE 2 DIABETES
Not getting enough physical activity can raise a person's risk of developing type 2 diabetes. Physical activity helps control blood sugar (glucose), weight, and blood pressure and helps raise "good" cholesterol and lower "bad" cholesterol. Adequate physical activity—at least 150 minutes of moderate activity a week—can also help reduce the risk of heart disease and nerve damage, which are often problems for people with diabetes.

CANCER
Getting the recommended amount of physical activity can lower the risk of many cancers, including cancers of the breast, colon, and uterus. Regular physical activity is one of the most important things people can do to improve their health. Moving more and sitting less have tremendous benefits for everyone, regardless of age, sex, race, ethnicity, or current fitness level.

The Health Benefits of Physical Activity

Physical activity is one of the best things people can do for their health. The *Physical Activity Guidelines for Americans, Second Edition* presents new findings on the benefits of regular physical activity, which include:
- improved sleep
- increased ability to perform everyday activities
- improved cognitive ability and a reduced risk of dementia
- improved bone and musculoskeletal health

Emerging research also suggests that physical activity may help our immune systems protect our bodies from infection and disease.

EXCESSIVE ALCOHOL USE

Excessive alcohol use is a leading preventable cause of death in the United States, shortening the lives of those who die by an average of 26 years. Excessive alcohol use includes:
- binge drinking, which is defined as consuming four or more drinks on an occasion for a woman or five or more drinks on an occasion for a man
- heavy drinking, which is defined as 8 or more drinks per week for a woman or 15 or more drinks per week for a man
- any alcohol use by pregnant women or anyone younger than the age of 21

A small percentage of adults who drink account for half of the 35 billion total drinks consumed by U.S. adults each year. The CDC estimates that one in six U.S. adults binge drinks, with 25 percent doing so at least weekly, on average, and 25 percent consuming at least eight drinks during a binge occasion. Binge drinking is responsible for more than 40 percent of the deaths and three-quarters of the costs due to excessive alcohol use. States and communities can prevent binge drinking by supporting effective policies and programs, such as those recommended by the Community Preventive Services Task Force (CPSTF).

Each year in the United States, excessive alcohol use is responsible for:
- 140,000 deaths shortening lives by an average of 26 years
- one in five deaths among adults aged 20–49
- more than $249 billion in economic costs or $2.05 a drink

The Health Effects of Excessive Alcohol Use
CHRONIC HEALTH EFFECTS
Over time, excessive alcohol use can lead to chronic diseases and other serious problems, including alcohol use disorder (AUD) and problems with learning, memory, and mental health. There are other chronic health conditions linked to excessive alcohol use.

HIGH BLOOD PRESSURE, HEART DISEASE, AND STROKE
Binge drinking and heavy drinking can cause heart disease, including cardiomyopathy (disease of the heart muscle), as well as irregular heartbeat, HBP, and stroke.

LIVER DISEASE
Excessive alcohol use takes a toll on the liver and can lead to fatty liver disease (steatosis), hepatitis, fibrosis, and cirrhosis.

CANCER
Drinking alcoholic beverages of any kind, including wine, beer, and liquor, can contribute to cancers of the mouth and throat, larynx (voice box), esophagus, colon and rectum, liver, and breast (in women). For some cancers, even less than one drink in a day can increase risk. The less alcohol a person drinks, the lower the risk of these types of cancer.

IMMEDIATE HEALTH EFFECTS
Excessive alcohol use has immediate effects that increase the risk of many harmful health conditions.

INJURIES, VIOLENCE, AND POISONINGS
Drinking too much alcohol increases the risk of injuries, including those from motor vehicle crashes, falls, drownings, and burns. It increases the risk of violence, including homicide, suicide, and sexual assault. Alcohol also contributes to poisonings or overdoses from opioids and other substances.

UNINTENDED PREGNANCY AND SEXUALLY TRANSMITTED INFECTIONS
People who binge drink are more likely to have unprotected sex and multiple sex partners. These activities increase the risk of unintended pregnancy and sexually transmitted infections (STIs), including human immunodeficiency virus (HIV).

POOR PREGNANCY OUTCOMES
There is no known safe amount of alcohol use during pregnancy. Alcohol use during pregnancy can cause fetal alcohol spectrum disorders (FASDs). It may also increase the risk of miscarriage, premature birth, stillbirth, and SIDS.[1]

---

[1] National Center for Chronic Disease Prevention and Health Promotion (NCCDPHP), "About Chronic Diseases," Centers for Disease Control and Prevention (CDC), July 21, 2022. Available online. URL: www.cdc.gov/chronicdisease/about/index.htm. Accessed February 12, 2024.

Chapter 4 | Family Health History

Chapter Contents
Section 4.1—What Is Family Health History?..............................25
Section 4.2—Family Health History and Chronic Disease.........26

Section 4.1 | What Is Family Health History?

Family health history is a record of the diseases and health conditions in your family. You and your family members share genes. You may also have behaviors in common, such as exercise habits and what you like to eat. You may live in the same area and come into contact with similar things in the environment. Family history includes all of these factors, any of which can affect your health.

HOW CAN YOU COLLECT YOUR FAMILY HEALTH HISTORY?

You may know a lot about your family health history or only a little. To get the complete picture, use family gatherings as a time to talk about health history. If possible, look at death certificates and family medical records. Collect information about your parents, sisters, brothers, half sisters, half brothers, children, grandparents, aunts, uncles, nieces, and nephews. Include information on major medical conditions, causes of death, age at disease diagnosis, age at death, and ethnic background. Be sure to update the information regularly and share what you have learned with your family and with your doctor.

WHY IS FAMILY HEALTH HISTORY IMPORTANT FOR YOUR HEALTH?

Most people have a family health history of at least one chronic disease, such as cancer, heart disease, and diabetes. If you have a close family member with a chronic disease, you may be more likely to develop that disease yourself, especially if more than one close relative has (or had) the disease or a family member got the disease at a younger age than usual.

Collect your family health history information before visiting the doctor and take it with you. Even if you do not know all of your family health history information, share what you do know. Family health history information, even if incomplete, can help your doctor decide which screening tests you need and when those tests should start.

HOW CAN YOU USE YOUR FAMILY HEALTH HISTORY TO IMPROVE YOUR HEALTH?

You cannot change your genes, but you can change unhealthy behaviors, such as smoking, not exercising or being active, and poor eating habits. If you have a family health history of disease, you may have the most to gain from lifestyle changes and screening tests. In many cases, healthy habits can reduce your risk for diseases that run in your family. Screening tests, such as blood sugar testing, mammograms, and colorectal cancer screening, help find early signs of disease. Finding disease early can often mean better health in the long run.

Knowing Is Not Enough: Act on Your Family Health History

Has your mother or sister had breast cancer? Talk with your doctor about whether having a mammogram earlier is right for you.

Does your mom, dad, sister, or brother have diabetes? Ask your doctor how early you should be screened for diabetes.

Did your mom, dad, brother, or sister get colorectal (colon) cancer before the age of 50? Talk with your doctor about whether you should start getting colonoscopies earlier or have them done more often.[1]

Section 4.2 | Family Health History and Chronic Disease

If you have a family health history of chronic diseases such as cancer, heart disease, diabetes, or osteoporosis, you are more likely to get that disease yourself. Share your family health history with your doctor, who can help you take steps to prevent disease and catch it early if it develops.

---

[1] "Family Health History: The Basics," Centers for Disease Control and Prevention (CDC), May 5, 2023. Available online. URL: www.cdc.gov/genomics/famhistory/famhist_basics.htm. Accessed February 14, 2024.

Family Health History

BREAST AND OVARIAN CANCERS AND FAMILY HEALTH HISTORY

If you are a woman with a family health history of breast cancer or ovarian cancer, you may be more likely to get these cancers yourself. Collecting your family health history of breast, ovarian, and other cancers and sharing this information with your doctor can help you find out if you are at higher risk. If you have had breast, ovarian, or other cancers, make sure your family members know about your diagnosis.

Your doctor might consider your family health history in deciding when you should start mammography screening for breast cancer. If you are a woman with a parent, sibling, or child with breast cancer, you are at higher risk for breast cancer. Based on the recommendations, you should consider talking to your doctor about starting mammography screening in your 40s. In some cases, your doctor might recommend that you have genetic counseling, and a genetic counselor might recommend genetic testing based on your family health history. Breast, ovarian, and other cancers are sometimes caused by inherited mutations in breast cancer gene 1 (*BRCA1*), breast cancer gene 2 (*BRCA2*), and other genes. The genetic counselor can help determine which genetic mutations you should be tested for, based on your personal and family health history of cancer, ancestry, and other factors.

Do the following when collecting your family health history:
- Include your parents, sisters, brothers, children, grandparents, aunts, uncles, nieces, and nephews.
- List any cancers that each relative had and at what age he or she was diagnosed. For relatives who have died, list the age and cause of death.
- Remember that breast and ovarian cancer risk does not just come from your mother's side of the family—your father's relatives with breast, ovarian, and other cancers matter, too.
- Update your family health history on a regular basis and let your doctor know about any new cases of breast, ovarian, or other cancer.

If you are concerned about your personal or family health history of breast, ovarian, or other cancers, talk to your doctor.

Whether or not you have a family health history of breast or ovarian cancer, you can take steps to help lower your risk of breast cancer and ovarian cancer.

COLORECTAL CANCER AND FAMILY HEALTH HISTORY

Having a family health history of colorectal cancer makes you more likely to get colorectal (colon) cancer yourself.

Knowing your family health history of colorectal cancer and sharing this information with your doctor can help you take steps to lower your risk. If you have multiple relatives who have been diagnosed with colorectal cancer or relatives who have been diagnosed at a young age (before the age of 50), your doctor may change your medical management to prevent colorectal cancer or catch it as early as possible. If you have been diagnosed with colorectal cancer, it is important to tell your family members.

Precancerous colorectal polyps are abnormal growths in the colon or rectum that can turn into cancer if they are not removed. However, not all polyps turn into cancer. If you have been diagnosed with certain types of colorectal polyps, your doctor may recommend starting colonoscopy screening earlier. Be sure to let your family members know about your history of colorectal polyps.

Based on the recommendations, most people start colorectal cancer screening at the age of 45, but if you have a family history, your doctor may recommend the following:
- colonoscopy starts at the age of 40 or 10 years before the age that the immediate family member was diagnosed with cancer
- more frequent screening
- colonoscopy only instead of other tests
- in some cases, genetic counseling

Do the following when collecting your family health history:
- Include your parents, sisters, brothers, children, grandparents, aunts, uncles, nieces, and nephews.
- Make sure to document both your mother's side of the family and your father's side of the family.

Family Health History

- Document which relatives have had cancer, the type(s) of cancer they have had, and the ages at which they were diagnosed.
- Report any history of polyps that each relative has had.
- List the age and cause of death for relatives who have died.
- Share your family health history with your doctor.
- Update your family health history regularly and alert your doctor to any new diagnosis.

LYNCH SYNDROME AND FAMILY HEALTH HISTORY

Having a family health history of Lynch syndrome makes you more likely to have Lynch syndrome yourself. Lynch syndrome is an inherited genetic condition that makes you more likely to get colorectal (colon) and other types of cancer.

If someone in your family has been diagnosed with Lynch syndrome, share this information with your doctor. Your doctor may refer you for genetic counseling or genetic testing. If you have Lynch syndrome, let your family members know. Note that not all inherited colorectal cancers are due to Lynch syndrome, and not everyone with Lynch syndrome will get colorectal cancer.

Lynch syndrome is hereditary, meaning that it is caused by an inherited genetic change or mutation, that can be passed from parent to child. If you have Lynch syndrome, your parents, children, sisters, and brothers have a 50 percent chance of having Lynch syndrome. Once a mutation that causes Lynch syndrome is found in one person in a family, other members can then be tested for that mutation to find out if they have Lynch syndrome.

Tell your doctor if you have:
- a first-degree relative (parents, sisters, brothers, and children) with Lynch syndrome
- a first-degree relative with colorectal or endometrial cancer diagnosed before the age of 50
- a first-degree relative with colorectal or endometrial cancer and another Lynch syndrome-related cancer occurring either at the same time or at a different time (Lynch syndrome-related cancers include colorectal

(colon), uterine (endometrial), stomach, liver, kidney, brain, and some skin cancers.)
- two or more first- or second-degree relatives (grandparents, aunts, uncles, and half-siblings) with Lynch syndrome-related cancers and at least one that was diagnosed before the age of 50
- three or more first- or second-degree relatives with Lynch syndrome-related cancers at any age

DIABETES AND FAMILY HEALTH HISTORY

If you have a mother, father, sister, or brother with diabetes, you are more likely to get diabetes yourself. You are also more likely to have prediabetes. Talk to your doctor about your family health history of diabetes. Your doctor can help you take steps to prevent or delay diabetes and reverse prediabetes if you have it.

Over 37 million people in the United States have diabetes. People with diabetes have levels of blood sugar that are too high. The different types of diabetes include type 1 diabetes, type 2 diabetes, and gestational diabetes. Diabetes can cause serious health problems, including heart disease, kidney problems, stroke, blindness, and the need for lower leg amputations.

People with prediabetes have levels of blood sugar that are higher than normal but not high enough for them to be diagnosed with diabetes. People with prediabetes are more likely to get type 2 diabetes. About 96 million people in the United States have prediabetes, but most of them do not know they have it. If you have prediabetes, you can take steps to reverse it and prevent or delay diabetes—but not if you do not know that you have it.

If you have a family health history of diabetes, you are more likely to have prediabetes and develop diabetes. You are also more likely to get type 2 diabetes if you have had gestational diabetes, are overweight or obese, or are African American, American Indian, Asian American, Pacific Islander, or Hispanic. Learning about your family health history of diabetes is an important step in finding out if you have prediabetes and knowing if you are more likely to get diabetes.

Family Health History

Even if you have a family health history of diabetes, you can prevent or delay type 2 diabetes by eating healthier, being physically active, and maintaining or reaching a healthy weight. This is especially important if you have prediabetes, and taking these steps can reverse prediabetes.

HEREDITARY HEMOCHROMATOSIS AND FAMILY HEALTH HISTORY
Hereditary hemochromatosis is a genetic disorder that can cause severe liver disease and other health problems. Early diagnosis and treatment are critical to prevent complications from the disorder. If you have a family health history of hemochromatosis, talk to your doctor about testing for hereditary hemochromatosis.

What Is Hemochromatosis?
Hemochromatosis is a disorder in which the body can build up too much iron in the skin, heart, liver, pancreas, pituitary gland, and joints. Too much iron is toxic to the body, and over time, high levels of iron can damage tissues and organs and lead to:
- cirrhosis (liver damage)
- hepatocellular carcinoma (liver cancer)
- heart problems
- arthritis (joint pain)
- diabetes

What Causes Hereditary Hemochromatosis?
Hereditary hemochromatosis is most commonly caused by certain variants in the hemochromatosis (*HFE*) gene. If you inherit two of these variants, one from each parent, you have hereditary hemochromatosis and are at risk for developing high iron levels. If you have a family member, especially a sibling, who is known to have hereditary hemochromatosis, talk to your doctor about genetic testing.

In the United States, about 1 in 300 non-Hispanic White people has hereditary hemochromatosis, with lower rates among people of other races and ethnicities. Many people with hereditary hemochromatosis do not know they have it. Early symptoms of hemochromatosis, such as feeling tired or weak, are common and can cause it to be confused with a variety of other diseases. Men with hereditary hemochromatosis are more likely to develop complications often at an earlier age. An estimated 9 percent (about 1 in 10) of men with hereditary hemochromatosis will develop severe liver disease. However, most people with hereditary hemochromatosis never develop symptoms or complications.

What Are the Symptoms of Hemochromatosis?

A blood test can be used to screen people who may have hemochromatosis by measuring how much iron is in their blood. Affected people with or without a known family history of hemochromatosis can be diagnosed through blood tests for iron followed by genetic testing if they are symptomatic or have complications. Symptoms of hemochromatosis include the following:

- feeling of tiredness or weakness
- weight loss
- joint pain
- bronze or gray skin color
- abdominal pain
- loss of sex drive

How Can You Prevent Complications from Hemochromatosis?

If you or your family members have hemochromatosis, your doctor may suggest ways to lower the amount of iron in your body. The earlier hemochromatosis is diagnosed, the less likely you are to develop serious complications—many of which can cause permanent problems. If you are diagnosed with hemochromatosis, regularly scheduled blood removal is the most effective way to lower the amount of iron in your body. Your doctor may also recommend:

- annual blood tests to check your iron levels
- liver biopsy to check for cirrhosis
- iron chelation therapy, if you cannot have blood removed (This involves medicine taken either orally or injected to lower the amount of iron in your body.)

Family Health History

- dietary changes, such as avoiding multivitamins, vitamin C supplements, and iron supplements, which can increase iron throughout your body
- no alcohol use (because alcohol increases the risk of liver damage)
- steps to prevent infections, including not eating uncooked fish and shellfish and getting recommended vaccinations, including those against hepatitis A and B

OSTEOPOROSIS AND FAMILY HEALTH HISTORY

If one of your parents has had a broken bone, especially a broken hip, you may need to be screened earlier for osteoporosis. This is a medical condition where bones become weak and are more likely to break. Share your family health history with your doctor. Your doctor can help you take steps to strengthen weak bones and prevent broken bones.

How Can Osteoporosis Affect Your Health?

People with osteoporosis are more likely to break bones, most often in the hip, forearm, wrist, and spine. While most broken bones are caused by falls, osteoporosis can weaken bones to the point that a break can occur more easily, for example, by coughing or bumping into something. As you get older, you are more likely to have osteoporosis, and recovering from a broken bone becomes harder. Broken bones can have lasting effects, including pain that does not go away. Osteoporosis can cause the bones in the spine to break and begin to collapse so that some people with it get shorter and are not able to stand up straight. Broken hips are especially serious—afterward, many people are not able to live on their own and are more likely to die sooner.

How Can You Find Out If You Have Osteoporosis?

Osteoporosis is more common in women. It affects almost 20 percent (one in five) of women aged 50 and over and almost 5 percent (1 in 20) of men aged 50 and over. Many people with osteoporosis do not know they have it until they break a bone. Screening is important to find these people before this happens, so they can take steps to decrease the effects of osteoporosis.

Screening for osteoporosis is recommended for women who are aged 65 or older and for women who are aged 50–64 and have certain risk factors, which include having a parent who has broken a hip.

Screening for osteoporosis is commonly done using a type of low-level x-rays called "dual-energy x-ray absorptiometry" (DXA). Screening can also show if you have low bone mass, meaning your bones are weaker than normal and are likely to develop osteoporosis.

How Can You Improve Your Bone Health If You Have Osteoporosis?

There are steps you can take to improve your bone health and strengthen weak bones:
- Take medications to strengthen your bones and avoid medications that can make your bones weaker.
- Eat a healthy diet that includes adequate amounts of calcium and vitamin D.
- Perform weight-bearing exercises regularly.
- Do not smoke.
- Limit alcohol use.

Do not wait until you have a broken bone to take steps to improve your bone health—you can start at any age. You can also take steps to prevent falls, including doing exercises to improve your leg strength and balance, having your eyes checked, and making your home safer.

HEART DISEASE AND FAMILY HEALTH HISTORY

If you have a family health history of heart disease, you are more likely to develop heart disease yourself.

Different types of heart disease and related conditions, such as high blood pressure (HBP) and high blood cholesterol, can run in families. Knowing your family health history of heart disease and

Family Health History

related conditions is one of the first steps you can take to prevent heart disease and heart attacks in the future.

Tell your doctor if your parents, sisters, brothers, children, grandparents, grandchildren, aunts, uncles, nieces, or nephews have or have had:
- heart disease, including:
  - coronary artery disease (CAD) or atherosclerosis
  - heart attack
  - high blood cholesterol
  - angina (pressure or squeezing pain in the chest)
  - arrhythmias, such as atrial fibrillation
  - cardiomyopathy
  - congenital heart defects
  - heart failure
  - other heart-related conditions
- aortic aneurysm
- stroke
- diabetes
- HBP
- pacemaker
- percutaneous coronary intervention (PCI; also called "coronary angioplasty") with or without stent
- heart bypass or other heart surgery

Based on this information, your doctor may suggest steps to prevent or treat heart disease. If you have been diagnosed with heart disease or related conditions, it is important to tell your family members.

Act on Your Family History of Heart Attacks

If your father, mother, brother, or sister had a heart attack before the age of 50, your risk of heart disease, heart attack, and stroke is increased.

Many with a family history of early heart attacks also:
- are overweight/have obesity
- smoke
- are not physically active

- do not choose healthy foods and drinks
- have high cholesterol
- have HBP
- have diabetes

Tips on Collecting Your Family Health History
Do the following when collecting your family health history:
- Include your parents, sisters, brothers, children, grandparents, grandchildren, aunts, uncles, nieces, and nephews.
- Make sure you include both your mother's and father's sides of the family.
- Note which relatives have had heart disease, related conditions, or procedures and the age at which they were diagnosed or treated.
- List the age and cause of death for relatives who have died.
- Share your family health history with your doctor and family members.
- Update your family health history regularly and alert your doctor to any new diagnosis, condition, or procedure.

If you are concerned about your personal or family health history of heart disease, talk to your doctor.

FAMILIAL HYPERCHOLESTEROLEMIA AND FAMILY HEALTH HISTORY
Having a family health history of familial hypercholesterolemia (FH), high cholesterol, makes you more likely to have FH yourself. Most people with FH do not know they have it. Finding out if you have FH is important so that you can take steps to prevent having an early heart attack or heart disease. Family health history is important for diagnosing FH, so be sure to collect your family health history of high cholesterol, heart attacks, and heart disease.

Family Health History

Tell your doctor if you have:
- a family member with FH
- a family health history of low-density lipoprotein (LDL) cholesterol levels higher than 190 mg/dL in adults or higher than 160 mg/dL in children
- a father, brother, son, or other male family member who had heart disease or a heart attack before the age of 50
- a mother, sister, daughter, or other female family members who had heart disease or a heart attack before the age of 60[2]

---

[2] "Family Health History and Chronic Disease," Centers for Disease Control and Prevention (CDC), May 5, 2023. Available online. URL: www.cdc.gov/genomics/famhistory/famhist_chronic_disease.htm. Accessed February 14, 2024.

Chapter 5 | **Preventing Chronic Diseases**

Many chronic diseases are caused by key risk behaviors. By making healthy choices, you can reduce your likelihood of getting a chronic disease and improve your quality of life (QOL). The following are few tips to prevent chronic diseases:

- **Quit smoking**. Stopping smoking (or never starting) lowers the risk of serious health problems, such as heart disease, cancer, type 2 diabetes, and lung disease, as well as premature death—even for longtime smokers. Take the first step and call 800-QUIT-NOW (800-7848-669) for free support.
- **Eat healthy**. Eating healthy helps prevent, delay, and manage heart disease, type 2 diabetes, and other chronic diseases. A balanced, healthy dietary pattern includes a variety of fruits, vegetables, whole grains, lean protein, and low-fat dairy products and limits added sugars, saturated fats, and sodium.
- **Get regular physical activity**. Regular physical activity can help you prevent, delay, or manage chronic diseases. Aim for moderate-intensity physical activity (such as brisk walking or gardening) for at least 150 minutes a week, with muscle-strengthening activities two days a week.
- **Avoid drinking too much alcohol**. Over time, excessive drinking can lead to high blood pressure (HBP), various cancers, heart disease, stroke, and liver disease. By not drinking too much, you can reduce these health risks.

- **Get screened.** To prevent chronic diseases or catch them early, visit your doctor and dentist regularly for preventive services.
- **Take care of your teeth.** Oral diseases—which range from cavities and gum disease to oral cancer—cause pain and disability for millions of Americans. To help prevent these problems, drink fluoridated water, brush with fluoride toothpaste twice a day, and floss daily. Visit your dentist at least once a year, even if you have no natural teeth or have dentures.
- **Get enough sleep.** Insufficient sleep has been linked to the development and poor management of diabetes, heart disease, obesity, and depression. Adults should get at least seven hours of sleep daily.
- **Know your family history.** If you have a family history of a chronic disease, such as cancer, heart disease, diabetes, or osteoporosis, you may be more likely to develop that disease yourself. Share your family health history with your doctor, who can help you take steps to prevent these conditions or catch them early.
- **Make healthy choices in school and at work.** By making healthy behaviors part of your daily life, you can prevent conditions such as HBP or obesity, which raise your risk of developing the most common and serious chronic diseases.[1]

---

[1] National Center for Chronic Disease Prevention and Health Promotion (NCCDPHP), "How You Can Prevent Chronic Diseases," Centers for Disease Control and Prevention (CDC), October 26, 2023. Available online. URL: www.cdc.gov/chronicdisease/about/prevent/index.htm. Accessed February 15, 2024.

Chapter 6 | Common Screening and Diagnostic Tests

Chapter Contents
Section 6.1—Screening Tests: What You Need to Know............43
Section 6.2—Screening Tests for Women 45
Section 6.3—Screening Tests for Men 48
Section 6.4—Laboratory-Developed Tests..................................51
Section 6.5—Home-Use Tests..52
Section 6.6—Direct-to-Consumer Genetic Testing....................55
Section 6.7—Biomarkers 60

Section 6.1 | Screening Tests: What You Need to Know

THE BENEFITS AND HARMS OF SCREENING TESTS

Catching chronic health conditions early—even before you have symptoms—seems like a great idea. That is what screening tests are designed to do. Some screenings can reduce your risk of dying from the disease. But sometimes experts say, a test may cause more harm than good. Before you get a test, talk with your doctor about the possible benefits and harms to help you decide what is best for your health.

Screening tests are given to people who seem healthy to try to find unnoticed problems. They are done before you have any signs or symptoms of the disease. They come in many forms. Your doctor might take your health history and perform a physical exam to look for signs of health or disease. They can also include lab tests of blood, tissue, or urine samples or imaging procedures that look inside your body.

"I wouldn't say that all people should just simply get screening tests," says Dr. Barnett S. Kramer, a cancer prevention expert at the National Institutes of Health (NIH). "Patients should be aware of both the potential benefits and the harms when they're choosing what screening tests to have and how often."

Teams of experts regularly look at all the evidence about the balance of benefits and harms of different screening tests. They develop guidelines for who should be screened and how often.

Choosing whether you should be screened for a health condition is not always easy. Screening suggestions are often based on your age, family health history, and other factors. You might be screened for many conditions, including diabetes, sexually transmitted infections (STIs), heart disease, osteoporosis, obesity, depression, pregnancy issues, and cancers.

Every screening test comes with its own risks. Some procedures can cause problems such as bleeding or infection. A positive screening test can lead to further tests that come with their own risks.

"Most people who feel healthy are healthy," says Dr. Kramer. "So a negative test to confirm that you're healthy doesn't add much new information." But mistakenly being told that you do or do not have a disease can be harmful. It is called a "misdiagnosis."

A false negative means that you are told you do not have the disease, but you do. This can cause problems if you do not pay attention to symptoms that appear later on because you think you do not have the disease. A false positive means that you are told you may have the disease, but you do not. This can lead to unnecessary worry and potentially harmful tests and treatments that you do not need.

Even correctly finding a disease may not improve your health or help you live longer. You may learn you have an untreatable disease long before you would have. Or find a disease that never would have caused a problem. This is called "overdiagnosis." Some cancers, for example, never cause symptoms or become life-threatening. But if found by a screening test, it is likely to be treated. Cancer treatments can have harsh and long-lasting side effects. There is no way to know if the treatment will help you live longer.

An effective screening test may decrease your chances of dying of the condition. Most have not been shown to lengthen your overall life expectancy, Dr. Kramer explains. Their usefulness varies and may depend on your risk factors, age, or treatment options.

If you are at risk for certain health conditions—because of a family history or lifestyle exposures, such as smoking—you may choose to have screenings more regularly. If you are considering a screening, talk with your health-care provider.

ASK YOUR DOCTOR ABOUT SCREENING TESTS

You may ask the following questions to your doctor about screening tests:
- What is my chance of dying of the condition if I do or do not have the screening?
- What are the harms of the test? How often do they occur?
- How likely are false positive or false negative results?
- What are the possible harms of the diagnostic tests if I get a positive screening result?

Common Screening and Diagnostic Tests

- What is the chance of finding a disease that would not have caused a problem?
- How effective are the treatment options?
- Am I healthy enough to take the therapy if you discover a disease?
- What are other ways to decrease my risk of dying of this condition? How effective are they?[1]

Section 6.2 | Screening Tests for Women

Screenings are tests that look for diseases before you have symptoms. Blood pressure checks and mammograms are examples of screenings. You can get some screenings, such as blood pressure readings, at your doctor's office. Others, such as mammograms, need special equipment, so you may need to go to a different office. After a screening test, ask when you will see the results and who to talk to about them.

SCREENINGS WOMEN NEED
The following are some diseases and conditions for which women need to get screened:
- **Breast cancer.** Talk with your health-care team about whether you need a mammogram.
- *BRCA1* **(breast cancer gene 1) and** *BRCA2* **(breast cancer gene 2) genes**. If you have a family member with breast, ovarian, or peritoneal cancer, talk with your doctor or nurse about your family history. Women with a strong family history of certain cancers may benefit from genetic counseling and *BRCA* (breast cancer gene) genetic testing.

---

[1] *NIH News in Health*, "To Screen or Not to Screen?—The Benefits and Harms of Screening Tests," National Institutes of Health (NIH), March 2017. Available online. URL: https://newsinhealth.nih.gov/2017/03/screen-or-not-screen. Accessed February 15, 2024.

- **Cervical cancer.** Starting at the age of 21, get a Pap smear every three years until you are 65 years old. Women aged 30 or older may choose to switch to a combination Pap smear and human papillomavirus (HPV) test every five years until the age of 65. If you are older than 65 or have had a hysterectomy, talk with your doctor or nurse about whether you still need to be screened.
- **Colon cancer.** Between the ages of 50 and 75, get a screening test for colorectal cancer. Several tests—for example, a stool test or a colonoscopy—can detect this cancer. Your health-care team can help you decide which is best for you. If you are between the ages of 76 and 85, talk with your doctor or nurse about whether you should continue to be screened.
- **Depression.** Your emotional health is as important as your physical health. Talk to your health-care team about being screened for depression, especially if during the last two weeks:
  - you have felt down, sad, or hopeless
  - you have felt little interest or pleasure in doing things
- **Diabetes.** Get screened for diabetes (high blood sugar) if you have high blood pressure (HBP) or if you take medication for HBP. Diabetes can cause problems with your heart, brain, eyes, feet, kidneys, nerves, and other body parts.
- **Hepatitis C virus (HCV).** Get screened one time for HCV infection if:
  - you were born between 1945 and 1965
  - you have ever injected drugs
  - you received a blood transfusion before 1992

  If you currently are an injection drug user, you should be screened regularly.
- **High blood cholesterol.** Have your blood cholesterol checked regularly with a blood test if:
  - you use tobacco
  - you are overweight or obese

Common Screening and Diagnostic Tests

- you have a personal history of heart disease or blocked arteries
- a male relative in your family had a heart attack before the age of 50 or a female relative before the age of 60
- **High blood pressure (HBP).** Have your blood pressure checked at least every two years. HBP can cause strokes, heart attacks, kidney and eye problems, and heart failure.
- **Human immunodeficiency virus (HIV).** If you are 65 or younger, get screened for HIV. If you are older than 65, talk to your doctor or nurse about whether you should be screened.
- **Lung cancer.** Talk to your doctor or nurse about getting screened for lung cancer if you are between the ages of 55 and 80, have a 30-pack-year smoking history, and smoke now or have quit within the past 15 years. (Your pack-year history is the number of packs of cigarettes smoked per day times the number of years you have smoked.) Know that quitting smoking is the best thing you can do for your health.
- **Overweight and obesity.** The best way to learn if you are overweight or obese is to determine your body mass index (BMI). You can determine your BMI by entering your height and weight into a BMI calculator. A BMI between 18.5 and 25 indicates a normal weight. Persons with a BMI of 30 or higher may be obese. If you are obese, talk to your doctor or nurse about getting intensive behavioral counseling and help to lose weight. Overweight and obesity can lead to diabetes and cardiovascular disease (CVD).
- **Osteoporosis (bone thinning).** Have a screening test at the age of 65 to make sure your bones are strong. The most common test is a dual-energy x-ray absorptiometry (DEXA) scan—a low-dose x-ray of the spine and hip. If you are under the age of 65 and at high risk for bone fractures, you should also be screened.

Talk with your health-care team about your risk for bone fractures.
- **Sexually transmitted infections (STIs).** STIs can make it hard to get pregnant, may affect your baby, and can cause other health problems. Get screened for chlamydia and gonorrhea infections if you are 24 or younger and sexually active. If you are older than 24, talk to your doctor or nurse about whether you should be screened. Ask your doctor or nurse whether you should be screened for other STIs.[2]

Section 6.3 | Screening Tests for Men

Screenings are tests that look for diseases before you have symptoms. Blood pressure checks and tests for high blood cholesterol are examples of screenings. You can get some screenings, such as blood pressure readings, in your doctor's office. Others, such as a colonoscopy (a test for colon cancer), need special equipment, so you may need to go to a different office.

SCREENINGS MEN NEED

The following are some diseases and conditions for which men need to get screened:
- **Abdominal aortic aneurysm (AAA).** If you are between the ages of 65 and 75 and have ever been a smoker (smoked 100 or more cigarettes in your lifetime), get screened once for AAA. AAA is a bulging in your abdominal aorta, your largest artery. An AAA may burst, which can cause dangerous bleeding and death. An ultrasound, a painless procedure in which you lie on a table while a technician slides a medical

---

[2] Agency for Healthcare Research and Quality (AHRQ), "Women: Stay Healthy at Any Age," U.S. Department of Health and Human Services (HHS), May 2014. Available online. URL: www.ahrq.gov/sites/default/files/publications/files/healthy-women.pdf. Accessed February 15, 2024.

Common Screening and Diagnostic Tests

device over your abdomen, will show whether an aneurysm is present.
- **Colon cancer.** If you are between the ages of 50 and 75, get a screening test for colorectal cancer. Several different tests—for example, a stool test or a colonoscopy—can detect this cancer. Your healthcare team can help you decide which is best for you. If you are between the ages of 76 and 85, talk with your doctor or nurse about whether you should continue to be screened.
- **Depression.** Your emotional health is as important as your physical health. Talk to your doctor or nurse about being screened for depression, especially if during the last two weeks:
  - you have felt down, sad, or hopeless
  - you have felt little interest or pleasure in doing things
- **Diabetes.** Get screened for diabetes (high blood sugar) if you have high blood pressure (HBP) or if you take medication for HBP. Diabetes can cause problems with your heart, brain, eyes, feet, kidneys, nerves, and other body parts.
- **Hepatitis C virus (HCV).** Get screened one time for HCV infection if:
  - you were born between 1945 and 1965
  - you have ever injected drugs
  - you received a blood transfusion before 1992

  If you currently are an injection drug user, you should be screened regularly for the following conditions:
- **High blood cholesterol.** If you are 35 or older, have your blood cholesterol checked regularly with a blood test. High cholesterol increases your chance of heart disease, stroke, and poor circulation. Talk to your doctor or nurse about having your cholesterol checked starting at the age of 20 if:
  - you use tobacco
  - you are overweight or obese

- you have diabetes or HBP
- you have a history of heart disease or blocked arteries
- a man in your family had a heart attack before the age of 50 or a woman before the age of 60
- **High blood pressure (HBP).** Have your blood pressure checked at least every two years. HBP can cause strokes, heart attacks, kidney and eye problems, and heart failure.
- **Human immunodeficiency virus (HIV).** If you are 65 or younger, get screened for HIV. If you are older than 65, ask your doctor or nurse whether you should be screened.
- **Lung cancer.** Talk to your doctor or nurse about getting screened for lung cancer if you are between the ages of 55 and 80, have a 30-pack-year smoking history, and smoke now or have quit within the past 15 years. (Your pack-year history is the number of packs of cigarettes smoked per day times the number of years you have smoked.) Know that quitting smoking is the best thing you can do for your health.
- **Overweight and obesity.** The best way to learn if you are overweight or obese is to determine your body mass index (BMI). You can determine your BMI by entering your height and weight into a BMI calculator. A BMI between 18.5 and 25 indicates a normal weight. Persons with a BMI of 30 or higher may be obese. If you are obese, talk to your doctor or nurse about getting intensive behavioral counseling and help to lose weight. Overweight and obesity can lead to diabetes and cardiovascular disease (CVD).[3]

---

[3] Agency for Healthcare Research and Quality (AHRQ), "Men: Stay Healthy at Any Age," U.S. Department of Health and Human Services (HHS), March 2014. Available online. URL: www.ahrq.gov/sites/default/files/wysiwyg/patients-consumers/patient-involvement/healthy-men/healthy-men.pdf. Accessed February 15, 2024.

Common Screening and Diagnostic Tests

Section 6.4 | **Laboratory-Developed Tests**

Laboratory-developed tests (LDTs) play an important role in health care. LDTs are in vitro diagnostic products (IVDs) that are intended for clinical use and are designed, manufactured, and used within a single clinical laboratory that meets certain laboratory requirements. Specifically, such laboratories must be certified under the Clinical Laboratory Improvement Amendments of 1988 (CLIA) and meet the regulatory requirements under the CLIA to perform high-complexity testing.

IVDs are intended for use in the collection, preparation, and examination of specimens taken from the human body, such as blood, saliva, or tissue. LDTs, like other IVDs, can be used to measure or detect a wide variety of substances, analytes, or markers in the human body, such as proteins, glucose, cholesterol, or deoxyribonucleic acid (DNA), to provide information about a patient's health, including to diagnose, monitor, or determine treatment for diseases and conditions.

IVDs offered as LDTs are used in a growing number of healthcare decisions, and concerns about the safety and effectiveness of these tests have been raised for many years.

Although historically the U.S. Food and Drug Administration (FDA) has generally exercised enforcement discretion over most LDTs, meaning that the agency generally has not enforced applicable requirements with respect to most LDTs, the risks associated with most modern LDTs are much greater than the risks that were associated with LDTs used decades ago. In the 1970s and 1980s, many LDTs were lower risk, small volume, and used for specialized needs of a local patient population. Since then, due to changes in business practices and the increasing ability to ship patient specimens across the country quickly, many LDTs are now used more widely, for a larger and more diverse population, with large laboratories accepting specimens from across the country. LDTs are also increasingly relying on high-tech instrumentation and software, being performed in large volumes, and being used more frequently to help guide critical health-care decisions.

INCREASED U.S. FOOD AND DRUG ADMINISTRATION OVERSIGHT TO HELP ENSURE SAFETY AND EFFECTIVENESS OF LABORATORY-DEVELOPED TESTS

Due to the evolution and proliferation of LDTs, as well as the increasing concerns regarding their safety and effectiveness, the FDA has engaged in discussions regarding increased oversight of LDTs for many years, including holding a workshop in 2010, proposing draft guidance documents in 2014, issuing a discussion paper in 2017, and engaging with congressional and industry stakeholders. Throughout this time, the FDA has maintained that patients and health-care providers need assurances that the tests they are using are safe and effective to make good health-care decisions. These assurances are lacking for IVDs offered as LDTs without active FDA oversight. False test results or false claims regarding the meaning of test results can lead to significant patient harm.

On September 29, 2023, the FDA announced a proposed rule aimed at helping ensure the safety and effectiveness of these tests. The proposed rule seeks to amend the FDA's regulations to make explicit that IVDs are devices under the Federal Food, Drug, and Cosmetic Act (FD&C Act), including when the manufacturer of the IVD is a laboratory. Along with this amendment, the FDA is proposing a policy under which the FDA intends to provide greater oversight of LDTs through a phaseout of its general enforcement discretion approach for most LDTs.[4]

Section 6.5 | Home-Use Tests

Home-use tests allow you to test for some diseases or conditions at home. These tests are cost-effective, quick, and confidential. Home-use tests can help:
- detect possible health conditions when you have no symptoms so that you can get early treatment and

[4] "Laboratory Developed Tests," U.S. Food and Drug Administration (FDA), January 18, 2024. Available online. URL: www.fda.gov/medical-devices/in-vitro-diagnostics/laboratory-developed-tests. Accessed February 15, 2024.

lower your chance of developing later complications (i.e., cholesterol testing and hepatitis testing)
- detect specific conditions when there are no signs so that you can take immediate action (i.e., pregnancy testing)
- monitor conditions to allow frequent changes in treatment (i.e., glucose testing to monitor blood sugar levels in diabetes)

Despite the benefits of home testing, you should take the following precautions when using home-use tests:
- **See your health-care provider regularly.** Home-use tests are intended to help you with your health care, but they should not replace periodic visits to your doctor.
  - Most tests are best evaluated together with your medical history, a physical exam, and other testing.
  - Always see your doctor if you are feeling sick or are worried about a possible medical condition or if the test instructions recommend you do so.
- **Always use new test strips that are authorized for sale in the United States.** The U.S. Food and Drug Administration (FDA) has issued a safety communication warning about the risks of using previously owned test strips or test strips that are not authorized for sale in the United States.[5]

Follow the tips listed here to use home-use tests as safely and effectively as possible:
- Read the label and instructions carefully. Review all instructions and pictures carefully to make sure you understand how to perform the test. Be sure you know:
  - what the test is for and what it is not for
  - how to store the test before you use it
  - how to collect and store the sample

---

[5] "Home Use Tests," U.S. Food and Drug Administration (FDA), June 21, 2022. Available online. URL: www.fda.gov/medical-devices/in-vitro-diagnostics/home-use-tests. Accessed February 15, 2024.

- when and how to run the test, including timing instructions
- how to interpret the test
- what might interfere with the test
- the manufacturer's phone number if you have questions
- Use only tests regulated by the FDA. There are several ways to find out if the FDA regulates a home-use test. You can ask your pharmacist or the vendor selling the test. If the FDA does not regulate the test, the U.S. government has not determined that the test is reasonably safe or effective or substantially equivalent to another legally marketed device.
- Follow all instructions. You must follow all test instructions to get an accurate result. Most home tests require specific timing, materials, and sample amounts. You should also check the expiration dates and storage conditions before performing a test to make sure the components still work correctly.
- Keep good records of your testing.
- Call the "800" telephone number listed on your home-use test if you have any questions.
- When in doubt, contact your doctor. All tests can give false results. You should see your doctor if you believe your test results are wrong.
- Do not change medications or dosages based on a home-use test without talking to your doctor.[6]

---

[6] "How You Can Get the Best Results with Home Use Tests," U.S. Food and Drug Administration (FDA), December 28, 2017. Available online. URL: www.fda.gov/medical-devices/home-use-tests/how-you-can-get-best-results-home-use-tests. Accessed February 15, 2024.

Section 6.6 | Direct-to-Consumer Genetic Testing

Most of the time, genetic testing is done through health-care providers such as physicians, nurse practitioners, or genetic counselors. Health-care providers determine which test is needed, order the test from a laboratory, collect the deoxyribonucleic acid (DNA) sample, send the DNA sample to the lab for testing and interpretation, and share the results with the patient. Often, a health insurance company covers part or all of the cost of testing. This type of testing is known as "clinical genetic testing."

Direct-to-consumer genetic testing is different: These genetic tests are marketed directly to customers via television, radio, print advertisements, or the Internet, and the tests can be bought online or in stores. After purchasing a test kit, customers send the company a DNA sample and receive their results directly from a secure website or app or in a written report. Direct-to-consumer genetic testing provides people access to their genetic information without necessarily involving a health-care provider or health insurance company in the process.

Many companies offer direct-to-consumer genetic tests for a variety of purposes. The most popular tests use a limited set of genetic variations to make predictions about certain aspects of health, provide information about common traits, and offer clues about a person's ancestry. The number of companies providing direct-to-consumer genetic testing is growing, along with the range of health information provided by these tests. Because there is little regulation of direct-to-consumer genetic testing services, it is important to assess the quality of available services before pursuing any testing.

WHAT KINDS OF DIRECT-TO-CONSUMER GENETIC TESTS ARE AVAILABLE?

With direct-to-consumer genetic testing companies offering a variety of tests, it can be challenging to determine which tests will be most informative and helpful to you. When considering testing, think about what you hope to get out of the test. Some direct-to-consumer genetic tests are very specific (such as paternity tests), while other services provide a broad range of health, ancestry, and lifestyle information.

MAJOR TYPES OF DIRECT-TO-CONSUMER GENETIC TESTS
Disease Risk and Health

The results of these tests estimate your genetic risk of developing several common diseases that are caused by environmental factors and multiple variants in several genes. These common diseases include such as celiac disease, Parkinson disease (PD), and Alzheimer disease (AD). Some companies also include a person's carrier status for less common conditions, including cystic fibrosis (CF) and sickle cell disease (SCD). A carrier is someone who has a gene variant in one copy of the gene that, when present in both copies of the gene, causes a genetic disorder. The tests may also look for certain genetic variations that could be related to other health-related traits, such as weight and metabolism (how a person's body converts the nutrients from food into energy). These tests may also provide information about how a person may respond to certain drugs (pharmacogenomics).

Lifestyle

The results of these tests claim to provide information about lifestyle factors, such as nutrition, fitness, weight loss, skincare, sleep, and even wine preferences, based on variations in your DNA. Many of the companies that offer this kind of testing also sell services, products, or programs that they customize based on your test results.

Before choosing a direct-to-consumer genetic test, find out what kinds of health, ancestry, or other information will be reported to you. Most direct-to-consumer genetic tests do not sequence whole genes but look at only a subset of variants within the genes associated with the conditions or traits they report on. For more comprehensive genetic testing, see a genetics professional. Think about whether there is any information you would rather not know. In some cases, you can decline to find out specific information if you tell the company before it delivers your results.

HOW IS DIRECT-TO-CONSUMER GENETIC TESTING DONE?

For most types of direct-to-consumer genetic testing, the process involves the following.

Purchasing a Test

Test kits can be purchased online (and are shipped to your home) or at a store. The price of some test kits includes the analysis and interpretation, while in other cases, this information is purchased separately.

Collecting the Sample

Collection of the DNA sample usually involves spitting saliva into a tube or swabbing the inside of your cheek and putting that swab into a tube. The test kit will include step-by-step instructions, so be sure you understand them before you begin. If you have questions, contact the company before collecting your sample. You then mail the sample as directed by the company. In some cases, you will need to visit a health clinic to have blood drawn.

Analyzing the Sample

A laboratory will analyze the sample to look for particular genetic variations. The variations included in the test depend on the purpose of the test.

Receiving Results

In most cases, you will be able to access your results on a secure website or app. (You will likely need to create an account on the testing company website to access results.) Other test companies share results in the mail or over the phone. The results usually include an interpretation of what specific genetic variations may mean for your health. At some companies, you can request additional explanation from a genetic counselor or other health-care provider. This additional service may or may not involve an extra cost. Some testing companies may update your results over time based on new scientific information, such as a new genetic variant associated with a trait on their test.

WHAT ARE THE BENEFITS AND RISKS OF DIRECT-TO-CONSUMER GENETIC TESTING?

Direct-to-consumer genetic testing has both benefits and limitations, as they are somewhat different from those of genetic testing ordered by a health-care provider.

The benefits of direct-to-consumer genetic testing include the following:

- Direct-to-consumer genetic testing promotes awareness of genetic diseases.
- It provides personalized information about your health, disease risk, and other traits.
- It may help you be more proactive about your health.
- It does not require approval from a health-care provider or health insurance company.
- As results are provided directly to the individual, they are not in your insurance or medical record (unless you share results with your health-care professional).
- It is often less expensive than genetic testing obtained through a health-care provider, which can make testing more accessible to people with no or limited health insurance.
- DNA sample collection is usually simple and noninvasive, and results are available quickly.
- Your anonymous data are added to a large database that can be used to further medical research. Depending on the company, the database may represent up to several million participants.

Risks and limitations of direct-to-consumer genetic testing include the following:

- Tests may not be available for the health conditions or traits that interest you.
- This type of testing cannot tell definitively whether you will or will not get a particular disease. Results often

- need to be confirmed with genetic tests administered by a health-care professional.
- The tests look only at a subset of variants within genes, so disease-causing variants can be missed.
- Unexpected information that you receive about your health may be stressful or upsetting.
- As testing is done outside a health-care clinic, individuals often are not provided with genetic counseling or thorough informed consent.
- People may make important decisions about disease treatment or prevention based on inaccurate, incomplete, or misunderstood information from their test results.
- There is little oversight or regulation of testing companies.
- Unproven or invalid tests can be misleading. There may not be enough scientific evidence to link a particular genetic variation with a given disease or trait.
- Genetic privacy may be compromised if testing companies use your genetic information in an unauthorized way or if your data are stolen.
- The results of genetic testing may affect your ability to obtain life, disability, or long-term care insurance.

Direct-to-consumer genetic testing provides only partial information about your health. Other genetic and environmental factors, lifestyle choices, and family medical history also affect the likelihood of developing many disorders. These factors would be discussed during a consultation with a doctor or genetic counselor, but in many cases, they are not addressed when using at-home genetic tests.

HOW MUCH DOES DIRECT-TO-CONSUMER GENETIC TESTING COST, AND IS IT COVERED BY HEALTH INSURANCE?

The price of direct-to-consumer genetic testing ranges from under a hundred dollars to thousands of dollars. The cost depends on how many genetic variations are analyzed (and it will cost more if whole genome or whole exome sequencing is used), how extensive the interpretation of results is, and whether other products, programs, or services are included. Some companies charge separately for the sample collection kit and the analysis, while others offer the sample collection and analysis as part of a package. In some cases, consultation with a health-care professional (such as a genetic counselor) is included in the cost of testing; in others, it can be added for an additional fee. Before you proceed with testing, make sure you know the total cost for all the results, support, and other services you expect to receive.

Direct-to-consumer genetic tests, even tests that provide information about health and disease risk, are not covered by most health insurance plans. Because this testing is done without a referral from a health-care provider and is not considered "diagnostic" (i.e., it cannot be used to diagnose any disease or condition), health insurance companies generally will not pay for it. However, the tests may be eligible for reimbursement through flexible spending accounts (FSAs) or health spending accounts (HSAs) if the testing includes health information. If you decide to share your results with your health-care provider and he or she recommends additional testing or management, that follow-up care may be covered by insurance.

Direct-to-consumer genetic tests that are unrelated (or indirectly related) to health, such as ancestry testing and paternity testing, are typically not covered by FSAs, HSAs, or health insurance plans.[7]

Section 6.7 | Biomarkers

A biomarker (short for biological marker) is an objective measure that captures what is happening in a cell or an organism at a given moment. Biomarkers can serve as early warning systems for your

---

[7] MedlinePlus, "What Is Direct-to-Consumer Genetic Testing?" National Institutes of Health (NIH), June 21, 2022. Available online. URL: https://medlineplus.gov/genetics/understanding/dtcgenetictesting/directtoconsumer. Accessed February 15, 2024.

Common Screening and Diagnostic Tests

health. For example, high levels of lead in the bloodstream may indicate a need to test for nervous system and cognitive disorders, especially in children. High cholesterol levels are a common biomarker for heart disease risk.

Many biomarkers come from simple measurements made during a routine doctor visit, such as blood pressure or body weight. Other biomarkers are based on laboratory tests of blood, urine, or tissues. Some capture changes at the molecular and cellular level by looking at genes or proteins.

Biomarkers play an important role in illuminating relationships among environmental exposures, human biology, and disease. Scientists can use biomarkers to better understand fundamental biological processes, advance exposure science, and turn research findings into practical medical and public health applications.[8]

WHAT IS BIOMARKER TESTING FOR CANCER TREATMENT?

Biomarker testing is a way to look for genes, proteins, and other substances (called "biomarkers" or "tumor markers") that can provide information about cancer. Each person's cancer has a unique pattern of biomarkers. Some biomarkers affect how certain cancer treatments work. Biomarker testing may help you and your doctor choose a cancer treatment for you.

There are also other kinds of biomarkers that can help doctors diagnose and monitor cancer during and after treatment.

Biomarker testing is for people who have cancer. People with solid tumors and people with blood cancer can get biomarker testing.

Biomarker testing for cancer treatment may also be called as follows:
- tumor testing
- tumor genetic testing
- genomic testing or genomic profiling
- molecular testing or molecular profiling
- somatic testing
- tumor subtyping

---

[8] "Biomarkers," National Institute of Environmental Health Sciences (NIEHS), August 2, 2023. Available online. URL: www.niehs.nih.gov/health/topics/science/biomarkers. Accessed February 15, 2024.

A biomarker test may be called a "companion diagnostic test" if it is paired with a specific treatment.

Biomarker testing is different from genetic testing that is used to find out if someone has inherited mutations that make them more likely to get cancer. Inherited mutations are those you are born with. They are passed on to you by your parents.

HOW ARE BIOMARKER TESTS USED TO SELECT CANCER TREATMENT?

Biomarker tests can help you and your doctor select a cancer treatment for you. Some cancer treatments, including targeted therapies and immunotherapies, may only work for people whose cancers have certain biomarkers.

For example, people with cancer that has certain genetic changes in the epidermal growth factor receptor (*EGFR*) gene can get treatments that target those changes, called "EGFR inhibitors." In this case, biomarker testing can find out whether someone's cancer has an *EGFR* gene change that can be treated with an EGFR inhibitor.

Biomarker testing could also help you find a study of a new cancer treatment (a clinical trial) that you may be able to join. Some studies enroll people based on the biomarkers in their cancer, instead of where in the body the cancer started growing. These are sometimes called "basket trials."

For some other clinical trials, biomarker testing is part of the study. For example, studies such as the National Cancer Institute Molecular Analysis for Therapy Choice (NCI-MATCH) and National Cancer Institute-Children's Oncology Group (NCI-COG) Pediatric MATCH are using biomarker tests to match people to treatments based on the genetic changes in their cancers.

HOW IS BIOMARKER TESTING DONE?

If you and your health-care providers decide to make biomarker testing part of your care, they will take a sample of your cancer cells. If you have a solid tumor, they may take a sample during surgery. If you are not having surgery, you may need to have a biopsy of your tumor.

Common Screening and Diagnostic Tests

If you have blood cancer or are getting a biomarker test known as a "liquid biopsy," you will need to have a blood draw. You might get a liquid biopsy test if you cannot safely get a tumor biopsy, for example, because your tumor is hard to reach with a needle.

Your samples will be sent to a special lab where they will be tested for certain biomarkers. The lab will create a report that lists the biomarkers in your cancer cells and if there are any treatments that might work for you. Your health-care team will discuss the results with you to decide on a treatment.

For some biomarker tests that analyze genes, you will also need to give a sample of your healthy cells. This is usually done by collecting your blood, saliva, or a small piece of your skin. These tests compare your cancer cells with your healthy cells to find genetic changes (called "somatic mutations") that arose during your lifetime. Somatic mutations cause most cancers and cannot be passed on to family members.

ARE THERE DIFFERENT TYPES OF BIOMARKER TESTS?

There are many types of biomarker tests that can help select cancer treatment. Most biomarker tests used to select cancer treatment look for genetic markers. But some look for proteins or other kinds of markers.

Some tests check for a single biomarker. Others check for many biomarkers at the same time and may be called "multigene tests" or "panel tests." One example is the Oncotype DX test, which looks at the activity of 21 different genes to predict whether chemotherapy is likely to work for someone with breast cancer.

Some tests are for people with a certain type of cancer, such as melanoma. Other tests look for biomarkers that are found in many cancer types, and such tests can be used by people with different kinds of cancer.

Some tests, called "whole exome sequencing," look at all the genes in your cancer. Others, called "whole genome sequencing," look at all the deoxyribonucleic acid (DNA; both genes and outside of genes) in your cancer.

Still, other biomarker tests look at the number of genetic changes in your cancer (known as "tumor mutational burden").

This information can help figure out if a type of immunotherapy known as "immune checkpoint inhibitors" may work for you.

Biomarker tests known as "liquid biopsies" look in blood or other fluids for biomarkers from cancer cells. There are two liquid biopsy tests approved by the U.S. Food and Drug Administration (FDA), called "Guardant360 CDx" and "FoundationOne Liquid CDx."

WHAT DO THE RESULTS OF A BIOMARKER TEST MEAN?

The results of a biomarker test could show that your cancer has a certain biomarker that is targeted by a known therapy. That means that the therapy may work to treat your cancer. The matching therapy may be available as an FDA-approved treatment, an off-label treatment, or through participation in a clinical trial.

The results could also show that your cancer has a biomarker that may prevent a certain therapy from working. This information could spare you from getting a treatment that would not help you.

In many cases, biomarker testing may find changes in your cancer that would not help your doctor make treatment decisions. For example, genetic changes that are thought to be harmless (benign) or whose effects are not known (variant of unknown significance) are not used to make treatment decisions.

Based on your test results, your health-care provider may recommend a treatment that is not FDA-approved for your cancer type but is approved for the treatment of a different type of cancer that has the same biomarker as your cancer. This means the treatment would be used off-label, but it may work for you because your cancer has the biomarker that the treatment targets.

Some biomarker tests can find genetic changes that you may have been born with (inherited) that increase your risk of cancer or other diseases. These genetic changes are also called "germline mutations." If such a change is found, you may need to get another genetic test to confirm whether you truly have an inherited mutation that increases cancer risk.

Finding out that you have an inherited mutation that increases cancer risk may affect you and your family. For that reason, your health-care provider may recommend that you speak with a genetic

Common Screening and Diagnostic Tests

health-care provider (such as a genetic counselor, clinical geneticist, or certified genetic nurse) to help you understand what the test results mean for you and your family.[9]

---

[9] "Biomarker Testing for Cancer Treatment," National Cancer Institute (NCI), December 14, 2021. Available online. URL: www.cancer.gov/about-cancer/treatment/types/biomarker-testing-cancer-treatment. Accessed February 15, 2024.

Chapter 7 | After Your Diagnosis: Getting Support

Here are a few basic tips to help you cope with your diagnosis, make decisions, and get on with your life.

TAKE THE TIME YOU NEED
A Diagnosis Can Change Your Life
You might be feeling some of the following emotions after getting your diagnosis:
- afraid
- alone
- angry
- anxious
- ashamed
- confused
- depressed
- helpless
- in denial
- numb
- overwhelmed
- panicky
- powerless
- relieved (that you finally know what is wrong)
- sad

- shocked
- stressed

It is perfectly normal to have these feelings. It is also normal, and very common, to have trouble taking in and understanding information after you receive the news—especially if the diagnosis was a surprise. And it can be even harder to make decisions about treating or managing your disease or condition.

Take Time to Make Your Decisions

No matter how the news of your diagnosis has affected you, do not rush into a decision. In most cases, you do not need to take action right away. Ask your doctor how much time you can safely take.

Taking the time you need to make decisions can help you:
- feel less anxious and stressed
- avoid depression
- cope with your condition
- feel more in control of your situation
- play a key role in decisions about your treatment

GET THE SUPPORT YOU NEED

Sometimes the emotional side of illness can be just as hard to deal with as the physical side. You may have fears or concerns. You may feel overwhelmed. No matter what your situation, having other people to turn to will help you know you are not alone. Here are the kinds of support you might want to seek.

Family and Friends

Talking to family and friends you feel close to can help you cope with your illness or condition. Just knowing that someone is there can be a comfort.

Sometimes it is hard to ask for help. And sometimes your family and friends want to help, but they do not want to intrude, or they do not know how to ask or what to offer. Think about specific ways

After Your Diagnosis: Getting Support

people can help you. One idea is to ask someone to come with you to a doctor's appointment to help ask questions, take notes, and talk with you afterward.

If you do not have family or friends who can provide support, other people or groups can.

Support or Self-Help Groups

Support groups are made up of people with the same disease or condition who get together to share information and concerns and to help one another.

Support groups may or may not be led by experts. Self-help groups are similar to support groups but usually are led by the participants. The names "support group" and "self-help group" sometimes are used to refer to either kind.

Research on support groups shows that participants feel less anxious, experience less depression, have a better quality of life (QOL), and have more success coping with their disease or condition. Similar findings have been reported for self-help groups.

Online Support or Self-Help Groups

The Internet has support or self-help groups for people whose concerns and situations may be similar to yours. You can also find "message boards," where you can post questions and get answers. These online communities can help you connect with people who can give you support and provide information.

But be careful. Not every idea or treatment you come across in these groups will be scientifically proven to be safe and effective. If you read about something interesting and new, check it out with your doctor.

Counselor or Therapist

A good counselor or therapist can help you cope with sadness, depression, and feelings of being overwhelmed. If you think this kind of help might be right for you, ask your doctor or other healthcare professional to recommend someone in your area.

Meet People Like You

You might want to meet and talk with someone in your own situation. Someone who has been there can talk about the real-life outcomes of their treatment choices as well as how they have learned to live with their disease or condition. Some advocacy or support groups can help you make this kind of contact.[1]

---

[1] Agency for Healthcare Research and Quality (AHRQ), "Next Steps after Your Diagnosis," U.S. Department of Health and Human Services (HHS), November 2020. Available online. URL: www.ahrq.gov/questions/resources/diagnosis/index.html. Accessed February 15, 2024.

Part 2 | Treatment and Management of Common Diseases

Chapter 8 |
Respiratory Diseases

When the respiratory system is mentioned, people generally think of breathing, but breathing is only one of the activities of the respiratory system. The body cells need a continuous supply of oxygen for the metabolic processes that are necessary to maintain life. The respiratory system works with the circulatory system to provide oxygen and remove the waste products of metabolism. It also helps regulate the pH of the blood.

Respiration is the sequence of events that results in the exchange of oxygen and carbon dioxide between the atmosphere and the body cells. Every three to five seconds, nerve impulses stimulate the breathing process, or ventilation, which moves air through a series of passages into and out of the lungs. After this, there is an exchange of gases between the lungs and the blood. This is called "external respiration." The blood transports the gases to and from the tissue cells. The exchange of gases between the blood and tissue cells is called "internal respiration." Finally, the cells utilize the oxygen for their specific activities. This is called "cellular metabolism," or "cellular respiration." Together, these activities constitute respiration.[1]

The treatment and management options for some common diseases of the respiratory system are as follows.

---

[1] Surveillance, Epidemiology, and End Results (SEER) Program, "Introduction to the Respiratory System," National Cancer Institute (NCI), June 30, 2002. Available online. URL: https://training.seer.cancer.gov/anatomy/respiratory. Accessed February 12, 2024.

ASTHMA

Asthma is a chronic (long-term) lung disease. It affects your airways, the tubes that carry air in and out of your lungs. When you have asthma, your airways can become inflamed and narrowed. This can cause wheezing, coughing, and tightness in your chest. When these symptoms get worse than usual, it is called an "asthma attack" or "flare-up."

If you have asthma, you will work with your health-care provider to create a treatment plan. The plan will include ways to manage your asthma symptoms and prevent asthma attacks. It will include the following:

- **Strategies to avoid triggers**. For example, if tobacco smoke is a trigger for you, you should not smoke or allow other people to smoke in your home or car.
- **Short-term relief medicines**. Also called "quick-relief medicines," they help prevent symptoms or relieve symptoms during an asthma attack. They include an inhaler to carry with you all the time. It may also include other types of medicines that work quickly to help open your airways.
- **Control medicines**. You take them every day to help prevent symptoms. They work by reducing airway inflammation and preventing the narrowing of the airways.

If you have a severe attack and the short-term relief medicines do not work, you will need emergency care.

Your provider may adjust your treatment until asthma symptoms are controlled.

Sometimes asthma is severe and cannot be controlled with other treatments. If you are an adult with uncontrolled asthma, in some cases, your provider might suggest bronchial thermoplasty. This is a procedure that uses heat to shrink the smooth muscle in the lungs. Shrinking the muscle reduces your airway's ability to tighten and allows you to breathe more easily. The procedure has some risks, so it is important to discuss them with your provider.[2]

BRONCHITIS

Bronchitis is a condition that develops when the airways in the lungs, called "bronchial tubes," become inflamed and cause coughing, often with mucus production. Bronchitis can be acute (short-term) or chronic (long-term).

Acute Bronchitis

Acute bronchitis, which is very common, usually results, from an infection, and may be contagious. Most people recover after a few days or weeks.

Acute bronchitis often goes away on its own without treatment. However, you can take steps at home to feel better.
- Use over-the-counter (OTC) medicines containing dextromethorphan or guaifenesin to possibly relieve cough symptoms or to loosen mucus.
- Drink hot tea or water with honey.
- Suck on throat lozenges.
- Keep a humidifier nearby.
- Use inhaled medicines such as albuterol if prescribed. They may relieve symptoms.

Health-care providers typically prescribe antibiotics only if they find that you have a bacterial infection, which is more common in young children. If you are taking any prescribed medicines or have other diseases, talk to your health-care provider before taking any OTC medicines.

Chronic Bronchitis

Chronic bronchitis is defined as lasting for at least three months and returning at least two years in a row. In chronic bronchitis,

---

[2] MedlinePlus, "Asthma," National Institutes of Health (NIH), January 24, 2024. Available online. URL: https://medlineplus.gov/asthma.html. Accessed February 12, 2024.

breathing can be more difficult because the airway lining stays inflamed, which leads to swelling and more mucus production.

The goal of the treatment for chronic bronchitis is to help you breathe better and control your symptoms. Your health-care provider may talk to you about:
- quitting smoking
- taking medicines to help clear your airways or prevent symptoms from getting worse
- oxygen therapy to help you breathe better
- pulmonary rehabilitation to learn breathing techniques such as pursed-lip breathing and to help you prevent symptoms from getting worse[3]

CHRONIC OBSTRUCTIVE PULMONARY DISEASE

Chronic obstructive pulmonary disease (COPD) is a group of lung diseases that make it hard to breathe and get worse over time. COPD includes two main types:
- **Emphysema**. It affects the air sacs in your lungs, as well as the walls between them. They become damaged and are less elastic.
- **Chronic bronchitis**. In this, the lining of your airways is constantly irritated and inflamed. This causes the lining to swell and make mucus.

Most people with COPD have both emphysema and chronic bronchitis, but how severe each type is can be different from person to person.

There is no cure for COPD. However, treatments can help with symptoms, slow the progress of the disease, and improve your ability to stay active. There are also treatments to prevent or treat complications of the disease. Treatments include:
- Lifestyle changes
  - If you are a smoker, quit smoking.
  - Avoid secondhand smoke and places where you might breathe in other lung irritants.

[3] "Bronchitis," National Heart, Lung, and Blood Institute (NHLBI), December 2, 2022. Available online. URL: www.nhlbi.nih.gov/health/bronchitis. Accessed February 12, 2024.

Respiratory Diseases

- Ask your health-care provider for an eating plan that will meet your nutritional needs and how much physical activity you can do. Physical activity can strengthen the muscles that help you breathe and improve your overall wellness.
- Medicines
  - Bronchodilators, which relax the muscles around your airways, help open your airways and make breathing easier. Most bronchodilators are taken through an inhaler. In more severe cases, the inhaler may also contain steroids to reduce inflammation.
  - Vaccines for the flu and pneumococcal pneumonia, since people with COPD are at higher risk for serious problems from these diseases.
  - Antibiotics are prescribed if you get a bacterial or viral lung infection.
- **Oxygen therapy**. If you have severe COPD and low levels of oxygen in your blood, oxygen therapy can help you breathe better. You may need extra oxygen all the time or only at certain times.
- **Pulmonary rehabilitation**. This is a program that helps improve the well-being of people who have chronic breathing problems. It may include:
  - an exercise program
  - disease management training
  - nutritional counseling
  - psychological counseling
- **Surgery**. This is usually a last resort for people who have severe symptoms that have not gotten better with medicines.
  - For COPD that is mainly related to emphysema, there are surgeries that:
    - remove damaged lung tissue
    - remove large air spaces (bullae, which can interfere with breathing) that can form when air sacs are destroyed
  - For severe COPD, some people may need a lung transplant.

If you have COPD, it is important to know when and where to get help for your symptoms. You should get emergency care if you have severe symptoms, such as trouble catching your breath or talking. Call your health-care provider if your symptoms are getting worse or if you have signs of an infection, such as a fever.[4]

PNEUMONIA

Pneumonia is an infection in one or both of your lungs. It causes the air sacs of your lungs to fill up with fluid or pus. Pneumonia can range from mild to severe, depending on what caused it, your age, and your overall health.

Treatment for pneumonia depends on the type of pneumonia, which germ is causing it, and how severe it is:
- Antibiotics treat bacterial pneumonia.
- In some cases, your provider may prescribe antiviral medicines for viral pneumonia.
- Antifungal medicines treat fungal pneumonia.

You may need to be treated in a hospital if your symptoms are severe or if you are at risk for complications. While there, you may get additional treatments. For example, if your blood oxygen level is low, you may receive oxygen therapy.

It may take time to recover from pneumonia. Some people feel better within a week. For other people, it can take a month or more.[5]

TUBERCULOSIS

Tuberculosis (TB) is a bacterial disease that usually attacks the lungs. But it can also attack other parts of the body, including the kidneys, spine, and brain. TB is found in the United States, but it is more common in certain other countries.

---

[4] MedlinePlus, "COPD," National Institutes of Health (NIH), October 5, 2021. Available online. URL: https://medlineplus.gov/copd.html. Accessed February 12, 2024.
[5] MedlinePlus, "Pneumonia," National Institutes of Health (NIH), December 8, 2023. Available online. URL: https://medlineplus.gov/pneumonia.html. Accessed February 12, 2024.

Respiratory Diseases

Not everyone infected with TB bacteria (germs) becomes sick. So there are two types of TB conditions:
- **Latent tuberculosis infection.** The TB germs live in your body but do not make you sick.
- **Tuberculosis disease (active TB).** A condition in which you get sick from the TB germs. TB disease can almost always be cured with antibiotics. But if it is not treated properly, it can be fatal.

The treatment for both latent TB infection and TB disease is antibiotics. To make sure you get rid of all the TB germs in your body, it is very important to follow the directions for taking your medicine.

If you do not follow the directions, the TB germs in your body could change and become antibiotic-resistant. That means the medicine may stop working, and your TB may become hard to cure.
- **For latent tuberculosis infections.** You usually take medicines for three to nine months. Treatment helps make sure you do not get TB disease in the future.
- **For active tuberculosis disease.** You usually need to take medicines for 6–12 months. Treatment will almost always cure you if you take your pills the right way.
- **For tuberculosis disease in your lungs or throat.** You will need to stay home for a few weeks, so you do not spread the disease to other people. You can protect the people you live with by:
  - covering your nose and mouth
  - opening windows when possible
  - not getting too close to them

By following medical advice for TB testing and treatment, you can keep yourself healthy and help stop the spread of TB.[6]

---

[6] MedlinePlus, "Tuberculosis," National Institutes of Health (NIH), August 8, 2022. Available online. URL: https://medlineplus.gov/tuberculosis.html. Accessed February 12, 2024.

Chapter 9 | Cardiovascular Diseases

The cardiovascular system is sometimes called the "blood-vascular system," or simply the "circulatory system." It consists of the heart, which is a muscular pumping device, and a closed system of vessels called "arteries," "veins," and "capillaries." As the name implies, blood contained in the circulatory system is pumped by the heart around a closed circle or circuit of vessels as it passes again and again through the various circulations of the body.[1]

The treatment and management options for some common diseases of the cardiovascular system are as follows.

CARDIAC ARREST

Cardiac arrest occurs when the heart suddenly and unexpectedly stops pumping. If this happens, blood stops flowing to the brain and other vital organs. Cardiac arrests are caused by certain types of arrhythmias that prevent the heart from pumping blood.

A cardiac arrest is fatal unless treatment begins immediately. Most cardiac arrests occur outside of hospitals. This means that emergency care of the affected person depends on family, friends, or people in the community.

It is important for everyone to know the symptoms of cardiac arrest and to act if they see someone having one. Important steps include calling 911 first, performing cardiopulmonary resuscitation (CPR), and using an automated external defibrillator (AED).

---

[1] Surveillance, Epidemiology, and End Results (SEER) Program, "Introduction to the Cardiovascular System," National Cancer Institute (NCI), April 27, 2009. Available online. URL: https://training.seer.cancer.gov/anatomy/cardiovascular. Accessed February 15, 2024.

If no one else is around—for example, if a cardiac arrest occurs at home—a family member or caregiver can call 911 while performing CPR.

AEDs are special defibrillators that untrained bystanders can use. They are often available in public places such as airports, office buildings, gyms, and shopping centers. AEDs give an electric shock if they detect a dangerous arrhythmia, such as ventricular fibrillation. The devices talk to the user to give step-by-step instructions.

Emergency Treatment

Steps to help a person having a cardiac arrest are:

- **If you see someone collapse, check to see whether the person responds to shouting and tapping on their body.** Check for breathing and a pulse. If the person is not breathing normally and if they do not respond, call 911 for help.
- **Start CPR.**
- **Locate an AED.** Follow the AED's verbal instructions to deliver a shock to restart the heart of the affected person.
- **Naloxone should be given as part of emergency treatment for cardiac arrest possibly caused by opioid overdose.** First responders carry naloxone. If the person is known to be at risk of opioid overdose and you are trained to give naloxone, you can treat them before first responders arrive.
- **Continue CPR until first responders arrive and take over.** First responders will continue CPR and may use an AED to give more shocks to restore the affected person's heart rhythm. They may also give medicines through an intravenous (IV) line.

Hospital Treatment after Surviving Cardiac Arrest

If you survive a cardiac arrest, you will be admitted to a hospital for ongoing care and treatment. In the hospital, health-care providers

Cardiovascular Diseases

closely monitor your heart. Hospital treatment focuses on preventing organ damage, especially to the brain.
- **Targeted temperature management (TTM).** TTM is necessary for all patients who cannot follow commands after their heartbeat returns. TTM helps protect the brain by lowering the body temperature using cooling blankets, cooling helmets, ice packs, or other methods.
- **Oxygen therapy.** This can help get enough oxygen into your lungs, so your organs can keep functioning as you recover.
- **Extracorporeal membrane oxygenation (ECMO).** ECMO treatment pumps blood through an artificial lung to add oxygen and remove carbon dioxide before returning the blood to your body.

While you are in the hospital, your medical team will try to find out what caused your cardiac arrest. If you are diagnosed with coronary heart disease, treatments may include medicines and surgical heart procedures such as bypass surgery and percutaneous coronary intervention (PCI; also known as "coronary angioplasty"), a procedure that may also include placing a stent. These procedures help restore blood flow through narrowed or blocked coronary arteries.

Cardioverter Devices Can Prevent Another Cardiac Arrest

Having one cardiac arrest means you are at risk for another one. Cardioverter devices are defibrillators that your doctor can implant in your body or that you can wear to help keep you safe. The devices can detect serious rhythm problems and use electric pulses or shocks to help control dangerous arrhythmias. Your health-care provider may recommend one of the following devices:
- **Implantable cardioverter defibrillator (ICD).** An ICD is a device that is surgically placed under the skin in your chest or abdomen. It has a battery and connects to your heart with wires called "leads." If the ICD detects a dangerous arrhythmia, it can act

as a pacemaker or give your heart an electric shock to restore a normal rhythm. Risks include infections, lead-related problems, cardiac tamponade, and rarely, perforations leading to complications such as pneumothorax.
- **Subcutaneous cardioverter device (SCD).** An SCD may be better than an ICD for some people, especially if they have a high risk of infection because of diabetes or other conditions. SCDs may also be safer for younger, active people who have a higher risk of cardiac arrest caused by a malfunction of the ICD (called "lead failure"). SCDs are not right for people who need pacemaker support.
- **Wearable cardioverter device (WCD).** A WCD may help people as they wait for a procedure to implant an ICD or SCD or for a heart transplant. If your provider needs to replace your ICD or SCD because of an infection, they may recommend a WCD until the infection heals. WCDs can also help keep people safe if they recently had bypass surgery or just started medical treatment for severe cardiomyopathy.[2]

CORONARY HEART DISEASE

Coronary heart disease is a type of heart disease where the arteries of the heart cannot deliver enough oxygen-rich blood to the heart. It is also sometimes called "coronary artery disease" (CAD) or "ischemic heart disease."

Your treatment for coronary heart disease depends on how serious your symptoms are and any other health conditions you have. If you are having a heart attack, for example, you may need emergency treatment. If your health-care provider diagnoses you with coronary heart disease, your treatment may include heart-healthy lifestyle changes in combination with medicines to prevent a heart attack or other health problems. Your provider will consider your

---

[2] "Cardiac Arrest," National Heart, Lung, and Blood Institute (NHLBI), May 19, 2022. Available online. URL: www.nhlbi.nih.gov/health/cardiac-arrest. Accessed February 15, 2024.

Cardiovascular Diseases

10-year risk calculation and work with you to determine how best to treat your coronary heart disease.

Heart-Healthy Lifestyle Changes
Your provider may recommend adopting lifelong heart-healthy lifestyle changes, such as the following:
- **Choose heart-healthy foods**. A heart-healthy eating plan includes fruits, vegetables, and whole grains and limits saturated fats, sodium (salt), added sugars, and alcohol. Your health-care provider may recommend following the Dietary Approaches to Stop Hypertension (DASH) eating plan or Therapeutic Lifestyle Changes (TLC) Program.
- **Be physically active**. Routine physical activity can help manage coronary heart disease risk factors such as high blood cholesterol, high blood pressure (HBP), or overweight and obesity. Before starting any exercise program, ask your provider what level of physical activity is right for you.
- **Quit smoking**. Smoking can damage and tighten your blood vessels. For free help and support to quit smoking, you can call the Smoking Quitline at 877-44U-QUIT (877-448-7848) of the National Cancer Institute (NCI). Talk to your provider if you vape. There is scientific evidence that nicotine and flavorings found in vaping products may damage your heart and lungs.
- **Get enough good quality sleep**. During sleep, your body can work to repair your heart and blood vessels. Not getting enough hours of sleep or good quality sleep can raise your risk for heart disease and other health problems. The recommended amount for adults is seven to nine hours of sleep a day.
- **Aim for a healthy weight**. Reaching and maintaining a healthy body weight can help you manage some coronary heart disease risk factors, such as high blood cholesterol, diabetes, and HBP. You can work with

your provider to create a weight-loss plan that is right for you.
- **Get your blood pressure and cholesterol checked.** Your provider can help you get your blood pressure and blood cholesterol to a healthy range.
- **Control your blood sugar.** High levels of glucose (sugar in your blood) can damage your blood vessels. You can work with your provider to limit how many calories you get each day from added sugars to help lower your risk of heart disease.
- **Manage stress.** Learning how to manage stress, relax, and cope with problems can improve your emotional and physical health.

Medicines

Some medicines can reduce or prevent chest pain and manage other medical conditions that may contribute to your coronary heart disease. Tell your health-care provider about all the medicines you take and any complementary health strategies you use, such as dietary supplements for lowering your cholesterol or meditation for managing your HBP. Together, you and your provider can make a treatment plan that is right for you.

As part of your treatment plan, your provider may prescribe you medicines that widen your blood vessels and help your heart beat with less force:

- **Angiotensin-converting enzyme (ACE) inhibitors and beta-blockers.** These medicines help lower blood pressure and decrease how hard your heart is working.
- **Calcium channel blockers.** These medicines lower blood pressure by allowing blood vessels to relax.
- **Nitrates.** Medicines such as nitroglycerin dilate your coronary arteries and relieve or prevent angina (chest pain).
- **Ranolazine.** These medicines treat coronary microvascular disease and the chest pain it may cause.

Cardiovascular Diseases

Your provider may also prescribe medicines to help manage the levels of cholesterol in your blood:
- **Statins**. Medicines such as atorvastatin and rosuvastatin can help control high blood cholesterol and slow down plaque buildup. You may need statin therapy if you have a high risk of coronary heart disease or stroke or if you have diabetes and are between the ages of 40 and 75. Your provider may stop the treatment if you are pregnant or planning a pregnancy.
- **Nonstatins**. These medicines can help lower your cholesterol levels if you cannot take statins or require additional cholesterol lowering. Your provider may also prescribe them in combination with a statin if statins alone are not enough to manage your cholesterol. Ezetimibe and bile acid sequestrants can lower the amount of cholesterol and fat you absorb from food. Proprotein convertase subtilisin/kexin type 9 (PCSK9) inhibitors, such as alirocumab and evolocumab, are nonstatins that you inject under your skin every two to four weeks to help remove cholesterol from your blood.
- **Medicines that lower your blood triglycerides**. These medicines can also help manage your cholesterol in combination with a heart-healthy diet. Your provider may prescribe fibrates (such as gemfibrozil or fenofibrate), omega-3 fatty acids, or niacin to help lower your triglyceride levels. However, this type of nonstatin is less effective in lowering your risk of coronary heart disease.

Some medicines can help manage other risk factors for heart disease, such as high blood sugar, overweight and obesity, or diabetes:
- **Medicines to control blood sugar**. Drugs such as empagliflozin, canagliflozin, metformin, and liraglutide can help lower the risk of complications for people with coronary heart disease and diabetes.

- **Medicines for weight management.** Drugs such as orlistat, semaglutide, and liraglutide can help lower the risk of coronary heart disease for people with overweight or obesity. To be effective, these medicines should be combined with a healthy diet and regular physical activity.

Procedures

You may need a procedure or heart surgery to treat coronary heart disease that is more serious:
- **Percutaneous coronary intervention.** This procedure opens coronary arteries that are narrowed or blocked by the buildup of plaque. During the procedure, your health-care provider may use shock waves to break up the hardened plaque and may also implant a small mesh tube, or stent, in your artery to prevent it from narrowing again. This can help relieve angina, or chest pain, which happens when the heart cannot get enough oxygen-rich blood. However, this procedure does not protect you from serious complications of coronary heart disease, such as heart failure or cardiac arrest.
- **Coronary artery bypass grafting (CABG).** A procedure that improves blood flow to the heart by using healthy arteries from the chest wall and veins from the legs to bypass the blocked arteries. Surgeons typically use CABG to treat people who have severe CAD in multiple coronary arteries. Your provider may recommend this surgery to lower your risk of having a heart attack and other complications.
- **Transmyocardial laser revascularization (TMR).** Also called "coronary endarterectomy," this procedure treats severe angina linked to coronary heart disease when other treatments are too risky or do not work.
- **Bariatric surgery.** This is a surgery that can help lower the risk of coronary heart disease and other problems that affect the blood vessels of people with obesity, especially for people who also have diabetes. Before

Cardiovascular Diseases

choosing this procedure, it is important to talk with your health-care provider about the benefits and risks of this approach.[3]

HEART ATTACK

A heart attack, also known as a "myocardial infarction," happens when the flow of blood that brings oxygen to a part of your heart muscle suddenly becomes blocked. Your heart cannot get enough oxygen. If blood flow is not restored quickly, the heart muscle will begin to die.

Your doctor or emergency medical personnel may start treatment even before they confirm that you are having a heart attack. Early treatment to remove the blood clot or plaque can prevent or limit damage to your heart, help your heart work better, and save your life.

Medicines

- **Aspirin**. These medicines can prevent more blood clots from forming. In some people, aspirin may cause bleeding in the stomach.
- **Nitroglycerin**. Also called "nitrates," these medicines can make it easier for your heart to pump blood and improve blood flow through your coronary arteries. Nitroglycerin also treats chest pain. You may also be given other medicines for chest pain. Side effects of this medicine include nausea, vomiting, weakness, a slow heartbeat, and low blood pressure.
- **Thrombolytic medicines**. Also called "clot busters," these medicines can help dissolve blood clots that are blocking your coronary arteries. These medicines may cause bleeding problems. You may be given these if you were unable to reach a hospital that can do a PCI quickly enough.

---

[3] "Coronary Heart Disease," National Heart, Lung, and Blood Institute (NHLBI), December 20, 2023. Available online. URL: www.nhlbi.nih.gov/health/coronary-heart-disease. Accessed February 15, 2024.

Oxygen Therapy

Oxygen therapy is a treatment that delivers oxygen gas for you to breathe. You can receive oxygen therapy from tubes resting in your nose, a face mask, or a tube placed in your trachea (windpipe). You may need oxygen therapy if you have a condition that causes your blood oxygen levels to be too low.

Oxygen therapy can be given for a short or long period of time in the hospital, another medical setting, or at home. Oxygen poses a fire risk, so you should never smoke or use flammable materials when using oxygen. You may experience side effects from this treatment, such as a dry or bloody nose, tiredness, and morning headaches. Oxygen therapy is generally safe.

Procedures

You may need one of the following procedures at the hospital or later to help restore blood flow to your heart. These procedures are often done as soon as your health-care team confirms that you are having a heart attack.

PERCUTANEOUS CORONARY INTERVENTION

PCI is a nonsurgical procedure that improves blood flow to your heart. Doctors use PCI to open blood vessels to the heart that are narrowed or blocked by a buildup of plaque. PCI requires cardiac catheterization.

A cardiologist, a doctor who specializes in the heart, performs PCI in a hospital cardiac catheterization laboratory. Live x-rays help your doctor guide a catheter through your blood vessels into your heart, where a special contrast dye is injected to highlight any blockage. To open a blocked artery, your doctor will insert another catheter over a guidewire and inflate a balloon at the tip of that catheter. Your doctor may also put a small mesh tube called a "stent" in your artery to help keep the artery open.

You may develop a bruise and soreness where the catheters are inserted. It is also common to have discomfort or bleeding where the catheters are inserted. You will recover in a special unit of the hospital for a few hours or overnight. You will get instructions on how much activity you can do and what medicines to take. You will need a ride home because of the medicines and anesthesia you received. Your doctor will check your progress during a follow-up visit. If a stent is implanted, you will have to take certain anticlotting medicines exactly as prescribed, usually for at least 6–12 months.

Serious complications during a PCI procedure or as you are recovering after one are rare, but they can happen. This might include:
- bleeding
- blood vessel damage
- treatable allergic reaction to the contrast dye
- need for emergency CABG during the procedure
- arrhythmias, or irregular heartbeats
- damaged arteries
- kidney damage
- heart attack
- stroke
- blood clots

Sometimes chest pain can occur during PCI because the balloon briefly blocks blood supply to the heart. Restenosis, when tissue regrows where the artery was treated, may occur in the months after a PCI. This may cause the artery to become narrow or blocked again. The risk of complications from this procedure is higher if you are older, have chronic kidney disease, are experiencing heart failure at the time of the procedure, or have extensive heart disease and more than one blockage in your coronary arteries.

Stenting
A stent is a small mesh tube that holds open passages in the body, such as weak or narrow arteries. Stenting is a minimally invasive procedure. The most common complication after a stenting procedure is a blockage or blood clot in the stent. You may need to take certain medicines, such as aspirin and other antiplatelet medicines, for a year or longer after receiving a stent in your artery to prevent serious complications such as blood clots.

Coronary Artery Bypass Grafting

CABG is a procedure to improve poor blood flow to the heart. It may be needed when the arteries supplying blood to heart tissue, called "coronary arteries," are narrowed or blocked. This surgery may lower the risk of serious complications for people who have a type of heart disease called "obstructive CAD." CABG may also be used in an emergency, such as a severe heart attack.[4]

HEART FAILURE

Heart failure, also known as "congestive heart failure" (CHF), is a condition that develops when your heart does not pump enough blood for your body's needs. This can happen if your heart cannot fill up with enough blood. It can also happen when your heart is too weak to pump properly. The term "heart failure" does not mean that your heart has stopped. However, heart failure is a serious condition that needs medical care.

Heart failure has no cure. But treatment can help you live a longer, more active life with fewer symptoms. Treatment depends on the type of heart failure you have and how serious it is.

Your health-care providers may include a cardiologist (a doctor who specializes in treating heart conditions), nurses, your primary care provider (PCP), pharmacists, a dietitian, physical therapists and other members of a cardiac rehabilitation team, and social workers.

Healthy Lifestyle Changes

Your provider may recommend these heart-healthy lifestyle changes alone or as part of a cardiac rehabilitation plan:
- Lower your sodium (salt) intake.
- Aim for a healthy weight.
- Get regular physical activity.
- Quit smoking.
- Avoid or limit alcohol.

---

[4] "Heart Attack," National Heart, Lung, and Blood Institute (NHLBI), March 24, 2022. Available online. URL: www.nhlbi.nih.gov/health/heart-attack. Accessed February 15, 2024.

Cardiovascular Diseases

- Manage contributing risk factors.
- Manage stress.
- Get good quality sleep.

Medicines
LEFT-SIDED HEART FAILURE
The following medicines are commonly used to treat heart failure with reduced ejection fraction.
- **Medicines that remove extra sodium and fluid from your body.** Diuretics and aldosterone antagonists, such as spironolactone, lower the amount of blood that the heart must pump. Very high doses of diuretics may cause low blood pressure, kidney disease, and worsening heart failure symptoms. Side effects of aldosterone antagonists can include kidney disease and high potassium levels.
- **Medicines to relax your blood vessels.** These medicines make it easier for your heart to pump blood. Examples include ACE inhibitors and angiotensin receptor blockers (ARBs). Possible side effects include cough, low blood pressure, and short-term reduced kidney function.
- **Medicines to slow your heart rate.** Medicines such as beta-blockers and ivabradine make it easier for your heart to pump blood and can help prevent long-term heart failure from getting worse. Possible side effects include a slow or irregular heart rate, HBP, fuzzy vision, or seeing bright halos.
- **Newer medicines.** Two new groups of medicines are approved to lower blood sugar in patients with diabetes, called "sodium-glucose cotransporter-2 (SGLT-2) inhibitors" and "glucagon-like peptide (GLP) agonists." They may also reduce heart failure hospitalizations. Their use in treating heart failure is currently being studied.
- **Digoxin.** This medicine makes your heart beat stronger and pumps more blood and is mostly used to treat

serious heart failure when other medicines do not help improve your symptoms. Side effects may include digestive problems, confusion, and vision problems.

The main treatments for heart failure with preserved ejection fraction are diuretics. Your doctor may also prescribe blood pressure medicines to help relieve your symptoms.

RIGHT-SIDED HEART FAILURE
If you have right-sided heart failure, your doctor may prescribe two types of medicines:
- **Medicines that remove extra sodium and fluid from your body.** Diuretics and aldosterone antagonists (such as spironolactone) lower the amount of blood that the heart must pump. Very high doses of diuretics may cause low blood pressure, kidney disease, and worsening heart failure symptoms. Side effects of aldosterone antagonists can include kidney disease and high potassium levels.
- **Medicines to relax your blood vessels.** These medicines make it easier for your heart to pump blood. Examples include ACE inhibitors and ARBs. Possible side effects include cough, low blood pressure, and short-term reduced kidney function.

Procedures and Surgeries
If you have heart failure with reduced ejection fraction and it worsens, you may need one of the following medical devices:
- **Biventricular pacemaker.** Also called "cardiac resynchronization therapy" (CRT), this device can help both sides of your heart contract at the same time to relieve your symptoms.
- **Mechanical heart pump.** A ventricular assist device or a total artificial heart may be used until you have surgery or as a long-term treatment.
- **Implantable cardioverter defibrillator (ICD).** An ICD checks your heart rate and uses electrical pulses to

Cardiovascular Diseases

correct irregular heart rhythms that can cause sudden cardiac arrest.

You may also need heart surgery to repair a congenital heart defect or damage to your heart. If your heart failure is life-threatening and other treatments have not worked, you may need a heart transplant.

For people with heart failure and preserved ejection fraction, there are no currently approved devices or procedures to improve symptoms.[5]

HEART VALVE DISEASE

Heart valve diseases are problems affecting one or more of the four valves in the heart. Heart valves open and shut with each heartbeat to keep blood flowing in the right direction. Problems with heart valves can occur if the valves are leaky (a condition called "regurgitation"), too narrow (stenosis), or do not have a proper opening (atresia).

Heart valve disease is a lifelong condition. However, many people have heart valve defects or disease but do not have symptoms. The condition may stay the same throughout your life and not cause any problems. Or the condition may slowly get worse until you start to notice symptoms. If not treated, heart valve disease can cause heart failure or other life-threatening conditions.

Your health-care provider may recommend healthy lifestyle changes or medicine first to treat symptoms, which may delay problems. Eventually, you may need to have your faulty heart valve repaired or replaced. After repair or replacement, you will still need certain medicines and regular checkups with your doctor.

Heart-Healthy Lifestyle Changes
Healthy lifestyle changes include:
- choosing heart-healthy foods
- aiming for a healthy weight
- managing stress

---

[5] "Heart Failure," National Heart, Lung, and Blood Institute (NHLBI), March 24, 2022. Available online. URL: www.nhlbi.nih.gov/health/heart-failure. Accessed February 15, 2024.

- getting regular physical activity
- quitting smoking

Before starting any exercise program, ask your doctor about what level of physical activity is right for you.

Medicines

Your doctor may prescribe medicines to relieve the symptoms of your heart valve disease, prevent it from getting worse, or treat other heart problems that can affect your heart valves. These may include:
- medicines to control HBP, such as diuretics and vasodilators, to ease pressure on the heart and reduce the amount of work the heart must do to pump blood
- medicines to control the heart rate
- blood thinners to treat or prevent blood clots
- antibiotics to treat infections that cause heart inflammation or prevent rheumatic fever
- prostaglandin for newborns to keep certain pathways of the heart open and maintain blood flow to the body

Heart Valve Repair

Your doctor may recommend heart valve repair if you have new symptoms of heart valve disease or your current symptoms get worse.

The various ways that heart surgeons repair heart valves are listed subsequently. While most require surgery, some minimally invasive options are becoming available.
- **Fixing valve flaps**. Surgeons may sew flaps together, reshape flaps, patch tears, reattach loose flaps, or split apart flaps that have fused. These procedures are called "valvuloplasty."
- **Inflating a balloon**. This allows blood to pump blood through a valve or stretch a valve opening. Valvuloplasty may also involve a balloon.
- **Placing a stent**. This allows blood to flow or plugs into a leaking valve.

- **Implanting a device to treat mitral valve regurgitation.** This can be used for people who should not have open-heart surgery.
- **Removing calcium deposits.** Obstructions such as clumps of bacteria or tumors can also be removed.
- **Repairing supporting structures.** Replacing or shortening the cords that give the valve support, allows the valve to close properly.
- **Tightening or strengthening the valve base.** This prevents the tissue from sagging or leaking. Surgeons may attach a plastic ring. These procedures are called "annuloplasty."

Heart valve repair can improve symptoms, but sometimes problems return.

Possible complications of heart valve repairs include valve damage or leakage, blood vessel injury, cardiac compression, and stroke.

Heart Valve Replacement

Sometimes faulty or diseased heart valves cannot be repaired and must be replaced.

Your surgeon will replace the faulty or diseased valve with either a mechanical or a biological heart valve. Your team of doctors will work with you to determine whether a mechanical or a biological valve is best for you, depending on your age, risk factors, and other medical conditions.

- **Biological valves.** Also called "tissue valves," these are made from animal tissue and may have human-made parts as well. Although tissue valves do not require blood thinners, they do not last as long and may have to be replaced.
- **Mechanical valves.** These valves are made from carbon or other sturdy material, so they last longer than biological valves and usually do not have to be replaced. However, mechanical valves require you to take blood-thinning medicines for the rest of your life. These valves may also carry additional risks during pregnancy.

Valves can be replaced during open heart surgery or with a minimally invasive procedure using a catheter—a thin tube threaded through a blood vessel to the heart. A common example of the procedure using a catheter is transcatheter aortic valve replacement (TAVR). TAVR, which is sometimes called "transcatheter aortic valve implantation" (TAVI), replaces the aortic valve to treat aortic stenosis.

The risks of heart valve replacement include stroke, blood clots, damage and bleeding where the catheters were inserted, and injury to the kidneys or the heart. Sometimes the new valve leaks because it does not fit well.[6]

---

[6] "Heart Valve Diseases," National Heart, Lung, and Blood Institute (NHLBI), March 24, 2022. Available online. URL: www.nhlbi.nih.gov/health/heart-valve-diseases. Accessed February 15, 2024.

Chapter 10 | Gastrointestinal Diseases

The digestive system includes the digestive tract and its accessory organs, which process food into molecules that can be absorbed and utilized by the cells of the body. Food is broken down, bit by bit, until the molecules are small enough to be absorbed, and the waste products are eliminated. The digestive tract, also called the "alimentary canal" or "gastrointestinal (GI) tract," consists of a long continuous tube that extends from the mouth to the anus. It includes the mouth, pharynx, esophagus, stomach, small intestine, and large intestine. The tongue and teeth are accessory structures located in the mouth. The salivary glands, liver, gallbladder, and pancreas are major accessory organs that have a role in digestion. These organs secrete fluids into the digestive tract.[1]

The treatment and management options for some common diseases of the digestive system are as follows.

CELIAC DISEASE
Celiac disease is a chronic (long-term) digestive and immune disorder that damages your small intestine. The damage may prevent your body from absorbing vitamins, minerals, and other nutrients from the food you eat. This can lead to malnutrition and other serious health problems. Celiac disease is triggered by eating foods that contain gluten.

---

[1] Surveillance, Epidemiology, and End Results (SEER) Program, "Introduction to the Digestive System," National Cancer Institute (NCI), June 30, 2002. Available online. URL: https://training.seer.cancer.gov/anatomy/digestive. Accessed February 12, 2024.

The treatment for celiac disease is following a gluten-free diet for the rest of your life. Sticking with a gluten-free diet will treat or prevent many of the symptoms and other health problems caused by celiac disease. In most cases, it can also heal damage in the small intestine and prevent more damage.

Your provider may refer you to a registered dietician (a nutrition expert) who can help you learn how to eat a healthy diet without gluten. You will also need to avoid all hidden sources of gluten, such as certain supplements, cosmetics, toothpaste, and so on. Reading product labels can sometimes help you avoid gluten. If a label does not tell you what is in a product, check with the company that makes the product for an ingredients list. Do not just assume that a product is gluten-free if it does not mention it.[2]

CROHN'S DISEASE

Crohn's disease is a chronic (long-lasting) disease that causes inflammation in your digestive tract. It can affect any part of your digestive tract, which runs from your mouth to your anus. But it usually affects your small intestine and the beginning of your large intestine.

There is no cure for Crohn's disease, but treatments can decrease inflammation in your intestines, relieve symptoms, and prevent complications. Treatments include medicines, bowel rest, and surgery. No single treatment works for everyone. You and your provider can work together to figure out which treatment is best for you:

- **Medicines**. Drugs for Crohn's disease include various medicines that decrease inflammation. Many of these medicines do this by reducing the activity of your immune system. Certain medicines can also help with symptoms or complications, such as nonsteroidal antiinflammatory drugs (NSAIDs) and antidiarrheal medicines. If your Crohn's disease causes an infection, you may need antibiotics.

---

[2] MedlinePlus, "Celiac Disease," National Institutes of Health (NIH), August 7, 2023. Available online. URL: https://medlineplus.gov/celiacdisease.html. Accessed February 12, 2024.

Gastrointestinal Diseases

- **Bowel rest**. This involves drinking only certain liquids or not eating or drinking anything. This allows your intestines to rest. You may need to do this if your Crohn's disease symptoms are severe. You get your nutrients through drinking a liquid, a feeding tube, or an intravenous (IV) tube. You may need to do bowel rest in the hospital, or you may be able to do it at home. It will last for a few days or up to several weeks.
- **Surgery**. This can treat complications and reduce symptoms when other treatments are not helping enough. The surgery will involve removing a damaged part of your digestive tract to treat:
  - fistulas
  - bleeding that is life-threatening
  - intestinal obstructions
  - side effects from medicines when they threaten your health
  - symptoms when medicines do not improve your condition

Changing your diet can help reduce symptoms. Your provider may recommend that you make changes to your diet, such as:
- avoiding carbonated drinks
- avoiding popcorn, vegetable skins, nuts, and other high-fiber foods
- drinking more liquids
- eating smaller meals more often
- keeping a food diary to help identify foods that cause problems

In some cases, your provider may ask you to go on a special diet, such as a diet that is:
- high calorie
- lactose-free
- low fat
- low fiber
- low salt

If you are not absorbing enough nutrients, you may need to take nutritional supplements and vitamins.[3]

GASTRITIS AND GASTROPATHY

Gastritis and gastropathy are conditions that affect the stomach lining, also known as the "mucosa." In gastritis, the stomach lining is inflamed. In gastropathy, the stomach lining is damaged, but little or no inflammation is present.

Your doctor will recommend treatments based on the type of gastritis or gastropathy you have and its cause. Treating gastritis and gastropathy can improve symptoms, if present, and lower your chance of complications.

Helicobacter pylori Gastritis

Doctors treat *Helicobacter pylori* gastritis with a combination of medicines to kill *H. pylori* bacteria. These medicines most often include:
- two or more antibiotics
- a proton pump inhibitor (PPI)
- in some cases, bismuth subsalicylate

Your doctor may avoid prescribing antibiotics you have taken in the past because the *H. pylori* bacteria may have developed antibiotic resistance to those antibiotics.

If you are given medicines, take all doses exactly as your doctor prescribes. If you stop taking your medicine early, some bacteria may survive and reinfect you. In other words, *H. pylori* bacteria may develop antibiotic resistance.

To find out if medicines have worked, your health-care professional may recommend testing you for *H. pylori* at least four weeks after you have finished taking medicines. If you still have an *H. pylori* infection, your doctor may prescribe a different combination of antibiotics and other medicines to treat the infection.

---

[3] MedlinePlus, "Crohn's Disease," National Institutes of Health (NIH), October 18, 2023. Available online. URL: https://medlineplus.gov/crohnsdisease.html. Accessed February 12, 2024.

Making sure that all the *H. pylori* bacteria have been killed is important to prevent further complications of the infection.

Reactive Gastropathy

If long-term use of NSAIDs leads to reactive gastropathy, your doctor may recommend that you stop taking NSAIDs, take a lower dose, or take a different medicine for pain. Doctors may also recommend taking a PPI along with NSAIDs to prevent or treat reactive gastropathy and its possible complications.

If bile reflux is causing reactive gastropathy, doctors may prescribe ursodiol, a medicine that contains bile acids and can help heal the stomach lining, or surgery to stop the flow of bile into the stomach.

Autoimmune Gastritis

If you have autoimmune gastritis, your doctor may recommend iron, folic acid, and vitamin B_{12} supplements to prevent pernicious anemia. If autoimmune gastritis leads to pernicious anemia, doctors may recommend vitamin B_{12} injections to treat this condition.

For safety reasons, talk with your doctor before using dietary supplements, such as vitamins, or any complementary or alternative medicines or medical practices.

Acute Erosive Gastropathy

For patients with severe injuries or critical illness, doctors may prescribe medicines, such as PPIs, H2 blockers, or sucralfate (Carafate), that reduce stomach acid to prevent or treat stress gastritis.

If an irritating substance is causing acute erosive gastropathy, treatment includes removing contact with the substance. Doctors may also prescribe PPIs or H2 blockers to reduce stomach acid.

If acute erosive gastropathy causes severe bleeding in the stomach, doctors may treat the bleeding during upper GI endoscopy or with surgery in severe cases.

Gastritis or Gastropathy due to Other Causes

To treat gastritis or gastropathy due to other causes, doctors may prescribe medicines to treat the underlying cause or improve symptoms. Doctors may recommend diet changes if gastritis is related to celiac disease or food allergies.[4]

GASTROESOPHAGEAL REFLUX OR GASTROESOPHAGEAL REFLUX DISEASE

Gastroesophageal reflux (GER) happens when your stomach contents come back up into your esophagus. Many people have GER once in a while, and GER often happens without causing symptoms. In some cases, GER may cause heartburn, also called "acid indigestion."

Gastroesophageal reflux disease (GERD) is a more severe and long-lasting condition in which GER causes repeated symptoms that are bothersome or lead to complications over time.

Your doctor may recommend that you make lifestyle changes and take medicines to manage symptoms of GER or GERD. In some cases, doctors may also recommend surgery.

Lifestyle Changes

Lifestyle changes may reduce your symptoms. Your doctor may recommend:
- losing weight if you are overweight or have obesity
- elevating your head during sleep by placing a foam wedge or extra pillows under your head and upper back to incline your body and raise your head off your bed, 6–8 inches
- quitting smoking, if you smoke
- changing your eating habits and diet

Over-the-Counter and Prescription Medicines

You can buy many GERD medicines over the counter. However, if you have symptoms that will not go away with over-the-counter

---

[4] "Gastritis & Gastropathy," National Institute of Diabetes and Digestive and Kidney Diseases (NIDDK), August 2019. Available online. URL: www.niddk.nih.gov/health-information/digestive-diseases/gastritis-gastropathy. Accessed February 12, 2024.

Gastrointestinal Diseases

(OTC) medicines, you should talk with your doctor. Your doctor may prescribe one or more medicines to treat GERD.

- **Antacids.** Doctors may recommend antacids to relieve mild heartburn and other mild GER and GERD symptoms. Antacids are available over the counter. Antacids can help relieve mild symptoms. However, you should not use these medicines every day or for severe symptoms, except after discussing your antacid use with your doctor. These medicines can have side effects, such as diarrhea or constipation.
- **H2 blockers.** These medicines lower the amount of acid your stomach makes. H2 blockers can help heal the esophagus but not as well as PPIs can. You can buy H2 blockers over the counter, or your doctor can prescribe one.
- **Proton pump inhibitors (PPIs).** PPIs lower the amount of acid your stomach makes. PPIs are better at treating GERD symptoms than H2 blockers, and they can heal the esophageal lining in most people with GERD. You can buy PPIs over the counter, or your doctor can prescribe one. Doctors may prescribe PPIs for long-term GERD treatment. PPIs are generally safe and effective. Side effects are uncommon and may include headache, diarrhea, and upset stomach. Research also suggests that taking PPIs may increase the chance of *Clostridioides difficile* (*C. diff*) infection. Experts are still studying the effects of taking PPIs for a long time or in high doses. Talk with your doctor about the risks and benefits of taking PPIs.
- **Other medicines.** If antacids, H2 blockers, and PPIs do not improve your symptoms, your doctor may recommend other medicines.

Surgery and Other Medical Procedures

Your doctor may recommend surgery if your GERD symptoms do not improve with lifestyle changes and medicines, or if you wish to stop taking long-term GERD medicines to manage symptoms.

You are more likely to develop complications from surgery than from medicines.
- **Fundoplication**. This is the most common surgery for GERD. In most cases, it leads to long-term improvement of GERD symptoms. During the operation, a surgeon sews the top of your stomach around the end of your esophagus to add pressure to the lower esophageal sphincter and help prevent reflux. Surgeons may perform fundoplication as laparoscopic or open surgery. In laparoscopic fundoplication, which is more common, surgeons make small cuts in the abdomen and insert special tools to perform the operation. Laparoscopic fundoplication leaves several small scars. In open fundoplication, surgeons make a larger cut in the abdomen.
- **Bariatric surgery**. If you have GERD and obesity, your doctor may recommend weight loss surgery, also called "bariatric surgery," most often gastric bypass surgery. Bariatric surgery can help you lose weight and reduce GERD symptoms.
- **Endoscopy**. In a small number of cases, doctors may recommend procedures that use endoscopy to treat GERD. For endoscopy, doctors insert an endoscope—a small, flexible tube with a light and camera—through your mouth and into your esophagus. Doctors may use endoscopic procedures to sew the top of your stomach around the lower esophageal sphincter or to deliver radiofrequency energy to the sphincter. Doctors do not use these procedures often.[5]

PEPTIC ULCERS

A peptic ulcer is a sore on the lining of your stomach or duodenum. Peptic ulcers are sometimes called "stomach ulcers," "duodenal ulcers," or "peptic ulcer disease."

---

[5] "Acid Reflux (GER & GERD) in Adults," National Institute of Diabetes and Digestive and Kidney Diseases (NIDDK), July 2020. Available online. URL: www.niddk.nih.gov/health-information/digestive-diseases/acid-reflux-ger-gerd-adults. Accessed February 12, 2024.

Gastrointestinal Diseases

To treat peptic ulcers, doctors typically recommend medicines to help the ulcer heal. They also look for the cause of ulcers and treat or manage the cause. Talk with your doctor about the best treatment plan for you.

Healing Peptic Ulcers
Medicines that doctors recommend or prescribe to treat peptic ulcers include:
- PPIs
- H2 blockers
- other medicines

Treating the Causes of Peptic Ulcers
H. pylori infection and taking NSAIDs are the two most common causes of peptic ulcers. Doctors treat the underlying causes of peptic ulcers to help the ulcers heal and prevent them from coming back.

NONSTEROIDAL ANTIINFLAMMATORY DRUGS
If you have a peptic ulcer caused by taking NSAIDs, your doctor may recommend changing your medicines. Depending on the reason you have been taking NSAIDs, your doctor may suggest stopping NSAIDs, taking a different NSAID, taking a lower-dose NSAID, or taking a different medicine for pain.

If you need to keep taking NSAIDs, your doctor may recommend you also take a PPI.

OTHER CAUSES
If your peptic ulcers are not caused by *H. pylori* infection or NSAIDs, doctors will check for uncommon causes. Depending on the cause, doctors may recommend additional treatments.[6]

---

[6] "Peptic Ulcers (Stomach or Duodenal Ulcers)," National Institute of Diabetes and Digestive and Kidney Diseases (NIDDK), September 2022. Available online. URL: www.niddk.nih.gov/health-information/digestive-diseases/peptic-ulcers-stomach-ulcers. Accessed February 12, 2024.

ULCERATIVE COLITIS

Ulcerative colitis is a chronic disease in which abnormal reactions of the immune system cause inflammation and ulcers on the inner lining of your large intestine.

Doctors treat ulcerative colitis with medicines and surgery. Each person experiences ulcerative colitis differently, and doctors recommend treatments based on how severe ulcerative colitis is and how much of the large intestine is affected. Doctors most often treat severe and fulminant ulcerative colitis in a hospital.

Medicines

Doctors prescribe medicines to reduce inflammation in the large intestine and to help bring on and maintain remission—a time when your symptoms disappear. People with ulcerative colitis typically need lifelong treatment with medicines unless they have surgery to remove the colon and rectum.

The medicines your doctor prescribes will depend on how severe ulcerative colitis is. Ulcerative colitis medicines that reduce inflammation in the large intestine include:

- **Aminosalicylates.** Doctors prescribe aminosalicylates to treat mild or moderate ulcerative colitis or to help people stay in remission.
- **Corticosteroids.** Also called "steroids," which doctors prescribe to treat moderate-to-severe ulcerative colitis and to treat mild-to-moderate ulcerative colitis in people who do not respond to aminosalicylates. Doctors typically do not prescribe corticosteroids for long-term use or to maintain remission. Long-term use may cause serious side effects.
- **Immunosuppressants.** Doctors may prescribe immunosuppressants to treat people with moderate-to-severe ulcerative colitis and help them stay in remission. Doctors may also prescribe immunosuppressants to treat severe ulcerative colitis in people who are hospitalized and do not respond to other medicines.

- **Biologics**. Doctors prescribe biologics to treat people with moderate-to-severe ulcerative colitis and help them stay in remission.
- **Novel small molecule medicines**. Doctors may prescribe these medicines for adults with moderate-to-severe ulcerative colitis who do not respond to other medicines or who have severe side effects with other medicines.

Surgery

Your doctor may recommend surgery if you have:
- colorectal cancer
- dysplasia, or precancerous cells that increase the risk for developing colorectal cancer
- complications that are life-threatening, such as severe rectal bleeding, toxic megacolon, or perforation of the large intestine
- symptoms that do not improve or stop after treatment with medicines
- symptoms that only improve with continuous treatment with corticosteroids, which may cause serious side effects when used for a long time

To treat ulcerative colitis, surgeons typically remove the colon and rectum and change how your body stores and passes stool. The most common types of surgery for ulcerative colitis are as follows:
- **Ileoanal reservoir surgery**. Surgeons create an internal reservoir, or pouch, from the end part of the small intestine, called the "ileum." Surgeons attach the pouch to the anus. Ileoanal reservoir surgery most often requires two or three operations. After the operations, the stool will collect in the internal pouch and pass through the anus during bowel movements.
- **Ileostomy**. Surgeons attach the end of your ileum to an opening in your abdomen called a "stoma." After an ileostomy, the stool will pass through the stoma.

You will use an ostomy pouch—a bag attached to the stoma and worn outside the body—to collect stool.

Surgery may be laparoscopic or open. In laparoscopic surgery, surgeons make small cuts in your abdomen and insert special tools to view, remove, or repair organs and tissues. In open surgery, surgeons make a larger cut to open your abdomen.

If you are considering surgery to treat ulcerative colitis, talk with your doctor or surgeon about what type of surgery might be right for you and the possible risks and benefits.[7]

---

[7] "Ulcerative Colitis," National Institute of Diabetes and Digestive and Kidney Diseases (NIDDK), September 2020. Available online. URL: www.niddk.nih.gov/health-information/digestive-diseases/ulcerative-colitis. Accessed February 12, 2024.

Chapter 11 | Muscle and Bone Diseases

The muscular system is composed of specialized cells called "muscle fibers." Their predominant function is contractibility. Muscles, attached to bones or internal organs and blood vessels, are responsible for movement. Nearly all movement in the body is the result of muscle contraction. Exceptions to this are the action of cilia, the flagellum on sperm cells, and the amoeboid movement of some white blood cells (WBCs).

The integrated action of joints, bones, and skeletal muscles produces obvious movements such as walking and running. Skeletal muscles also produce more subtle movements that result in various facial expressions, eye movements, and respiration.[1]

Humans are vertebrates, animals having a vertebral column or backbone. They rely on a sturdy internal frame that is centered on a prominent spine. The human skeletal system consists of bones, cartilage, ligaments, and tendons, and accounts for about 20 percent of the body weight.

Bones provide a rigid framework, known as the "skeleton," that supports and protects the soft organs of the body. The skeleton supports the body against the pull of gravity. The large bones of the lower limbs support the trunk when standing. The skeleton also protects the soft body parts. The fused bones of the cranium surround the brain to make it less vulnerable to injury. Vertebrae surround and protect the spinal cord and bones of the rib cage that help protect the heart and lungs of the thorax.

---

[1] Surveillance, Epidemiology, and End Results (SEER) Program, "Introduction to the Muscular System," National Cancer Institute (NCI), June 30, 2002. Available online. URL: https://training.seer.cancer.gov/anatomy/muscular. Accessed February 15, 2024.

Bones work together with muscles as simple mechanical lever systems to produce body movement.[2]

The treatment and management options for some common diseases of the musculoskeletal system are as follows.

FIBROMYALGIA

Fibromyalgia is a condition that causes pain all over the body, also called "widespread pain." Fibromyalgia also causes sleep problems, fatigue, and emotional and mental distress. People with fibromyalgia may be more sensitive to pain than people without fibromyalgia. This is called "abnormal pain perception processing."

Fibromyalgia should be treated by a health-care professional or a team of health-care professionals who specialize in the treatment of fibromyalgia and other types of arthritis. Doctors who have specialized knowledge about fibromyalgia are called "rheumatologists." Health-care providers usually treat fibromyalgia with a combination of treatments, which may include:

- medications, including prescription drugs and pain relievers
- aerobic exercise and muscle strengthening exercise
- patient education classes, usually in primary care or community settings
- stress management techniques such as meditation, yoga, and massage
- good sleep habits to improve the quality of sleep
- cognitive behavioral therapy (CBT) to treat underlying depression (CBT is a type of talk therapy meant to change the way people act or think.)[3]

OSTEOPOROSIS

Osteoporosis is a bone disease that develops when bone mineral density (BMD) and bone mass decrease or when the structure

---

[2] Surveillance, Epidemiology, and End Results (SEER) Program, "Introduction to the Skeletal System," National Cancer Institute (NCI), August 24, 2010. Available online. URL: https://training.seer.cancer.gov/anatomy/skeletal. Accessed February 15, 2024.

[3] "Fibromyalgia," Centers for Disease Control and Prevention (CDC), May 25, 2022. Available online. URL: www.cdc.gov/arthritis/types/fibromyalgia.htm. Accessed February 15, 2024.

and strength of bone change. This can lead to a decrease in bone strength that can increase the risk of fractures (broken bones).

The goals for treating osteoporosis are to slow or stop bone loss and to prevent fractures. Your health-care provider may recommend:
- proper nutrition
- lifestyle changes
- exercise
- fall prevention to help prevent fractures
- medications

People who develop osteoporosis from another condition should work with their health-care provider to identify and treat the underlying cause. For example, if you take a medication that causes bone loss, your doctor may lower the dose of that medication or switch you to another medication. If you have a disease that requires long-term glucocorticoid therapy, such as rheumatoid arthritis or chronic lung disease, you can also take certain medications approved for the prevention or treatment of osteoporosis.

Nutrition

An important part of treating osteoporosis is eating a healthy, balanced diet, which includes:
- plenty of fruits and vegetables
- an appropriate amount of calories for your age, height, and weight (Your health-care provider or doctor can help you determine the amount of calories you need each day to maintain a healthy weight.)
- foods and liquids that include calcium, vitamin D, and protein (These help minimize bone loss and maintain overall health. However, it is important to eat a diet rich in all nutrients to help protect and maintain bone health.)

CALCIUM AND VITAMIN D

Calcium and vitamin D are important nutrients for preventing osteoporosis and helping bones reach peak bone mass. If you do not take in enough calcium, the body takes it from the bones, which can lead to bone loss.

Vitamin D is necessary for the absorption of calcium from the intestine. It is made in the skin after exposure to sunlight. Some foods naturally contain enough vitamin D, including fatty fish, fish oils, egg yolks, and liver. Other foods that are fortified with vitamin D are a major source of the mineral, including milk and cereals.

If you have trouble getting enough calcium and vitamin D in your diet, you may need to take supplements. Talk to your healthcare provider about the type and amount of calcium and vitamin D supplements you should take. Your doctor may check your blood levels of vitamin D and recommend a specific amount.

Lifestyle

In addition to a healthy diet, a healthy lifestyle is important for optimizing bone health. You should:
- avoid secondhand smoke, and if you smoke, quit
- drink alcohol in moderation, no more than one drink a day for women and no more than two drinks a day for men
- visit your doctor for regular checkups and ask about any factors that may affect your bone health or increase your chance of falling, such as medications or other medical conditions

Exercise

Exercise is an important part of an osteoporosis treatment program. Research shows that the best physical activities for bone health include strength training or resistance training. Because bone is a living tissue, during childhood and adulthood, exercise can make bones stronger. However, for older adults, exercise no longer increases bone mass. Instead, regular exercise can help older adults:
- build muscle mass and strength and improve coordination and balance
- improve daily function and delay loss of independence

Although exercise is beneficial for people with osteoporosis, it should not put any sudden or excessive strain on your bones. If you

Muscle and Bone Diseases

have osteoporosis, you should avoid high-impact exercise. To help prevent injury and fractures, a physical therapist or rehabilitation medicine specialist can:
- recommend specific exercises to strengthen and support your back
- reach you safe ways of moving and carrying out daily activities
- recommend an exercise program that is tailored to your circumstances

Exercise specialists, such as exercise physiologists, may also help you develop a safe and effective exercise program.

Medications

Your doctor may prescribe medications for osteoporosis. Your health-care provider will discuss the best option for you, taking into consideration your age, sex, general health, and the amount of bone you have lost. No matter which medications you take for osteoporosis, it is still important that you get the recommended amounts of calcium and vitamin D. Also, exercising and maintaining other aspects of a healthy lifestyle are important.

Medications can cause side effects. If you have questions about your medications, talk to your doctor or pharmacist. The U.S. Food and Drug Administration (FDA) has approved the following medications for the prevention or treatment of osteoporosis:
- **Bisphosphonates**. Several bisphosphonates are approved to help preserve bone density and strength and to treat osteoporosis. This type of drug works by slowing down bone loss, which can lower the chance of fractures.
- **Calcitonin**. This medication is made from a hormone from the thyroid gland and is approved for the treatment of osteoporosis in postmenopausal women who cannot take or tolerate other medications for osteoporosis.
- **Estrogen agonist/antagonist**. An estrogen agonist/antagonist, also known as a "selective estrogen receptor

modulator" (SERM), and "tissue-selective estrogen complex" (TSEC), are both approved to treat and prevent osteoporosis in postmenopausal women. They are not estrogen, but they have estrogen-like effects on some tissues and estrogen-blocking effects on other tissues. This action helps improve bone density, lowering the risk for some fractures.

- **Estrogen and hormone therapy**. Estrogen and combined estrogen and progestin (hormone therapy) are approved to prevent osteoporosis and fractures in postmenopausal women. Because of potential side effects, researchers recommend that women use hormone therapy at the lowest dose for the shortest time if other medications are not helping. It is important to carefully consider the risks and benefits of estrogen and hormone therapy for the treatment of osteoporosis.
- **Parathyroid hormone (PTH) analog and parathyroid hormone related-protein (PTHrP) analog**. PTH is a form of human parathyroid hormone that increases bone mass and is approved for postmenopausal women and men with osteoporosis who are at high risk for fracture. PTHrP is a medication that is also a form of parathyroid hormone. It is an injection and is usually prescribed for postmenopausal women who have severe osteoporosis and a history of multiple fractures.
- **RANK ligand (RANKL) inhibitor**. This is an inhibitor that helps slow down bone loss and is approved to treat osteoporosis in:
  - postmenopausal women or men with osteoporosis who are at high risk for fracture
  - men who have bone loss and are being treated for prostate cancer with medications that cause bone loss
  - women who have bone loss and are being treated for breast cancer with medications that cause bone loss
  - men and women who do not respond to other types of osteoporosis treatment

- **Sclerostin inhibitor**. This is a medication that treats severe osteoporosis by blocking the effect of a protein, helping the body increase new bone formation, and slowing down bone loss.[4]

PAGET DISEASE

Paget disease of bone is a chronic bone disorder. Normally, there is a process in which your bones break down and then regrow. In Paget disease, this process is abnormal. There is excessive breakdown and regrowth of bone. Because the bones regrow too quickly, they are bigger and softer than normal. They may be misshapen and easily fractured (broken). Paget usually affects just one or a few bones.

To avoid complications, it is important to find and treat Paget disease early. The treatments include the following:
- **Medicines**. There are several medicines to treat Paget disease. The most common type is bisphosphonates. They help reduce bone pain and stop or slow down the progress of the disease.
- **Surgery**. Surgery is sometimes needed for certain complications of the disease. There are surgeries to:
  - allow fractures (broken bones) to heal in a better position
  - replace joints such as the knee and hip when there is severe arthritis
  - realign a deformed bone to reduce the pain in weight-bearing joints, especially the knees
  - reduce pressure on a nerve, if enlargement of the skull or spine injuries affects the nervous system

Diet and exercise do not treat Paget, but they can help keep your skeleton healthy. If you do not have kidney stones, you should make sure to get enough calcium and vitamin D through your diet and supplements. Besides keeping your skeleton healthy, exercise

---

[4] "Osteoporosis," National Institute of Arthritis and Musculoskeletal and Skin Diseases (NIAMS), December 2022. Available online. URL: www.niams.nih.gov/health-topics/osteoporosis. Accessed February 15, 2024.

can prevent weight gain and maintain the mobility of your joints. Talk with your health-care provider before you start a new exercise program. You need to make sure that the exercise does not put too much stress on the affected bones.[5]

SCOLIOSIS

Scoliosis is a sideways curve of the spine. Everyone has normal curves in the spine, and when looked at from behind, the spine appears straight. However, children and teens with scoliosis have an abnormal S-shaped or C-shaped curve of the spine. The curve can happen on either side of the spine and in different places in the spine. In most people, the cause of scoliosis is unknown.

Doctors recommend treatment for scoliosis based on:
- the locations of the curve
- if the curve is mild, moderate, or severe
- if the curve causes symptoms
- if your child or teen is still growing

The goals of your child's treatment may include to:
- stop or slow the curve in the spine from progressing
- prevent or decrease pain
- prevent or manage any respiratory problems that may develop due to the curve
- help improve posture
- help improve quality of life (QOL)

Your child's doctor may recommend the following treatments:
- **Observation**. If the curve is mild and your child's skeleton is still growing, the doctor may recommend monitoring the spine. This may include visits with the doctor every few months.
- **Bracing**. If the curve is moderate and your child or teen is still growing, your doctor may recommend using a brace to keep the curve from getting any worse.

---

[5] MedlinePlus, "Paget's Disease of Bone," National Institutes of Health (NIH), June 19, 2021. Available online. URL: https://medlineplus.gov/pagetsdiseaseofbone.html. Accessed February 15, 2024.

The goal of wearing a brace is to slow or stop the curves in the spine from increasing. The type of brace depends on the severity of the curve. The brace is fitted to your child or teen and should be worn every day for the full number of hours recommended by the doctor. Research shows that braces work well if your child or teen is still growing and they are worn as directed. Once your child or teen is done growing, your doctor may determine that the brace is no longer needed.
- **Surgery.** If your child or teen is still growing and the scoliosis continues to progress, your doctor may recommend surgery. The type of surgery depends on the location and severity of the curve. All surgeries have risks for complications. Talk to the surgeon about the risks and benefits of surgery. Types of procedures may include the following:
  - **Spinal fusion.** This is a procedure that joins two or more vertebrae of the spine together. This can help straighten the curve. The surgeon may use metal rods and screws to help keep the spine straight while the spine heals.
  - **Insertion of an expandable rod.** A surgeon may recommend this procedure if your child or teen is still growing. This rod is lengthened by the surgeon at scheduled times as your child grows.
- **Physical therapy.** The doctor may recommend physical therapy to help strengthen muscles.

Research shows that alternative therapies such as chiropractic treatment, nutritional supplements, and electric stimulation do not help manage scoliosis or keep the curve from getting worse.[6]

SPINAL STENOSIS
Spinal stenosis happens when the spaces in the spine narrow and create pressure on the spinal cord and nerve roots. The spinal cord

---
[6] "Scoliosis in Children and Teens," National Institute of Arthritis and Musculoskeletal and Skin Diseases (NIAMS), July 2023. Available online. URL: www.niams.nih.gov/health-topics/scoliosis. Accessed February 15, 2024.

is a bundle of nerves that comes out of the base of the brain and runs down the center of the spine. The nerve roots branch out from the cord. The narrowing usually occurs over time and involves one or more areas of the spine.

Doctors treat spinal stenosis with different options such as nonsurgical treatments, medications, and surgical treatments.

Nonsurgical Treatments

- **Physical therapy**. This treatment helps maintain the motion of the spine, strengthen abdominal and back muscles, and build endurance, all of which help stabilize the spine. You may be encouraged to try slowly progressive aerobic activity, such as swimming or using exercise bicycles. In addition, your physical therapist or health-care provider may recommend home exercises.
- **Brace**. A brace provides some support and helps you regain mobility. This approach is sometimes used for people with weak abdominal muscles or older patients with age-related changes at several levels of the spine.
- **Complementary and alternative treatments**. These treatments may help relieve pain. Some examples are as follows:
  - **Manipulation of the spine and nearby tissues**. Professionals use their hands to adjust and massage the spine and muscles.
  - **Acupuncture**. This is a Chinese practice that uses thin needles that may relieve pain in some patients.

Medications

Your doctor may prescribe one or more of the following medications to help manage the pain and inflammation caused by spinal stenosis:

- antiinflammatory medications to help relieve inflammation and pain
- OTC pain relievers taken by mouth or applied to the skin

- prescription pain relievers for severe or acute pain
- antiinflammatory or numbing injections for pain that radiates or travels due to nerve compression or irritation

Surgical Treatments

If, after trying nonsurgical treatments and medications, you still have symptoms, your doctor may recommend meeting with a surgeon to talk about surgery. However, doctors may recommend surgery right away if you have numbness or weakness that interferes with walking, impaired bowel or bladder function, or other neurological involvement.

The decision to have surgery depends on:
- how nonsurgical treatments have helped your symptoms
- the amount of pain you feel
- other diseases and conditions you may have
- your overall health
- whether your specific spinal anatomy is amenable to surgery

However, not everyone is a candidate for surgery, even if symptoms persist. In addition, your surgeon will review the risks and possible benefits of the surgery or procedure.

Surgeons can relieve pressure on the spinal cord and nerves and restore spine alignment and health by performing surgery. Possible surgeries include the following:
- **Laminectomy**. This is a type of surgery that doctors perform to treat spinal stenosis by removing the bony spurs and the bone walls of the vertebrae. This helps to open up the spinal column and remove the pressure on the nerves. Doctors may perform a discectomy during a laminectomy. A discectomy involves removing part of the herniated disk to relieve pressure on the spinal cord or nerve root. A facetectomy involves removing part or all of a facet joint to relieve pressure.
- **Spinal fusion**. This is a type of surgery that helps treat age-related changes to the spine and spondylolisthesis

by joining two or more vertebrae in the spine that have slipped from their normal position. During this procedure, the surgeon may remove the disk between the vertebrae and use bone grafts or metal devices to secure bones together.
- **Minimally invasive surgery.** This is a type of surgery that uses smaller incisions than standard surgery. Minimally invasive surgery may cause less scarring and damage to nearby muscles and other tissues. It can lead to less pain and faster recovery after surgery.

Removing and repairing the areas of the spine that are creating pressure usually helps decrease symptoms. Most people have less leg pain and can walk better after surgery. However, if nerves were badly damaged before surgery, there may be some remaining pain or numbness or no improvement. Also, the degenerative process may continue, and pain or limitation of activity may reappear after surgery.[7]

---

[7] "Spinal Stenosis," National Institute of Arthritis and Musculoskeletal and Skin Diseases (NIAMS), November 2023. Available online. URL: www.niams.nih.gov/health-topics/spinal-stenosis. Accessed February 15, 2024.

Chapter 12 | Urinary System Diseases

The principal function of the urinary system is to maintain the volume and composition of body fluids within normal limits. One aspect of this function is to rid the body of waste products that accumulate as a result of cellular metabolism, and because of this, it is sometimes referred to as the "excretory system."

The urinary system maintains an appropriate fluid volume by regulating the amount of water that is excreted in the urine. Other aspects of its function include regulating the concentrations of various electrolytes in the body fluids and maintaining the normal pH of the blood.

In addition to maintaining fluid homeostasis in the body, the urinary system controls red blood cell (RBC) production by secreting the hormone erythropoietin. The urinary system also plays a role in maintaining normal blood pressure by secreting the enzyme renin.[1]

The following are the treatment and management options for some common diseases of the urinary system.

BLADDER INFECTION

A bladder infection is an illness caused by bacteria. Bladder infections are the most common type of urinary tract infection (UTI). A UTI can develop in any part of your urinary tract, including your urethra, bladder, ureters, or kidneys.

---

[1] Surveillance, Epidemiology, and End Results (SEER) Program, "Introduction to the Urinary System," National Cancer Institute (NCI), April 27, 2009. Available online. URL: https://training.seer.cancer.gov/anatomy/urinary. Accessed February 15, 2024.

If you have a bladder infection caused by bacteria, a health-care professional is likely to prescribe antibiotics. If the diagnosis is not certain, based on your symptoms or lab test results, you may not need antibiotics. Instead, your health-care professional will work to find the cause and the best treatment for your symptoms.

Medicines

Which antibiotic you take is based on the type of bacteria causing your infection and any allergies you may have to antibiotics.

The length of treatment depends on:
- how severe the infection is
- whether your symptoms and infection go away
- whether you have repeated infections
- whether you have problems with your urinary tract

Men may need to take antibiotics longer because bacteria can move into the prostate gland, which surrounds the urethra. Bacteria can hide deep inside prostate tissue.

Follow your health-care professional's instructions carefully and completely when taking antibiotics. Although you may feel relief from your symptoms, make sure to take the entire antibiotic treatment.

If needed, a health-care professional may prescribe other medicines to relieve any pain or discomfort from your bladder infection.

At-Home Treatments

Drink a lot of liquids and urinate often to speed healing. Water is best. Talk with a health-care professional if you cannot drink a lot of liquids due to other health problems, such as urinary incontinence, urinary frequency, or heart or kidney failure.

A heating pad on your back or abdomen may help you manage pain from a bladder infection.[2]

---

[2] "Bladder Infection (Urinary Tract Infection—UTI) in Adults," National Institute of Diabetes and Digestive and Kidney Diseases (NIDDK), March 2017. Available online. URL: www.niddk.nih.gov/health-information/urologic-diseases/bladder-infection-uti-in-adults. Accessed February 15, 2024.

KIDNEY INFECTION

A kidney infection is a type of UTI. Most kidney infections are caused by bacteria or viruses that first infect your lower urinary tract, usually your bladder. Then, the infection moves upstream to one or both of your kidneys, which are part of the upper urinary tract.

If you have a kidney infection, a health-care professional will prescribe antibiotics. Even before your test results are in, the health-care professional may prescribe an antibiotic that fights the most common types of bacteria. Although you may feel relief from your symptoms, make sure to take the entire antibiotic treatment that your health-care professional prescribes.

Once your lab results are in, the health-care professional may switch the antibiotic to one that better treats the type of infection you have. You may take these antibiotics by mouth, through a vein in your arm called "intravenous" (IV), or both.

If you are very sick from your kidney infection, you may go to a hospital for bed rest. A health-care professional may give you fluids through an IV.[3]

KIDNEY STONES

Kidney stones are hard, pebble-like pieces of material that form in one or both of your kidneys when high levels of certain minerals are in your urine. Kidney stones rarely cause permanent damage if treated by a health-care professional. Health-care professionals usually treat kidney stones based on their size, location, and what type they are.

Small kidney stones may pass through your urinary tract without treatment. If you are able to pass a kidney stone, a health-care professional may ask you to catch the kidney stone in a special container. A health-care professional will send the kidney stone to a lab to find out what type it is. A health-care professional may advise you to drink plenty of liquids if you are able to help move a

---

[3] "Kidney Infection (Pyelonephritis)," National Institute of Diabetes and Digestive and Kidney Diseases (NIDDK), April 2017. Available online. URL: www.niddk.nih.gov/health-information/urologic-diseases/kidney-infection-pyelonephritis. Accessed February 15, 2024.

kidney stone along. The health-care professional may also prescribe pain medicine.

Larger kidney stones or kidney stones that block your urinary tract or cause great pain may need urgent treatment. If you are vomiting and dehydrated, you may need to go to the hospital and get fluids through an IV.

Kidney Stone Removal

A urologist can remove the kidney stone or break it into small pieces with the following treatments:

- **Shock wave lithotripsy.** The doctor can use a shock wave lithotripsy to blast the kidney stone into small pieces. The smaller pieces of the kidney stone then pass through your urinary tract. A doctor can give you anesthesia during this outpatient procedure.
- **Cystoscopy and ureteroscopy.** During cystoscopy, the doctor uses a cystoscope to look inside the urethra and bladder to find a stone in your urethra or bladder. During ureteroscopy, the doctor uses a ureteroscope, which is longer and thinner than a cystoscope, to see detailed images of the lining of the ureters and kidneys. The doctor inserts the cystoscope or ureteroscope through the urethra to see the rest of the urinary tract. Once the stone is found, the doctor can remove it or break it into smaller pieces. The doctor performs these procedures in the hospital with anesthesia. You can typically go home the same day.
- **Percutaneous nephrolithotomy.** The doctor uses a thin viewing tool, called a "nephroscope," to locate and remove the kidney stone. The doctor inserts the tool directly into your kidney through a small cut made in your back. For larger kidney stones, the doctor may also use a laser to break the kidney stones into smaller pieces. The doctor performs percutaneous nephrolithotomy in a hospital with anesthesia. You may have to stay in the hospital for several days after the procedure.

Urinary System Diseases

After these procedures, sometimes the urologist may leave a thin flexible tube, called a "ureteral stent," in your urinary tract to help urine flow or a stone to pass. Once the kidney stone is removed, your doctor sends the kidney stone or its pieces to a lab to find out what type it is.

The health-care professional may also ask you to collect your urine for 24 hours after the kidney stone has passed or been removed. The health-care professional can then measure how much urine you produce in a day, along with mineral levels in your urine. You are more likely to form stones if you do not make enough urine each day or have a problem with high mineral levels.[4]

PROSTATE PROBLEMS

The prostate is a walnut-shaped gland that is part of a man's sex organs, which also include the penis, scrotum, and testicles. The prostate makes fluid that goes into semen, which is a mix of sperm and prostate fluid. Prostate fluid is important for a man's ability to father children. Common prostate problems include:
- prostatitis—inflammation, or swelling, of the prostate
- benign prostatic hyperplasia (BPH)—an enlarged prostate due to something other than cancer
- prostate cancer

Treatment depends on the type of prostate problem you have.

Prostatitis
Treatment depends on the type of prostatitis.
- **Chronic prostatitis**. If you have chronic prostatitis, your doctor will try treatments to lessen pain, discomfort, and inflammation. Your doctor may give you a medicine called an "alpha-blocker" to relax the muscles in your prostate and part of your bladder. Tamsulosin (Flomax) and silodosin (Rapaflo) are

---

[4] "Kidney Stones," National Institute of Diabetes and Digestive and Kidney Diseases (NIDDK), May 2017. Available online. URL: www.niddk.nih.gov/health-information/urologic-diseases/kidney-stones. Accessed February 15, 2024.

two commonly used alpha-blockers. Warm baths, relaxation exercises, and physical therapy may help.
- **Bacterial prostatitis**. If you have bacterial prostatitis, your doctor will give you an antibiotic, a medicine that kills bacteria. Bacterial prostatitis generally clears up quickly after treatment with antibiotics. As part of treatment, your doctor may ask you to change your diet and drink more liquids.

Benign Prostatic Hyperplasia

Treatments for BPH include the following:
- **Watchful waiting**. If your symptoms do not bother you too much, you may choose to live with them rather than take medicines or have surgery. However, you should have regular checkups to make sure your condition is not getting worse. With watchful waiting, you can be ready to choose a treatment as soon as you decide to treat your BPH.
- **Lifestyle changes**. Your doctor may suggest changes to your lifestyle if your symptoms are mild and bother you only a little. Your symptoms may get better if you:
  - drink fewer liquids before going out or before going to sleep
  - avoid or drink fewer liquids that have caffeine or alcohol in them
  - avoid medicines that may affect your bladder, such as certain cold and allergy medicines
  - change the timing of your medicines, such as diuretics, also called "water pills," or those that treat high blood pressure (HBP)
- **Medicines**. Your doctor may prescribe medicines such as finasteride (Proscar) and dutasteride (Avodart). These medicines can stop prostate growth or actually shrink the prostate in some men. Your doctor may also prescribe an alpha-blocker such as doxazosin (Cardura) or tadalafil (Cialis), another medicine that relaxes prostate and bladder muscles.

Urinary System Diseases

- **Surgery**. If your prostate keeps growing or your symptoms get worse, your doctor may recommend surgery to shrink your prostate. Most of the surgeries are transurethral, which means your doctor inserts a thin tube into your urethra to reach the prostate. Your doctor performs the transurethral surgery in an outpatient center or a hospital. Your doctor will give you medicines to help you relax and stop you from feeling pain, or your doctor may give you medicine, so you are asleep during surgery. Most men can go home the same day as the surgery.

In most cases, surgery to shrink or remove prostate tissue offers long-term relief from problems due to BPH. In a few cases, the prostate may continue to grow, and problems may return. Surgery for BPH does not prevent cancer. You should continue to have your prostate checked after surgery to make sure your prostate has not grown larger.

In some cases, your doctor may recommend removing your prostate. Your doctor performs this surgery in a hospital. Your doctor will give you medicine, so you are asleep during surgery. You will need a hospital stay after your surgery.[5]

URINARY INCONTINENCE

Urinary incontinence is the loss of bladder control or being unable to control urination. It is a common condition. It can range from being a minor problem to something that greatly affects your daily life. In any case, it can get better with proper treatment.

Treatment depends on the type and cause of your urinary incontinence. You may need a combination of treatments. Your provider may first suggest self-care treatments, including:
- **Lifestyle changes**. These modifications include:
  - drinking the right amount of liquid at the right time
  - being physically active

---

[5] "Prostate Problems," National Institute of Diabetes and Digestive and Kidney Diseases (NIDDK), March 2016. Available online. URL: www.niddk.nih.gov/health-information/urologic-diseases/prostate-problems. Accessed February 15, 2024.

- staying at a healthy weight
- avoiding constipation
- not smoking
- **Bladder training**. This involves urinating according to a schedule. Your provider makes a schedule for you, based on information from your bladder diary. After you adjust to the schedule, you gradually wait a little longer between trips to the bathroom. This can help stretch your bladder, so it can hold more urine.
- **Doing exercises to strengthen your pelvic floor muscles**. Strong pelvic floor muscles hold in urine better than weak muscles. The strengthening exercises are called "Kegel exercises." They involve tightening and relaxing the muscles that control urine flow.

If these treatments do not work, your provider may suggest other options such as:
- **Medicines**. These can be used to:
  - relax the bladder muscles, to help prevent bladder spasms
  - block nerve signals that cause urinary frequency and urgency
  - shrink the prostate and improve urine flow (in men)
- **Medical devices**. These devices include:
  - **Catheter**. This is a tube to carry urine out of the body. You might use one a few times a day or all the time.
  - **Ring or a tampon-like device (for women)**. This device is inserted into the vagina. The device pushes up against your urethra to help decrease leaks.
- **Bulking agents**. These agents are injected into the bladder neck and urethra tissues to thicken them. This helps close your bladder opening, so you have less leaking.

Urinary System Diseases

- **Electrical nerve stimulation.** This involves changing your bladder's reflexes using pulses of electricity.
- **Surgery.** This is a surgical procedure to support the bladder in its normal position. This may be done with a sling that is attached to the pubic bone.[6]

---

[6] MedlinePlus, "Urinary Incontinence," National Institutes of Health (NIH), January 9, 2024. Available online. URL: https://medlineplus.gov/urinaryincontinence.html. Accessed February 15, 2024.

Chapter 13 | Nervous System Diseases

The nervous system is the major controlling, regulatory, and communicating system in the body. It is the center of all mental activity, including thought, learning, and memory. Together with the endocrine system, the nervous system is responsible for regulating and maintaining homeostasis. Through its receptors, the nervous system keeps us in touch with our environment, both external and internal.

Like other systems in the body, the nervous system is composed of organs, principally the brain, spinal cord, nerves, and ganglia. These, in turn, consist of various tissues, including nerve, blood, and connective tissue. Together, these carry out the complex activities of the nervous system.[1]

The treatment and management options for some common diseases of the nervous system are as follows.

ALZHEIMER DISEASE

Alzheimer disease (AD) is a brain disorder that slowly destroys memory and thinking skills, and eventually, the ability to carry out the simplest tasks. In most people with AD, symptoms first appear later in life.

AD is complex, and it is therefore unlikely that any one drug or other intervention will successfully treat it in all people living with

---

[1] Surveillance, Epidemiology, and End Results (SEER) Program, "Introduction to the Nervous System," National Cancer Institute (NCI), June 30, 2002. Available online. URL: https://training.seer.cancer.gov/anatomy/nervous. Accessed February 13, 2024.

the disease. In ongoing clinical trials, scientists are developing and testing several possible treatment interventions.

While there is currently no cure for AD, medications are emerging to treat the progression of the disease by targeting its underlying causes. There are also medications that may temporarily improve or stabilize memory and thinking skills in some people and may help manage certain symptoms and behavioral problems.

Additionally, people with AD may also experience sleeplessness, depression, anxiety, agitation, and other behavioral and psychological symptoms. Scientists continue to research why these symptoms occur and are exploring new medications and nondrug strategies to manage them. Research shows that treating these symptoms may make people with AD feel more comfortable and also help their caregivers.[2]

AMYOTROPHIC LATERAL SCLEROSIS

Amyotrophic lateral sclerosis (ALS), formerly known as "Lou Gehrig disease," is a neurological disorder that affects motor neurons, the nerve cells in the brain and spinal cord that control voluntary muscle movement and breathing. As motor neurons degenerate and die, they stop sending messages to the muscles, which causes the muscles to weaken, start to twitch (fasciculations), and waste away (atrophy). Eventually, in people with ALS, the brain loses its ability to initiate and control voluntary movements such as walking, talking, chewing, and other functions, as well as breathing. ALS is progressive, meaning the symptoms get worse over time.

There is no treatment to reverse damage to motor neurons or cure ALS at this time. However, some treatments may slow the progression of the disease, improve quality of life (QOL), and extend survival. New treatments have become available in the past several years, and researchers continue to explore diverse avenues to slow or stop the progression of ALS.

---

[2] National Institute on Aging (NIA), "Alzheimer's Disease Fact Sheet," National Institutes of Health (NIH), April 5, 2023. Available online. URL: www.nia.nih.gov/health/alzheimers-and-dementia/alzheimers-disease-fact-sheet. Accessed February 13, 2024.

Nervous System Diseases

Supportive health care is best provided by integrated, multidisciplinary teams of professionals that may include physicians, pharmacists, physical, occupational, speech, and respiratory therapists, nutritionists, social workers, clinical psychologists, and home care and hospice nurses. These teams can design an individualized treatment plan and provide special equipment aimed at keeping people as mobile, comfortable, and independent as possible.

Doctors may use the following medications approved by the U.S. Food and Drug Administration (FDA) to support a treatment plan for ALS:

- **Riluzole (Rilutek).** It is an oral medication believed to reduce damage to motor neurons by decreasing levels of glutamate, which transports messages between nerve cells and motor neurons. Clinical trials in people with ALS showed that riluzole may prolong survival by a few months. The thickened liquid form (Tiglutik) or the tablet (Exservan) that dissolves on the tongue may be preferred if the person has swallowing difficulties.
- **Edaravone (Radicava).** It is an antioxidant given either orally or intravenously and has been shown to slow functional decline in some people with ALS. RADICAVA ORS® is a form of edaravone that can be taken orally or via a feeding tube.
- **Sodium phenylbutyrate/taurursodiol (Relyvrio).** It is an oral medication that is believed to prevent nerve cell death by blocking stress signals in cells. It has been shown to slow functional decline and extend survival in some individuals with ALS.
- **Tofersen (Qalsody).** It is given through a spinal injection to ALS patients who have been determined to have a mutation in the superoxide dismutase type 1 (*SOD1*) gene. While the benefits of this drug are still under study, it may work by decreasing one of the markers of damage to neurons.

A doctor may prescribe other medications or treatments to help manage symptoms, including muscle cramps and stiffness, excessive saliva and phlegm, unwanted episodes of crying and/or laughing, or other emotional displays. Medications may also help with any pain, depression, sleep disturbances, or constipation.[3]

BELL PALSY

Bell palsy is a neurological disorder that causes paralysis or weakness on one side of the face. It occurs when one of the nerves that controls muscles in the face becomes injured or stops working properly. Bell palsy is the most common cause of facial paralysis.

Common treatments for the symptoms of Bell palsy include medications, eye protection, surgery, and other therapies.

Steroids may be prescribed for new-onset Bell palsy. In most instances, oral steroids should be started within three days of symptom onset to reduce inflammation and swelling and increase the probability of recovering facial nerve function. Some people with Bell palsy may not respond well to or be able to take steroids. In some cases, antiviral medications may be prescribed in addition to steroids to help increase the chance of recovering facial function. People experiencing pain with Bell palsy may find relief by taking analgesics such as aspirin, acetaminophen, or ibuprofen. To avoid dangerous drug interactions, if you are already taking prescription medications, talk with your doctor or pharmacist before taking over-the-counter (OTC) drugs.

If the person has trouble closing one or both eyelids, lubricating eye drops or eye patches can help keep the eye moist and protect it from debris or injury, especially while they are sleeping. Physical therapy, facial massage, or acupuncture may provide some improvement in facial nerve function and pain. In some cases, cosmetic or reconstructive surgery may be appropriate to fix a permanently crooked smile or an eyelid that will not close.[4]

---

[3] "Amyotrophic Lateral Sclerosis (ALS)," National Institute of Neurological Disorders and Stroke (NINDS), November 28, 2023. Available online. URL: www.ninds.nih.gov/health-information/disorders/amyotrophic-lateral-sclerosis-als. Accessed February 13, 2024.
[4] "Bell's Palsy," National Institute of Neurological Disorders and Stroke (NINDS), November 21, 2023. Available online. URL: www.ninds.nih.gov/health-information/disorders/bells-palsy. Accessed February 13, 2024.

Nervous System Diseases

CEREBRAL PALSY

Cerebral palsy (CP) refers to a group of neurological disorders that appear in infancy or early childhood and permanently affect body movement and muscle coordination. CP is caused by damage to or abnormalities inside the developing brain that disrupt the brain's ability to control movement and maintain posture and balance. The term "cerebral" refers to the brain; "palsy" refers to the loss or impairment of motor function.

CP cannot be cured, but treatment will often improve a child's capabilities. Many children are able to manage their disabilities; the earlier treatment begins, the better chance children have of overcoming developmental disabilities.

There is no standard therapy that works for every person with CP. Referrals to specialists such as a child neurologist, developmental pediatrician, ophthalmologist, or otologist aid in a more accurate diagnosis and help doctors develop a specific treatment plan. Once the diagnosis is made, a team of health-care professionals will work with the child and parents to identify specific impairments and needs, and then develop an appropriate plan to tackle the core disabilities that affect the child's QOL.

Therapies

- **Physical therapy.** This therapy, usually in the first few years of life, is a cornerstone of CP treatment. Specific sets of exercises such as stretching, resistive, or strength training programs and activities can maintain or improve muscle strength, balance, and motor skills, and prevent contractures. Special braces (orthotic devices) may be used to improve mobility and stretch spastic muscles.
- **Occupational therapy.** This is a type of therapy that focuses on optimizing upper body function, improving posture, and making the most of a child's mobility. Occupational therapists help individuals address new ways to meet everyday activities and routines at home, school, and in the community.

- **Recreation therapy.** A therapy that encourages participation in art and cultural programs, sports, and other events that help an individual expand physical and cognitive skills and abilities. Parents of children who participate in recreational therapies usually notice an improvement in their child's speech, self-esteem, and emotional well-being.
- **Speech and language therapy.** This therapy can improve a child's ability to speak, help with swallowing disorders, and learn new ways to communicate, such as using sign language, and/or special communication devices such as a computer with a voice synthesizer.
- **Treatments for problems with eating and drooling.** These treatments are often necessary when children with CP have difficulty eating and drinking because they have little control over the muscles that move their mouth, jaw, and tongue.

Drug Treatments

- **Oral medications.** Medications such as diazepam, baclofen, dantrolene sodium, and tizanidine are usually used as the first line of treatment to relax stiff, contracted, or overactive muscles. Some drugs have side effects such as drowsiness, changes in blood pressure, and risk of liver damage that require continuous monitoring. Oral medications are most appropriate for children who need only mild reduction in muscle tone or who have widespread spasticity.
- **Botulinum toxin (BT-A).** BT-A is injected locally into the muscles and has become a standard treatment for overactive muscles in children with spastic CP. BT-A relaxes contracted muscles by keeping nerve cells from overactivating muscles. The relaxing effects last approximately three months. Side effects include pain upon injection and occasionally mild flu-like symptoms. BT-A injections are most effective when followed by physical therapy and splinting. BT-A injections work

best for children who have some control over their motor movements and have a limited number of muscles to treat, none of which is fixed or rigid.
- **Intrathecal baclofen (ITB)**. ITB therapy uses an implantable pump to deliver baclofen, a muscle relaxant, into the fluid surrounding the spinal cord. Baclofen decreases the excitability of nerve cells in the spinal cord, which then reduces muscle spasticity throughout the body. The pump can be adjusted if muscle tone is worse at certain times of the day or night. The baclofen pump is most appropriate for individuals with chronic, severe stiffness or uncontrolled muscle movement throughout the body.

Surgery
- **Orthopedic surgery**. This surgery is often recommended when spasticity and stiffness are severe enough to make walking and moving about difficult or painful. Surgeons can lengthen muscles and tendons that are proportionately too short, which can improve mobility and lessen pain. Tendon surgery may help the symptoms for some children with CP but could also have negative long-term consequences. Orthopedic surgeries may be staggered at times appropriate to a child's age and level of motor development. Surgery can also correct or greatly improve spinal deformities.
- **Surgery to cut nerves, or selective dorsal rhizotomy (SDR)**. SDR is a surgical procedure recommended for cases of severe spasticity when all the more conservative treatments have not helped. A surgeon locates and selectively severs overactivated nerves at the base of the spinal column. SDR is most commonly used to relax muscles and decrease chronic pain in limbs. Potential side effects include sensory loss, numbness, or uncomfortable sensations.

Assistive Devices
Assistive devices such as computers, computer software, voice synthesizers, and picture books can greatly help some individuals with

CP improve their communication skills. Other devices make it easier for people with CP to adapt to activities of daily living (ADLs).
- Orthotic devices help to compensate for muscle imbalance and increase independent mobility.
- Braces and splints use external force to correct muscle abnormalities and improve function such as sitting or walking. Other orthotics help stretch muscles or the positioning of a joint.
- Braces, wedges, special chairs, and other devices can help people sit more comfortably.
- Wheelchairs, rolling walkers, and powered scooters can help individuals who are not independently mobile.
- Vision aids include glasses, magnifiers, large-print books, and computer typefaces. Some individuals with CP may need surgery to correct vision problems.
- Hearing aids and telephone amplifiers may help people hear more clearly.

Complementary and Alternative Therapies

Many children and adolescents with CP use some form of complementary or alternative medicine. Although there are anecdotal reports of some benefits in some children with CP, alternative therapies have not been approved by the FDA for the treatment of CP. Such therapies include hyperbaric oxygen treatment (HBOT), special clothing worn during resistance training, certain forms of electrical stimulation of muscles, and dietary supplements, such as herbal products. Most controlled clinical trials involving these therapies have been inconclusive or showed no benefit. Families of children with CP should discuss all therapies with their doctor.[5]

EPILEPSY AND SEIZURES

Epilepsy is a chronic brain disorder in which groups of nerve cells, or neurons, in the brain, sometimes send the wrong signals and

---

[5] "Cerebral Palsy," National Institute of Neurological Disorders and Stroke (NINDS), November 28, 2023. Available online. URL: www.ninds.nih.gov/health-information/disorders/cerebral-palsy. Accessed February 13, 2024.

cause seizures. Neurons normally generate electrical and chemical signals that act on other neurons, organs, and muscles to produce human thoughts, feelings, and actions.

During a seizure, many neurons send signals at the same time, much faster than normal. This surge of excessive electrical activity may cause involuntary movements, sensations, emotions, and/or behaviors. The disturbance of normal nerve cell activity may cause a loss of awareness. Some people recover immediately after a seizure, while others may take minutes to hours to feel like themselves again. During this time, they may feel tired, sleepy, weak, or confused.

Once epilepsy is diagnosed, it is important to begin treatment as soon as possible. There are many different ways to successfully control seizures. There are several treatment approaches that can be used, depending on the individual and the type of epilepsy.

Medications to Treat Seizures in Epilepsy

The most common approach to treating epilepsy is to prescribe antiseizure medications. More than 40 different antiseizure medications are available today, all with different benefits and side effects. Most seizures can be controlled with one drug. Combining medications may amplify side effects such as fatigue and dizziness, so doctors usually prescribe just one drug whenever possible. Combinations of drugs, however, are still sometimes necessary for some forms of epilepsy that do not respond to a single drug.

Which drug a person should be prescribed depends on many different factors, including:
- seizure type
- lifestyle and age
- seizure frequency
- drug side effects
- medicines for other conditions
- pregnancy

It may take several months to determine the best drug and dosage. If one treatment is unsuccessful, another may work better.

When starting any new antiseizure medication, a doctor will begin with a low dose and increase the dose as needed depending on how effective the drug is. Sometimes doctors monitor the level of the drug in a person's blood to help determine when the optimal dosage has been reached. It may take time to find a dose that gives the best seizure control while minimizing side effects.

Side effects are often worse when first starting a new medicine and get better over time. Talk with your doctor about any side effects you experience while on medications and make sure they are aware of any other prescription or OTC medications you are taking, including any herbs or supplements. Some antiseizure medications can affect how and whether other drugs work and can interact in harmful ways with other medications. Some may make hormonal birth control less effective in women. Some medications are harmful to the fetus, so women who plan to get pregnant should consult with their physician to be sure that they are using medications that are safe during pregnancy.

Discontinuing the medication should always be done with the supervision of a health-care professional. It is very important to continue taking antiseizure medication for as long as it is prescribed. Discontinuing medication too early is one of the major reasons people who have been seizure-free start having new seizures and can lead to status epilepticus, which is potentially life-threatening. Some people with epilepsy may be advised to discontinue their antiseizure drugs after two to three years have passed without a seizure. Others may be advised to wait for four to five years, depending on the cause of the seizures.

While antiseizure medications are effective for many people with epilepsy, some do not respond to or are not able to take medications. Those individuals may be candidates for surgery, dietary changes, or devices to stop their seizures.

Diet and Lifestyle Changes in Epilepsy
Some types of epilepsy may respond to changes in diet. A high-fat, high-protein, very low-carbohydrate ketogenic diet is sometimes used to treat medication-resistant epilepsies. The diet induces a state known as "ketosis," which means that the body shifts to

breaking down fats instead of carbohydrates to survive. A ketogenic diet effectively reduces seizures for some people, especially children, with certain forms of epilepsy.

The ketogenic diet can be difficult to maintain since it requires that a person only eat certain foods and avoid many common foods that contain sugars and carbohydrates. Individuals using this diet to manage their seizures should be monitored to make sure they are getting enough nutrients. One side effect of a ketogenic diet is a buildup of uric acid in the blood, which can lead to kidney stones. A doctor or nutritionist can help people on this diet make sure they are getting the nutrients they need and in the right amounts.

Sleep disorders are common among people with epilepsy, and sleep deprivation is a powerful trigger of seizures. Treating sleep problems can help reduce seizures. People with epilepsy should practice good sleep hygiene: going to bed and getting up at the same time each day, reducing distractions in the bedroom, and avoiding big meals and exercise within a few hours of bedtime.

Surgery for Epilepsy

Surgery is typically only considered after a person with epilepsy has unsuccessfully tried at least two medications to prevent seizures, or when doctors have found a brain lesion (an area of abnormal brain tissue) believed to be causing the seizures. When someone is found to be a good candidate, the surgery should be performed as soon as possible.

In considering a person's candidacy for surgery to prevent seizures, doctors will review:
- the seizure type
- the brain region involved
- the effect of the brain region on everyday function and behavior

Surgeons usually avoid operating in areas of the brain that are necessary for speech, movement, sensation, memory and thinking, or other important abilities.

While surgery can significantly reduce or even halt seizures for many people, any kind of surgery involves risk. Surgery for epilepsy does not always successfully reduce seizures, and it can result in cognitive or personality changes as well as physical disability, even in people who are excellent candidates for it. Nonetheless, when medications fail, several studies have shown that surgery is much more likely to make someone seizure-free compared to attempts to use other medications. Anyone thinking about surgery for epilepsy should be assessed at an epilepsy center experienced in surgical techniques and should discuss the surgery's risks and benefits with their health-care team.

Even when surgery completely ends a person's seizures, it is important to continue taking antiseizure medication for some time, as prescribed by your health-care provider. It is generally recommended that individuals continue medication for at least two years after a successful operation to avoid the recurrence of seizures.

Surgical procedures for treating epilepsy disorders include the following:

- **Surgery to remove a seizure focus**. This surgery involves removing the defined area of the brain where seizures originate. It is the most common type of surgery for epilepsy, which doctors may refer to as a lobectomy or lesionectomy, and is appropriate only for focal seizures that originate in just one area of the brain.
- **Multiple subpial transection**. This surgery may be performed when seizures originate in part of the brain that cannot be removed. It involves making a series of cuts that are designed to prevent seizures from spreading into other parts of the brain while leaving the person's normal abilities intact.
- **Corpus callosotomy**. Severing the network of neural connections between the right and left halves (hemispheres) of the brain is done primarily in children with severe seizures that start in one half of the brain and spread to the other side. Corpus callosotomy can end drop attacks and other generalized seizures. However, the procedure does not stop seizures in the side of the brain where they originate, and these focal seizures may get worse after surgery.

- **Hemispherectomy and hemispherotomy.** This surgery involves removing half of the brain's cortex, or outer layer. These procedures are used predominantly in children who have seizures that do not respond to medication because of damage that involves only half the brain.
- **Thermal ablation for epilepsy.** Also known as "laser interstitial thermal therapy" (LITT), this procedure directs energy to a specific, targeted brain region causing the seizures (the seizure focus). The energy, which is changed to thermal energy, destroys the brain cells causing the seizures. Laser ablation is less invasive than open brain surgery for treating epilepsy.

Devices

Neurostimulation devices are used to treat epilepsy. These devices deliver electrical stimulation to the brain to reduce seizure frequency:
- **Vagus nerve stimulation (VNS).** This involves surgically implanting a device under the skin of the chest. The device, which is attached by wire to the vagus nerve in the lower neck, delivers short bursts of electrical energy to the brain.
- **Responsive neurostimulation (RNS).** This uses an implanted device that analyzes brain activity patterns to detect a forthcoming seizure. Once detected, the device administers an intervention, such as electrical stimulation or a fast-acting drug, to prevent the seizure from occurring.
- **Deep brain stimulation (DBS).** This involves surgically implanting an electrode connected to a pulse generator (similar to a pacemaker) to deliver electrical stimulation to specific areas in the brain to regulate electrical signals in neural circuits.[6]

---

[6] "Epilepsy and Seizures," National Institute of Neurological Disorders and Stroke (NINDS), November 28, 2023. Available online. URL: www.ninds.nih.gov/health-information/disorders/epilepsy-and-seizures. Accessed February 13, 2024.

HUNTINGTON DISEASE

Huntington disease (HD) is an inherited disorder that causes nerve cells (neurons) in parts of the brain to gradually break down and die. The disease attacks areas of the brain that help control voluntary (intentional) movement, as well as other areas. People living with HD develop uncontrollable dance-like movements (chorea) and abnormal body postures, as well as problems with behavior, emotion, thinking, and personality.

There is no treatment that can stop or reverse HD, but some symptoms can be treated:

- The drugs tetrabenazine and deutetrabenazine can treat chorea associated with HD.
- Antipsychotic drugs may ease chorea and help control hallucinations, delusions, and violent outbursts. Some antipsychotic medications can have side effects that make muscle contraction symptoms of HD worse. Individuals using antipsychotic drugs for HD symptoms should be closely monitored for side effects.
- Drugs may be prescribed to treat depression and anxiety.

Side effects of drugs used to treat the symptoms of HD may include fatigue, sedation, decreased concentration, restlessness, or hyperexcitability. These drugs should be only used when HD symptoms create problems for the person living with HD.[7]

MOTOR NEURON DISEASES

Motor neuron diseases (MNDs) are a group of progressive neurological disorders that destroy motor neurons, the cells that control skeletal muscle activity such as walking, breathing, speaking, and swallowing. This group includes diseases such as ALS, progressive bulbar palsy (PBP), primary lateral sclerosis (PLS), progressive muscular atrophy (PMA), spinal muscular atrophy (SMA), Kennedy disease, and post-polio syndrome (PPS).

---

[7] "Huntington's Disease," National Institute of Neurological Disorders and Stroke (NINDS), December 4, 2023. Available online. URL: www.ninds.nih.gov/health-information/disorders/huntingtons-disease. Accessed February 13, 2024.

Nervous System Diseases

There is no cure or standard treatment for MNDs. Symptomatic and supportive treatment can help individuals be more comfortable while maintaining their QOL. Multidisciplinary clinics, with specialists in neurology, physical therapy, respiratory therapy, and social work, are particularly important in the care of individuals with MNDs.

Medications
- **Riluzole.** This is the first drug approved by the FDA to treat ALS; however, it cannot reverse the damage already done to motor neurons.
- **Edaravone.** This is an antioxidant approved by the FDA to treat ALS, slow down the decline of physical function, and prevent disease progression in people with ALS.
- **Nusinersen.** This is the first drug to treat children and adults with SMA approved by the FDA, which is a type of treatment called "antisense oligonucleotide (ASO) therapy" and works by increasing the survival motor neuron (SMN) protein necessary for the muscles and nerves to work normally.
- **Onasemnogene abeparovec-xioi (Zolgensma™).** This is a type of gene therapy that was approved by the FDA for children less than two years old who have infantile-onset SMA. A safe virus delivers a fully functional human SMN gene to the targeted motor neurons, which in turn improves muscle movement and function, and also improves survival.
- **Muscle relaxers.** Medications such as baclofen, tizanidine, and benzodiazepines may reduce muscle stiffness and help muscle spasms.
- **Botulinum toxin.** These injections may be used to treat muscle stiffness by weakening overactive muscles. They may be injected into the salivary glands to stop drooling. Excessive saliva can also be treated with medications such as amitriptyline, glycopyrrolate, and atropine.

Supportive Therapies
- **Physical therapy and rehabilitation.** This may help improve posture, prevent joint immobility, and slow muscle weakness and atrophy. Stretching and strengthening exercises may help reduce stiffness, as well as increase the range of motion and circulation. Some individuals require additional therapy for speech, chewing, and swallowing difficulties. Applying heat may relieve muscle pain. Assistive devices such as supports or braces, orthotics, speech synthesizers, and wheelchairs may help some people maintain independence.
- **Proper nutrition and a balanced diet.** These are essential to maintaining weight and strength. People who cannot chew or swallow may require a feeding tube.
- **Noninvasive positive pressure ventilation (NIPPV).** Also known as "ventilators," this can prevent sleep apnea at night. Some individuals may also require assisted ventilation during the day due to muscle weakness in the neck, throat, and chest.

The outlook for individuals with MNDs varies depending on the type and the age the symptoms begin. MNDs, such as PLS or Kennedy disease, are usually not fatal and progress slowly. People with SMA type III may be stable for long periods. Some forms of MND, such as the severe form of SMA and ALS, are fatal.[8]

MULTIPLE SCLEROSIS
Multiple sclerosis (MS) is the most common disabling neurological disease of young adults with symptom onset generally occurring between the ages of 20 and 40 years. In MS, the immune system cells that normally protect us from viruses, bacteria, and unhealthy cells mistakenly attack myelin in the central nervous system (CNS). Myelin is a substance that makes up the protective sheath (myelin sheath) that coats nerve fibers (axons).

---

[8] "Motor Neuron Diseases," National Institute of Neurological Disorders and Stroke (NINDS), November 28, 2023. Available online. URL: www.ninds.nih.gov/health-information/disorders/motor-neuron-diseases. Accessed February 13, 2024.

There is no cure for MS, but there are treatments that can reduce the number and severity of relapses and delay the long-term disability progression of the disease.
- **Corticosteroids**. Treatments such as intravenous (IV; infused into a vein) methylprednisolone are prescribed over the course of three to five days. IV steroids quickly and potently suppress the immune system and reduce inflammation. They may be followed by a tapered dose of oral corticosteroids. Clinical trials have shown that these drugs hasten recovery from MS attacks but do not alter the long-term outcome of the disease.
- **Plasma exchange (plasmapheresis)**. This can treat severe flare-ups in people with relapsing forms of MS who do not have a good response to methylprednisolone. Plasma exchange involves taking blood out of the body and removing components in the blood's plasma that are thought to be harmful. The rest of the blood, plus replacement plasma, is then transfused back into the body. This treatment has not been shown to be effective for secondary progressive or chronic progressive MS.

Disease-Modifying Treatments
Current therapies approved by the FDA for MS are designed to modulate or suppress the inflammatory reactions of the disease. They are most effective for relapsing-remitting MS at early stages of the disease.

INJECTABLE MEDICATIONS
- **Beta interferon drugs**. These are among the most common medications used to treat MS. Interferons are signaling molecules that regulate immune cells. Potential side effects of these drugs include flu-like symptoms (which usually fade with continued therapy), depression, or elevation of liver enzymes. Some individuals will notice a decrease in the effectiveness of the drugs

after 18–24 months of treatment. If flare-ups occur or symptoms worsen, doctors may switch treatment to alternative drugs.
- **Glatiramer acetate.** This changes the balance of immune cells in the body, but how it works is not entirely clear. Side effects are usually mild and consist of local injection site reactions or swelling.

INFUSION TREATMENTS
- **Natalizumab.** This treatment is administered intravenously once a month. It works by preventing cells of the immune system from entering the brain and spinal cord. It is very effective but is associated with an increased risk of a serious and potentially fatal viral infection of the brain called "progressive multifocal leukoencephalopathy" (PML). Natalizumab is generally recommended only for individuals who have not responded well to or who are unable to tolerate other first-line therapies.
- **Ocrelizumab.** This treatment is administered intravenously every six months and treats adults with relapsing or primary progressive forms of MS. It is the only FDA-approved disease-modifying therapy (DMT) for primary progressive MS. The drug targets the circulating immune cells that produce antibodies, which also play a role in the formation of MS lesions. Side effects include infusion-related reactions and an increased risk of infections. Ocrelizumab may increase the risk of cancer as well.
- **Alemtuzumab.** This treatment is administered for five consecutive days, followed by three days of infusions one year later. It targets proteins on the surface of immune cells. Because this drug increases the risk of autoimmune disorders, it is recommended for those who have had inadequate responses to two or more MS therapies.
- **Mitoxantrone.** This treatment is administered intravenously four times a year and has been approved for especially severe forms of relapsing-remitting and

Nervous System Diseases

secondary progressive MS. Side effects include the development of certain types of blood cancers in up to 1 percent of those with MS, as well as with heart damage. This drug should be considered as a last resort to treat people with a form of MS that leads to rapid loss of function and for whom other treatments did not work.

ORAL TREATMENTS
- **Fingolimod**. This is a once-daily medication that reduces the MS relapse rate in adults and children. It is the first FDA-approved drug to treat MS in adolescents and children aged 10 years and older. The drug prevents white blood cells (WBCs) called "lymphocytes" from leaving the lymph nodes and entering the blood, brain, and spinal cord. Fingolimod may result in a slow heart rate and eye problems when first taken. Fingolimod can also increase the risk of infections, such as herpes virus infections, or in rare cases, be associated with PML.
- **Dimethyl fumarate**. This is a twice-daily medication used to treat relapsing forms of MS. Its exact mechanism of action is not currently known. Side effects of dimethyl fumarate are flushing, diarrhea, nausea, and lowered WBC count.
- **Teriflunomide**. This is a once-daily medication that reduces the rate of proliferation of activated immune cells. Teriflunomide side effects can include nausea, diarrhea, liver damage, and hair loss.
- **Cladribine**. This is administered as two courses of tablets about one year apart. Cladribine targets certain types of WBCs that drive immune attacks in MS. The drug may increase the risk of developing cancer and should be considered for individuals who have not responded well to other MS treatments.
- **Diroximel fumarate**. This is a twice-daily drug similar to dimethyl fumarate (brand name Tecfidera) but with fewer gastrointestinal side effects. Scientists suspect these drugs, which have been approved to treat secondary progressive

MS, reduce damage to the brain and spinal cord by making the immune response less inflammatory although their exact mechanism of action is poorly understood.
- **Siponimod tablets (Mayzent).** These are taken orally and have a similar mechanism of action to fingolimod. Siponimod has been approved by the FDA to treat secondary progressive MS.

Clinical trials have shown that cladribine, diroximel fumarate, and dimethyl fumarate decrease the number of relapses, delay the progress of physical disability, and slow the development of brain lesions.[9]

NEUROFIBROMATOSIS

Neurofibromatosis is not a single medical disorder. It refers to three different conditions involving the development of tumors that may affect the brain, spinal cord, and the nerves that send signals between the brain and spinal cord and all other parts of the body. Most tumors are noncancerous (benign) although some may become cancerous (malignant). The conditions are:
- neurofibromatosis type 1 (NF1), also known as "von Recklinghausen disease"
- neurofibromatosis type 2 (NF2)
- schwannomatosis (SWN)

NF1 cannot be cured, but treatments can help manage signs and symptoms. Many people with NF1 will not require any prolonged treatment for any manifestation (disease signs or development) during their lives. People with NF1 should be evaluated periodically by an NF1 specialist, even if they are not experiencing symptoms, to evaluate for signs or symptoms that may indicate a need for treatment and to provide reassurance that treatment is not needed when appropriate.

---

[9] "Multiple Sclerosis," National Institute of Neurological Disorders and Stroke (NINDS), November 28, 2023. Available online. URL: www.ninds.nih.gov/health-information/disorders/multiple-sclerosis. Accessed February 13, 2024.

Nervous System Diseases

The FDA approved selumetinib (Koselugo) as a treatment for children aged two years and older with NF1. The drug helps stop tumor cells from growing.

Surgery may be used to remove tumors that develop symptoms or are of concern for cancer, as well as for tumors that cause significant discomfort. Several surgical options exist for many of the manifestations of NF1, but there is no general agreement among doctors about when surgery should be performed, or which surgical option is best. Some bone malformations, such as scoliosis, can be corrected surgically or by stabilizing the spine with a brace. Some malformations that affect blood vessels can be successfully addressed with surgery or nonsurgical procedures.

Chemotherapy may be used to treat optic pathways or other brain gliomas. The drug selumetinib (Koselugo®) has been approved by the FDA to treat children older than two years of age who have symptoms but inoperable plexiform neurofibromas. Chemotherapy regimens are a core part of treating cancers that may arise in the setting of NF1, including malignant peripheral nerve sheath tumor (MPNST) and breast cancer.

Treatments for other conditions associated with NF1 are aimed at controlling or relieving symptoms. Headaches and seizures are treated with medications. Because children with NF1 have a higher-than-average risk for a variety of learning disabilities, attention deficit hyperactivity disorder (ADHD), motor delays, and autism, they should be evaluated by a care team knowledgeable in NF1 and may be advised to have formal neuropsychological assessments to assist in creating individualized educational plans (IEPs) for school.

NF2 is best managed at a specialty clinic with an initial screening and annual follow-up evaluations (more frequent if the disease is severe). Improved diagnostic technologies, such as magnetic resonance imaging (MRI), can reveal tumors of the vestibular nerve as small as a few millimeters in diameter. Vestibular schwannomas grow slowly, but they can grow large enough to engulf one of the eight cranial nerves as well as cause brain stem compression and damage to surrounding cranial nerves.

Surgical options depend on tumor size and the extent of hearing loss. There is no general agreement among doctors about when surgery should be performed or which surgical option is best.

Individuals considering surgery should carefully weigh the risks and benefits of all options to determine which treatment is right for them.

There is no currently accepted medical treatment or drug for SWN. Surgery may help some people with growing tumors or symptoms that are directly referred to as individual schwannomas. However, the potential risk of nerve damage must be weighed carefully against the potential benefits of surgery.[10]

PARKINSON DISEASE

Parkinson disease (PD) is a brain disorder that causes unintended or uncontrollable movements, such as shaking, stiffness, and difficulty with balance and coordination.

Although there is no cure for PD, medicines, surgical treatment, and other therapies can often relieve some symptoms.

Medicines

Medicines can help treat the symptoms of PD by:
- increasing the level of dopamine in the brain
- having an effect on other brain chemicals, such as neurotransmitters, which transfer information between brain cells
- helping control nonmovement symptoms

The main therapy for PD is levodopa. Nerve cells use levodopa to make dopamine to replenish the brain's dwindling supply. Usually, people take levodopa along with another medication called "carbidopa." Carbidopa prevents or reduces some side effects of levodopa therapy—such as nausea, vomiting, low blood pressure, and restlessness—and reduces the amount of levodopa needed to improve symptoms.

People living with PD should never stop taking levodopa without telling their doctor. Suddenly stopping the drug may have

---

[10] "Neurofibromatosis," National Institute of Neurological Disorders and Stroke (NINDS), November 28, 2023. Available online. URL: www.ninds.nih.gov/health-information/disorders/neurofibromatosis. Accessed February 13, 2024.

serious side effects, such as being unable to move or having difficulty breathing.

The doctor may prescribe other medicines to treat PD symptoms, including:
- dopamine agonists to stimulate the production of dopamine in the brain
- enzyme inhibitors (e.g., monoamine oxidase B (MAO-B) inhibitors and catechol-O-methyltransferase (COMT) inhibitors) to increase the amount of dopamine by slowing down the enzymes that break down dopamine in the brain
- amantadine to help reduce involuntary movements
- anticholinergic drugs to reduce tremors and muscle rigidity

Deep Brain Stimulation

For people with PD who do not respond well to medications, the doctor may recommend DBS. During a surgical procedure, a doctor implants electrodes into part of the brain and connects them to a small electrical device implanted in the chest. The device and electrodes painlessly stimulate specific areas in the brain that control movement in a way that may help stop many of the movement-related symptoms of PD, such as tremors, slowness of movement, and rigidity.

Other Therapies

Other therapies that may help manage PD symptoms include:
- physical, occupational, and speech therapies, which may help with gait and voice disorders, tremors and rigidity, and decline in mental functions
- a healthy diet to support overall wellness
- exercises to strengthen muscles and improve balance, flexibility, and coordination
- massage therapy to reduce tension
- yoga and tai chi to increase stretching and flexibility[11]

---

[11] National Institute on Aging (NIA), "Parkinson's Disease: Causes, Symptoms, and Treatments," National Institutes of Health (NIH), April 14, 2022. Available online. URL: www.nia.nih.gov/health/parkinsons-disease/parkinsons-disease-causes-symptoms-and-treatments. Accessed February 13, 2024.

Chapter 14 | Immune System Diseases

The immune system consists of white blood cells (WBCs), the thymus, the spleen, lymph nodes, and lymph channels. It provides immunity to the body from bacteria, viruses, parasites, and tumors by producing B lymphocyte and T lymphocyte cells. Also, the immune system helps the body distinguish its own cells and tissues from foreign cells and substances. In this way, it plays a role in fighting cancer, developing autoimmunity, and rejecting transplanted organs.[1]

The following are the treatment and management options for some common diseases of the immune system.

HUMAN IMMUNODEFICIENCY VIRUS

Human immunodeficiency virus (HIV) is a virus that attacks cells that help the body fight infection, making a person more vulnerable to other infections and diseases. If left untreated, HIV can lead to the disease acquired immunodeficiency syndrome (AIDS).

HIV treatment involves taking highly effective medicines called "antiretroviral therapy" (ART) that work to control the virus. ART is recommended for everyone with HIV, and people with HIV should start ART as soon as possible after diagnosis, even on that same day.

People on ART take a combination of HIV medicines called an "HIV treatment regimen." A person's initial HIV treatment regimen

---

[1] "Immunological (Immune System)," Centers for Disease Control and Prevention (CDC), March 3, 2011. Available online. URL: wwwn.cdc.gov/tsp/substances/ToxOrganListing.aspx?toxid=16. Accessed February 13, 2024.

generally includes three HIV medicines from at least two different HIV drug classes that must be taken exactly as prescribed. There are several options that have two or three different HIV medicines combined into a once-daily pill. Long-acting injections of HIV medicine, given every two months, are also available if your healthcare provider determines that you meet certain requirements.

If taken as prescribed, HIV medicine reduces the amount of HIV in your blood (also called your "viral load") to a very low level, which keeps your immune system working and prevents illness. This is called "viral suppression," defined as having less than 200 copies of HIV per milliliter of blood.

HIV medicine can also make your viral load so low that a standard lab test cannot detect it. This is called having an "undetectable level viral load." Almost everyone who takes HIV medicine as prescribed can achieve an undetectable viral load, usually within six months after starting treatment. Many will bring their viral load to an undetectable level quickly, but it could take more time for a small portion of people just starting HIV medicine.

There are important health benefits to getting the viral load as low as possible. People with HIV who know their status, take HIV medicine as prescribed, and get and keep an undetectable viral load can live long and healthy lives.

There is also a major prevention benefit. People with HIV who take HIV medicine as prescribed and get and keep an undetectable viral load will not transmit HIV to their HIV-negative partners through sex.

HIV treatment is most likely to be successful when you know what to expect and are committed to taking your medicines exactly as prescribed. Working with your health-care provider to develop a treatment plan will help you learn more about HIV and manage it effectively.

If left untreated, HIV will attack your immune system and can allow different types of life-threatening infections and cancers to develop. If your immune system is not working well, you are at risk of getting an opportunistic infection. These are infections that do not normally affect people with healthy immune systems but that can affect people who are not on treatment and whose immune systems are weakened by HIV. Your health-care provider may prescribe medicines to prevent certain infections.

ART is not a cure and the virus remains in your body, even when your viral load is undetectable, so you need to keep taking your HIV medicine as prescribed. If you stop taking your HIV medicine, your viral load will quickly go back up.

If you have stopped taking your HIV medicine or are having trouble taking all the doses as prescribed, talk to your health-care provider as soon as possible. Your provider can help you get back on track and discuss the best strategies to prevent transmitting HIV to your sexual partners until your viral load is confirmed to be undetectable again.[2]

RHEUMATOID ARTHRITIS

Rheumatoid arthritis (RA) is a chronic (long-lasting) autoimmune disease that mostly affects joints. RA occurs when the immune system, which normally helps protect the body from infection and disease, attacks its own tissues. The disease causes pain, swelling, stiffness, and loss of function in joints.

Treatment of RA continues to improve, which can give many people relief from symptoms, improving their quality of life (QOL). Doctors may use the following options to treat RA:

- medications
- physical therapy and occupational therapy
- surgery
- routine monitoring and ongoing care
- complementary therapies

Your doctor may recommend a combination of treatments, which may change over time based on your symptoms and the severity of your disease. No matter which treatment plan your doctor recommends, the overall goals are to help:

- relieve pain
- decrease inflammation and swelling

---

[2] HIV.gov, "HIV Treatment Overview," U.S. Department of Health and Human Services (HHS), June 7, 2022. Available online. URL: www.hiv.gov/hiv-basics/staying-in-hiv-care/hiv-treatment/hiv-treatment-overview. Accessed February 13, 2024.

- prevent, slow, or stop joint and organ damage
- improve your ability to participate in daily activities

RA may start causing joint damage during the first year or two that a person has the disease. Once joint damage occurs, it generally cannot be reversed, so early diagnosis and treatment are very important.

Medications

Most people who have RA take medications. Studies show that early treatment with combinations of medications, instead of one medication alone, may be more effective in decreasing or preventing joint damage.

Many of the medications that doctors prescribe to treat RA help decrease inflammation and pain, and slow or stop joint damage. They may include:

- Antiinflammatory medications to provide pain relief and lower inflammation.
- Corticosteroids that can help decrease inflammation, provide some pain relief, and slow joint damage. Because they are potent drugs and have potential side effects, your doctor will prescribe the lowest dose possible to achieve the desired benefit.
- Disease-modifying antirheumatic drugs (DMARDs) that can help to slow or change the progression of the disease.
- Biologic response modifiers, which are also DMARDs, if your disease does not respond to initial therapies. These medications target specific immune messages and interrupt the signal, helping to decrease or stop inflammation.
- JAK inhibitors, which are also DMARDs, send messages to specific cells to stop inflammation from inside the cell. These medications may also be considered if your disease does not respond to initial therapies.

Physical Therapy and Occupational Therapy
Your doctor may recommend physical therapy and occupational therapy. Physical therapy can help you regain and maintain overall strength and target specific joints that bother you. Occupational therapy can help develop, recover, improve, as well as maintain the skills needed for daily living and working. Sometimes assistive devices or braces may be helpful to optimize movement, reduce pain, and help you maintain the ability to work.

Surgery
Your doctor may recommend surgery if you have permanent damage or pain that limits your ability to perform day-to-day activities. Surgery is not for everyone. You and your doctor can discuss the options and choose what is right for you.

Your doctor will consider the following before recommending surgery:
- your overall health
- the condition of the affected joint or tendon
- the risks and benefits of the surgery

Types of surgery may include joint repairs and joint replacements.

Routine Monitoring and Ongoing Care
Regular medical care is important because your doctor can:
- monitor how the disease is progressing
- determine how well the medications are working
- talk to you about any side effects from the medications
- adjust your treatment as needed

Monitoring typically includes regular visits to the doctor. It may also include blood and urine tests, and x-rays or other imaging tests. Having RA increases your risk of developing osteoporosis, particularly if you take corticosteroids. Osteoporosis is a bone disease that causes the bones to weaken and easily break. Talk to your doctor about your risk for the disease and the potential benefits of calcium and vitamin D supplements or other osteoporosis treatments.

Since RA can affect other organs, your doctor may also monitor you for cardiovascular or respiratory health. Many of the medications used to treat RA may increase the risk of infection. Doctors may monitor you for infections. Vaccines may be recommended to lower the risk and severity of infections.[3]

SEVERE COMBINED IMMUNODEFICIENCY

"Severe combined immunodeficiency" (SCID) is a term applied to a group of inherited disorders characterized by defects in both T- and B-cell responses, hence the term "combined." The most common type of SCID is called "X-linked severe combined immunodeficiency" (XSCID) because the mutated gene, which normally produces a receptor for activation signals on immune cells, is located on the X chromosome. Another form of SCID is caused by a deficiency of the enzyme adenosine deaminase (ADA), normally produced by a gene on chromosome 20.

The classic symptoms of SCID include an increased susceptibility to a variety of infections, including ear infections (acute otitis media or AOM), pneumonia or bronchitis, oral thrush (a type of yeast that multiplies rapidly, creating white, sore areas in the mouth), and diarrhea. Because children with SCID experience multiple infections, they fail to grow and gain weight as expected (i.e., failure to thrive). Children with untreated SCID rarely live past the age of two.

The most effective treatment for SCID is transplantation of blood-forming stem cells from the bone marrow of a healthy person. Bone marrow stem cells can live for a long time by renewing themselves as needed and can also produce a continuous supply of healthy immune cells. A bone marrow transplant from a tissue-matched sister or brother offers the greatest chance for curing SCID. However, most patients do not have a matched sibling donor, so transplants from a parent or unrelated matched donor are often

---

[3] "Rheumatoid Arthritis," National Institute of Arthritis and Musculoskeletal and Skin Diseases (NIAMS), November 2022. Available online. URL: www.niams.nih.gov/health-topics/rheumatoid-arthritis. Accessed February 13, 2024.

performed. These latter types of transplant succeed less often than do transplants from a matched, related donor. All transplants done in the first three months of life have the highest success rate.

In 1990, National Institutes of Health (NIH) researchers performed the first successful human gene therapy on two girls with ADA SCID. The treatments consisted of removing some of the girls' own T cells, inserting a normal copy of the ADA gene into the cells, expanding the T cells in a culture system and returning them to the girls' bodies through a vein. Repeated treatments led to normalization of T cell numbers. Although the girls have continued to rely on ADA enzyme injections for their primary management, they have developed normal immunity.

Following this pioneering work, scientists at National Human Genome Research Institute (NHGRI) and around the world have continued to conduct clinical research with ADA SCID and additional genetic forms of SCID. This work has led to breakthroughs for improving the efficiency of gene transfer as well as insights into the biology of XSCID and ADA SCID. NHGRI researchers are continuing to develop more effective gene therapy treatments, first in experimental animal models and then in very small numbers of humans. One particular discovery made by NHGRI investigators is the observation that in individuals in whom some cells naturally expressed normal levels of γc or ADA, the expressing cells tend to grow better than the defective cells. This discovery showed that gene transfers could be accomplished with relatively few stem cells that would then outgrow the defective cells and give rise to a full complement of corrected T and B cells, restoring the immune system.

Gene therapy trials for SCID were halted worldwide for a number of years when it was reported that children who had been treated for XSCID in a French gene-therapy experiment had developed a type of leukemia. It was soon discovered that the mechanism used to insert the corrective gene had placed it in a region of a receiving cell's chromosome that switched on a cancer-causing gene (oncogene). NHGRI researchers are evaluating insertion profiles of standard and novel gene delivery methods. A goal of this work is to find ways to achieve permanent correction of the deoxyribonucleic acid (DNA) in blood-forming stem cells while avoiding the activation of oncogenes.

NHGRI investigators are also studying approaches to improve the effectiveness of bone marrow transplantation for these conditions. A major limitation to bone marrow transplantation is that blood-forming stem cells are not well understood. They are few in number and cannot be purified or expanded outside the body for very long. NHGRI researchers are investigating the roles of genes that control the reproduction and differentiation of blood-forming stem cells in order to significantly increase the supplies of these life-saving cells for clinical use.[4]

SYSTEMIC LUPUS ERYTHEMATOSUS

Systemic lupus erythematosus (SLE), is the most common type of lupus. SLE is an autoimmune disease in which the immune system attacks its own tissues, causing widespread inflammation and tissue damage in the affected organs. It can affect the joints, skin, brain, lungs, kidneys, and blood vessels. There is no cure for lupus, but medical interventions and lifestyle changes can help control it.

Treating SLE often requires a team approach because of the number of organs that can be affected.

SLE treatment consists primarily of immunosuppressive drugs that inhibit activity of the immune system. Hydroxychloroquine and corticosteroids (e.g., prednisone) are often used to treat SLE. The U.S. Food and Drug Administration (FDA) approved belimumab in 2011, the first new drug for SLE in more than 50 years.

SLE may also occur with other autoimmune conditions that require additional treatments, such as Sjögren syndrome, antiphospholipid syndrome (APS), thyroiditis, hemolytic anemia, and idiopathic thrombocytopenia purpura (ITP).[5]

---

[4] "About Severe Combined Immunodeficiency," National Human Genome Research Institute (NHGRI), June 2, 2014. Available online. URL: www.genome.gov/Genetic-Disorders/Severe-Combined-Immunodeficiency. Accessed February 13, 2024.

[5] "Systemic Lupus Erythematosus (SLE)," Centers for Disease Control and Prevention (CDC), July 5, 2022. Available online. URL: www.cdc.gov/lupus/facts/detailed.html. Accessed February 13, 2024.

Immune System Diseases

TYPE 1 DIABETES

If you have type 1 diabetes, your pancreas does not make insulin or makes very little insulin. Type 1 diabetes was once called "insulin-dependent diabetes" or "juvenile diabetes," but it can develop at any age. Type 1 diabetes is less common than type 2 diabetes.

Unlike many health conditions, diabetes is managed mostly by you, with support from your health-care team:
- primary care doctor
- foot doctor
- dentist
- eye doctor
- registered dietitian nutritionist
- diabetes educator
- pharmacist

If you have type 1 diabetes, you will need to take insulin shots (or wear an insulin pump) every day. Insulin is needed to manage your blood sugar levels and give your body energy. You cannot take insulin as a pill. That is because the acid in your stomach would destroy it before it could get into your bloodstream. Your doctor will work with you to figure out the most effective type and dosage of insulin for you.

You will also need to do regular blood sugar checks. Ask your doctor how often you should check it and what your target blood sugar levels should be. Keeping your blood sugar levels as close to target as possible will help you prevent or delay diabetes-related complications.

Stress is a part of life, but it can make managing diabetes harder. Both managing your blood sugar levels and dealing with daily diabetes care can be tougher to do. Regular physical activity, getting enough sleep, and exercises to relax can help. Talk to your doctor and diabetes educator about these and other ways you can manage stress

Healthy lifestyle habits are really important too:
- making healthy food choices
- being physically active

- controlling your blood pressure
- controlling your cholesterol

Make regular appointments with your health-care team. They will help you stay on track with your treatment plan and offer new ideas and strategies if needed.[6]

---

[6] "What Is Type 1 Diabetes?" Centers for Disease Control and Prevention (CDC), September 5, 2023. Available online. URL: www.cdc.gov/diabetes/basics/what-is-type-1-diabetes.html. Accessed February 13, 2024.

Part 3 | Working with Health-Care Providers and the Health-Care System

Chapter 15 | Choosing Your Doctor

Finding a main doctor (often called your "primary doctor" or "primary care doctor") whom you feel comfortable talking to is the first step in good communication. How well you and your doctor talk to each other is one of the most important steps to getting good health care. This doctor gets to know you and what your health is normally like. He or she can help you make medical decisions that suit your values and daily habits and can keep in touch with the other medical specialists and health-care providers you may need.

Taking an active role in your health care puts the responsibility for good communication on both you and your doctor. This means asking questions if the doctor's explanations or instructions are unclear, bringing up problems even if the doctor does not ask, and letting the doctor know if you have concerns about a particular treatment or change in your daily life.

If you do not have a primary doctor or are not at ease with the one you currently see, now may be the time to find a new doctor. Whether you just moved to a new city, changed insurance providers, or had a bad experience with your doctor or medical staff, it is worthwhile to spend time finding a doctor you can trust.

People sometimes hesitate to change doctors because they worry about hurting their doctor's feelings. But doctors understand that different people have different needs. They know it is important for everyone to have a doctor with whom they are comfortable.

Primary care physicians frequently are family practitioners, internists, or geriatricians. A geriatrician is a doctor who specializes in older people, but family practitioners and internists may also have a lot of experience with older patients. Here are some suggestions that can help you find a doctor who meets your needs.

DECIDE WHAT YOU ARE LOOKING FOR IN A DOCTOR
A good first step is to make a list of qualities that matter to you. Do you care if your doctor is a man or a woman? Is it important that your doctor has evening office hours, is associated with a specific hospital or medical center, or speaks your language? Do you prefer a doctor who has an individual practice or one who is part of a group so you can see one of your doctor's partners if your doctor is not available? After you have made your list, go back over it and decide which qualities are most important and which are nice, but not essential.

MAKE A LIST OF SEVERAL POSSIBLE DOCTORS
Once you have a general sense of what you are looking for, ask friends and relatives, medical specialists, and other health professionals for the names of doctors with whom they have had good experiences. Rather than just getting a name, ask about the person's experiences.

If you belong to a managed care plan—a health maintenance organization (HMO) or preferred provider organization (PPO)—you may be required to choose a doctor in the plan, or else you may have to pay extra to see a doctor outside the network. Most managed care plans will provide information on their doctors' backgrounds and credentials. Some plans have websites with lists of participating doctors from which you can choose.

It may be helpful to develop a list of a few names you can choose from. As you find out more about the doctors on this list, you may rule out some of them. In some cases, a doctor may not be taking new patients, and you may have to make another choice.

What Are Health Maintenance Organizations and Preferred Provider Organizations?
Members of an HMO pay a set monthly fee no matter how many (or few) times they see a doctor. Usually, there are no deductibles or

claims forms, but you will have a co-payment for doctor visits and prescriptions. Each member chooses a primary care doctor from within the HMO network. The primary care doctor coordinates all care and, if necessary, refers members to specialists.

A PPO is a network of doctors and other health-care providers. The doctors in this network agree to provide medical services to PPO health plan members at discounted costs. Members can choose to see any doctor at any time. Choosing a non-PPO provider is called "going out of network" and will cost more than seeing a member of the PPO network.

GATHER INFORMATION FROM THE WEB

The Doctor Finder website of the American Medical Association (AMA; https://find-doctor.ama-assn.org) and the Certification Matters database of the American Board of Medical Specialties (ABMS; www.certificationmatters.org) can help you find doctors in your area. These websites do not recommend individual doctors, but they do provide a list of doctors you may want to consider. MedlinePlus, a website from the National Library of Medicine (NLM) at the National Institutes of Health (NIH), has a comprehensive list of directories (www.medlineplus.gov/directories), which may also be helpful. For a list of doctors who participate in Medicare, visit the Medicare.gov Physician Compare tool website (www.medicare.gov/care-compare/?redirect=true&providerType=Physician).

Do not forget to call your local or state medical society to check if complaints have been filed against any of the doctors you are considering.

What Is a "Board-Certified" Doctor?

Doctors who are board certified have extra training after regular medical school. They also have passed an exam certifying their expertise in specialty areas. Examples of specialty areas are general internal medicine, family medicine, geriatrics, gynecology, and orthopedics. The ABMS has a database of all board-certified physicians that is updated daily. Board certification is one way to learn about a doctor's medical expertise; it does not tell you about the doctor's communication skills.

COLLECT INFORMATION ABOUT THE DOCTORS YOU ARE CONSIDERING

Once you have narrowed your list to two or three doctors, call their offices. The office staff is a good source of information about the doctor's education and qualifications, office policies, and payment procedures. Pay attention to the office staff—you will have to communicate with them often.

You may want to set up an appointment to meet and talk with a doctor you are considering. He or she is likely to charge you for such a visit. After the appointment, ask yourself if this doctor is a person with whom you could work well. If you are not satisfied, schedule a visit with one of your other candidates.

When learning about a doctor, consider asking questions such as:
- Do you have many older patients?
- How do you feel about involving my family in care decisions?
- Can I call or email you or your staff when I have questions? Do you charge for telephone or email time?
- What telehealth services do you offer?
- What are your thoughts about complementary or alternative treatments?

CHOOSE A DOCTOR

When making a decision about which doctor to choose, you might want to ask yourself questions such as:
- Did the doctor give me a chance to ask questions?
- Was the doctor really listening to me?
- Could I understand what the doctor was saying? Was I comfortable asking him or her to say it again?

Once you have chosen a doctor, make your first actual care appointment. This visit may include a medical history and a

Choosing Your Doctor

physical exam. Be sure to bring your medical records or have them sent from your former doctor. Bring a list of your current medicines or put the medicines in a bag and take them with you. If you have not already met the doctor, ask for extra time during this visit to ask any questions you have about the doctor or the practice.[1]

---

[1] National Institute on Aging (NIA), "How to Choose a Doctor You Can Talk To," National Institutes of Health (NIH), February 1, 2020. Available online. URL: www.nia.nih.gov/health/medical-care-and-appointments/how-choose-doctor-you-can-talk. Accessed February 16, 2024.

Chapter 16 | Talking with Your Health-Care Provider before Making Decisions

Chapter Contents
Section 16.1—Why Being Able to Talk with Your Doctor Matters 177
Section 16.2—How to Prepare for a Doctor's Appointment 179
Section 16.3—Make the Most of Your Time at the Doctor's Office 183
Section 16.4—Be More Involved in Your Health Care 187

Chapter 16 | Talking with Your Health-Care Provider before Making Decisions

Section 16.1 | Why Being Able to Talk with Your Doctor Matters

YOUR DOCTOR IS YOUR PARTNER IN HEALTH CARE

You probably have many questions about your disease or condition. The first person to ask is your doctor.

It is fine to seek more information from other sources; in fact, it is important to do so. But consider your doctor your partner in health care—someone who can discuss your situation with you, explain your options, and help you make decisions that are right for you.

It is not always easy to feel comfortable around doctors. But research has shown that good communication with your doctor can actually be good for your health. It can help you:
- feel more satisfied with the care you receive
- have better outcomes (end results), such as reduced pain and better recovery from symptoms

Being an active member of your health-care team also helps reduce your chances of medical mistakes, and it helps you get high-quality care.

Of course, good communication is a two-way street. Here are some ways to help make the most of the time you spend with your doctor.

PREPARE FOR YOUR VISIT
- **Think about what you want to get out of your appointment**. Write down all your questions and concerns.
- **Prepare and bring to your doctor's visit a list of all the medicines you take**.
- **Consider bringing along a trusted relative or friend**. This person can help ask questions, take notes, and help you remember and understand everything once you leave the doctor's office.

GIVE INFORMATION TO YOUR DOCTOR
- Do not wait to be asked.
- Tell your doctor everything he or she needs to know about your health—even the things that might make you feel embarrassed or uncomfortable.
- Tell your doctor how you are feeling—both physically and emotionally.
- Tell your doctor if you are feeling depressed or overwhelmed.

GET INFORMATION FROM YOUR DOCTOR
- Ask questions about anything that concerns you. Keep asking until you understand the answers. If you do not, your doctor may think you understand everything that is said.
- Ask your doctor to draw pictures if that will help you understand something.
- Take notes.
- Tape-record your doctor visit, if that will be helpful to you. But, first, ask your doctor if this is okay.
- Ask your doctor to recommend resources such as websites, booklets, or tapes with more information about your disease or condition.

GET INFORMATION ABOUT NEXT STEPS
- Get the results of any tests or procedures. Discuss the meaning of these results with your doctor.
- Make sure you understand what will happen if you need surgery.
- Talk with your doctor about which hospital is best for your health-care needs.

Finally, if you are not satisfied with your doctor, you can do the following two things:
- Talk with your doctor and try to work things out.
- Switch doctors if you are able to.

It is very important to feel confident about your care.

Talking with Your Health-Care Provider before Making Decisions

Ten Important Questions to Ask Your Doctor after a Diagnosis

The following 10 questions can help you understand your disease or condition, how it might be treated, and what you need to know and do before making treatment decisions:

- What is the technical name of my disease or condition, and what does it mean in plain English?
- What is my prognosis (outlook for the future)?
- How soon do I need to make a decision about treatment?
- Will I need any additional tests, and if so, what kind and when?
- What are my treatment options?
- What are the pros and cons of my treatment options?
- Is there a clinical trial (research study) that is right for me?
- Now that I have this diagnosis, what changes will I need to make in my daily life?
- What organizations do you recommend for support and information?
- What resources (booklets, websites, audiotapes, videos, digital video discs (DVDs), etc.) do you recommend for further information?[1]

Section 16.2 | How to Prepare for a Doctor's Appointment

A basic plan can help you make the most of your appointment whether you are starting with a new doctor or continuing with the doctor you have seen for years. The following tips will make it easier for you and your doctor to cover everything you need to talk about.

---

[1] Agency for Healthcare Research and Quality (AHRQ), "Next Steps after Your Diagnosis—Step 3: Talk with Your Doctor," U.S. Department of Health and Human Services (HHS), November 2020. Available online. URL: www.ahrq.gov/questions/resources/diagnosis/step3.html. Accessed February 16, 2024.

MAKE A LIST AND PRIORITIZE YOUR CONCERNS
Make a list of what you want to discuss. For example, do you have a new symptom you want to ask the doctor about? Do you want to get a flu shot? Are you concerned about how a treatment is affecting your daily life? If you have more than a few items to discuss, put them in order and ask about the most important ones first. Do not put off the things that are really on your mind until the end of your appointment—bring them up right away.

TAKE INFORMATION WITH YOU TO THE DOCTOR
Some doctors suggest you put all your prescription drugs, over-the-counter (OTC) medicines, vitamins, and herbal remedies or supplements in a bag and bring them with you. Others recommend you bring a list of everything you take and the dose. You should also take your insurance cards, the names and phone numbers of other doctors you see, and your medical records if the doctor does not already have them.

CONSIDER BRINGING A FAMILY MEMBER OR FRIEND TO THE DOCTOR'S OFFICE
Sometimes it is helpful to bring a family member or close friend with you. Let your family member or friend know in advance what you want from your visit. Your companion can remind you what you planned to discuss with the doctor if you forget. He or she can take notes for you and can help you remember what the doctor said.

Do not let your companion take too strong a role. The visit is between you and the doctor. You may want some time alone with the doctor to discuss personal matters. If you are alone with the doctor during or right after the physical exam, this might be a good time to raise private concerns. Or you could ask your family member or friend to stay in the waiting room for part of the appointment. For the best results, let your companion know in advance how he or she can be most helpful.

Talking with Your Health-Care Provider before Making Decisions

GETTING STARTED WITH A NEW DOCTOR
Your first meeting is a good time to talk with the doctor and the office staff about some communication basics.
- **Introduce yourself.** When you see the doctor and office staff, introduce yourself and let them know by what name you prefer to be called.
- **Ask how the office runs.** Learn what days are busiest and what times are best to call. Ask what to do if there is an emergency or if you need a doctor when the office is closed.
- **Share your medical history.** Tell the doctor about your illnesses, operations, medical conditions, and other doctors you see. You may want to ask the doctor to send you a copy of the medical history form before your visit, so you can fill it out at home, where you have the time and information you need to complete it. If you have problems understanding how to fill out any of the forms, ask for help. Some community organizations provide this kind of help.
- **Share former doctors' names.** Give the new doctor all of your former doctors' names and addresses, especially if they are in a different city. This is to help your new doctor get copies of your medical records. Your doctor will ask you to sign a medical release form giving him or her permission to request your records.

KEEP YOUR DOCTOR UP-TO-DATE
Let your doctor know what has happened in your life since your last visit. If you have been treated in the emergency room or by a specialist, tell the doctor right away. Mention any changes you have noticed in your appetite, weight, sleep, or energy level. Also, tell the doctor about any recent changes in any medications you take or the effects they have had on you.

BE SURE YOU CAN SEE AND HEAR AS WELL AS POSSIBLE
Many older people use glasses or need aids for hearing. Remember to take your eyeglasses to the doctor's visit. If you have a hearing

aid, make sure that it is working well and wear it. Let the doctor and staff know if you have a hard time seeing or hearing. For example, you may want to say: "My hearing makes it hard to understand everything you're saying. It helps a lot when you speak slowly and face me when you're talking."

REQUEST AN INTERPRETER IF YOU NEED ONE

If the doctor you selected or were referred to does not speak your language, ask the doctor's office to provide an interpreter. Even though some English-speaking doctors know basic medical terms in Spanish or other languages, you may feel more comfortable speaking in your own language, especially when it comes to sensitive subjects, such as sexuality or depression. Call the doctor's office ahead of time, as they may need to plan for an interpreter to be available.

Always let the doctor, your interpreter, or the staff know if you do not understand your diagnosis or the instructions the doctor gives you. Do not let language barriers stop you from asking questions or voicing your concerns.

Using an Interpreter at the Doctor's Office

- Consider telling your interpreter what you want to talk about with your doctor before the appointment.
- If your language is spoken in multiple countries, such as Spanish, and your interpreter does not come from the same country or background as you, use universal terms to describe your symptoms and communicate your concerns.
- Make sure your interpreter understands your symptoms or condition so that he or she can correctly translate your message to the doctor. You do not want the doctor to prescribe the wrong medication.
- Do not be afraid to let your interpreter know if you did not understand something that was said, even if you need to ask that it be repeated several times.[2]

---

[2] National Institute on Aging (NIA), "How to Prepare for a Doctor's Appointment," National Institutes of Health (NIH), February 3, 2020. Available online. URL: www.nia.nih.gov/health/medical-care-and-appointments/how-prepare-doctors-appointment. Accessed February 16, 2024.

Talking with Your Health-Care Provider before Making Decisions

Section 16.3 | Make the Most of Your Time at the Doctor's Office

Have you ever left your doctor's office realizing you forgot to ask an important question? Or were you frustrated because you did not fully understand the doctor's instructions? The following tips may help.

DECIDE WHAT QUESTIONS ARE MOST IMPORTANT TO ASK THE DOCTOR

Before your appointment, pick three or four questions or concerns that you most want to talk about with the doctor. You can tell him or her what they are at the beginning of the appointment and then discuss each in turn. If you have time, you can then go on to other questions.

STAY FOCUSED ON WHY YOU ARE THERE

Although your doctor might like to talk with you at length, each patient is given a limited amount of time. To make the best use of your time, stick to the point. For instance, give the doctor a brief description of the symptom, when it started, how often it happens, and if it is getting worse or better.

BE HONEST WITH YOUR DOCTOR

It is tempting to say what you think the doctor wants to hear, for example, that you smoke less or eat a more balanced diet than you really do. While this is natural, it is not in your best interest. If you are lesbian, gay, bisexual, or transgender (LGBT), it is important to come out to your doctor, as people who are LGBT have unique health needs. Your doctor can suggest the best treatment only if you say what is really going on. For instance, you might say: "I have been trying to quit smoking, as you recommended, but I am not making much headway."

SHARE YOUR POINT OF VIEW ABOUT THE VISIT WITH YOUR DOCTOR

Tell the doctor if you feel rushed, worried, or uncomfortable. If necessary, you can offer to return for a second visit to discuss your concerns. Try to voice your feelings in a positive way. For example, you could say something like: "I know you have many patients to see, but I'm really worried about this. I'd feel much better if we could talk about it a little more."

REMEMBER, THE DOCTOR MAY NOT BE ABLE TO ANSWER ALL YOUR QUESTIONS

Even the best doctor may be unable to answer some questions. Most doctors will tell you when they do not have answers. They may also help you find the information you need or refer you to a specialist. If a doctor regularly brushes off your questions or symptoms as simply a part of aging, think about looking for another doctor.

Tips to Help You Remember the Doctor's Instructions

No matter what your age, it is easy to forget a lot of what your doctor says. Even if you are comfortable talking with your doctor, you may not always understand what he or she says. So, as your doctor gives you information, it is a good idea to check that you are following along. Ask about anything that does not seem clear. For instance, you might say: "I want to make sure I understand. Could you explain that a little more?" or "I did not understand that word. What does it mean?"

Another way to check is to repeat what you think the doctor means in your own words and ask, "Is this correct?" Here are some other ideas to help make sure you have all the information you need:

- **Take notes**. Take along a notepad and pen and write down the main points or ask the doctor to write them down for you. If you cannot write while the doctor is talking to you, make notes in the waiting room after the visit. Or bring an audio recorder along and (with the doctor's permission)

record what is said. Recording is especially helpful if you want to share the details of the visit with others.
- **Get written or recorded materials**. Ask if your doctor has any brochures, digital video discs (DVDs), or other materials about your health conditions or treatments. For example, if your doctor says that your blood pressure is high, he or she may give you brochures explaining what causes high blood pressure (HBP) and what you can do about it. Ask the doctor to recommend other sources, such as websites, disease management centers, nonprofit organizations, and government agencies that may have written or recorded information you can use.
- **Talk to other members of the health-care team**. Sometimes the doctor may want you to talk with other health professionals who can help you understand and carry out the decisions about how to manage your condition. Nurses, physician assistants, pharmacists, and occupational or physical therapists may be able to take more time with you than the doctor.
- **Call or email the doctor**. If you are uncertain about the doctor's instructions after you get home, call the office. A nurse or other staff member can check with the doctor and call you back. Ask if they have an email address or online health portal you can use to send questions.[3]

Talking about your health means sharing information about how you feel physically, emotionally, and mentally. Knowing how to describe your symptoms and bring up other concerns will help you become a partner in your health care. Use the worksheets available at www.nia.nih.gov/health/medical-care-and-appointments/talking-your-doctor-worksheets to organize your questions and information when talking with your doctor.

---

[3] National Institute on Aging (NIA), "Five Ways to Get the Most Out of Your Doctor's Visit," National Institutes of Health (NIH), February 3, 2020. Available online. URL: www.nia.nih.gov/health/medical-care-and-appointments/five-ways-get-most-out-your-doctors-visit. Accessed February 16, 2024.

SHARE ANY SYMPTOMS YOU HAVE

A symptom is evidence of a disease or disorder in the body. Examples of symptoms include pain, fever, a lump or bump, unexplained weight loss or gain, or having a hard time sleeping.

Be clear and concise when describing your symptoms. Your description helps the doctor identify the problem. A physical exam and medical tests provide valuable information, but your symptoms point the doctor in the right direction.

Your doctor will ask when your symptoms started, what time of day they happen, how long they last, how often they occur, if they seem to be getting worse or better, and if they keep you from going out or doing your usual activities.

Take the time to make some notes about your symptoms before you call or visit the doctor. Worrying about your symptoms is not a sign of weakness. Being honest about what you are experiencing does not mean that you are complaining. The doctor needs to know how you feel.

Questions to ask yourself about your symptoms:
- What exactly are my symptoms?
- Are the symptoms constant? If not, when do I experience them?
- Does anything I do make the symptoms better or worse?
- Do the symptoms affect my daily activities? Which ones? How?

TELL THE DOCTOR ABOUT YOUR HABITS

To provide the best care, your doctor must understand you as a person and know what your life is like. The doctor may ask about where you live, what you eat, how you sleep, what you do each day, what activities you enjoy, what your sex life is like, and if you smoke or drink. Be open and honest with your doctor. It will help him or her understand your medical conditions fully and recommend the best treatment choices for you.[4]

---

[4] National Institute on Aging (NIA), "What Do I Need to Tell the Doctor?" National Institutes of Health (NIH), February 3, 2020. Available online. URL: www.nia.nih.gov/health/medical-care-and-appointments/what-do-i-need-tell-doctor. Accessed February 16, 2024.

Talking with Your Health-Care Provider before Making Decisions

Section 16.4 | Be More Involved in Your Health Care

TIPS FOR PATIENTS

Here are some tips to use before, during, and after your medical appointment to make sure you get the best possible care.

One way you can make sure you get good quality health care is to be an active member of your health-care team.

Patients who ask questions and make sure they understand the answers tend to get more timely, accurate diagnoses and have better outcomes.

Before Your Appointment
- Bring all the medicines you take to your appointment. This includes:
  - prescription medicines
  - nonprescription medicines, such as aspirin or antacids
  - vitamins
  - dietary or herbal supplements
- Write down the questions you have for the visit.
- Know your current medical conditions, past surgeries, and illnesses.

During Your Appointment
- Explain your symptoms, health history, and any problems with medicines you have taken in the past.
- Ask questions to make sure you understand what your doctor is telling you.
- Let your doctor know if you are worried about being able to follow his or her instructions.
- If your doctor recommends a treatment, ask about options.
- If you need a test, ask:
  - how the test is done
  - how it will feel
  - what you need to do to get ready for it
  - how you will get the results

- If you need a prescription, tell your doctor if you are pregnant, are nursing, have reactions to medicines, or take vitamins or herbal supplements.
- Find out what to do next. Ask for:
  - written instructions
  - brochures
  - videos
  - websites

After Your Appointment

- Always follow your doctor's instructions.
- If you do not understand your doctor's instructions after you get home, call your doctor.
- Talk with your doctor or pharmacist before you stop taking any medicines that your doctor prescribed.
- Call your doctor if your symptoms get worse or if you have problems following the instructions.
- Make appointments to have tests done or see a specialist if you need to.
- Call your doctor's office to find out test results. Ask what you should do about the results.[5]

---

[5] Agency for Healthcare Research and Quality (AHRQ), "Be More Engaged in Your Healthcare," U.S. Department of Health and Human Services (HHS), December 2020. Available online. URL: www.ahrq.gov/questions/be-engaged/index.html. Accessed February 16, 2024.

Chapter 17 | Making Decisions with Your Doctor

FIND OUT ABOUT DIFFERENT TREATMENTS
You will benefit most from treatment when you know what is happening and are involved in making decisions. Make sure you understand what your treatment involves and what it will or will not do. Have the doctor give you directions in writing and feel free to ask questions. For example: "What are the pros and cons of having surgery at this stage?" or "Do I have any other choices?"

If your doctor suggests a treatment that makes you uncomfortable, ask if there are other treatments that might work. If cost is a concern, ask the doctor if less expensive choices are available. The doctor can work with you to develop a treatment plan that meets your needs.

Here are some things to remember when deciding on a treatment:

- **Discuss choices**. There are different ways to manage many health conditions, especially chronic conditions, such as high blood pressure (HBP) and cholesterol. Ask what your options are.
- **Discuss risks and benefits**. Once you know your options, ask about the pros and cons of each one. Find out what side effects might occur, how long the treatment would continue, and how likely it is that the treatment will work for you.

- **Consider your own values and circumstances.** When thinking about the pros and cons of a treatment, do not forget to consider its effects on your overall life. For instance, will one of the side effects interfere with a regular activity that means a lot to you? Is one treatment choice expensive and not covered by your insurance? Doctors need to know about these practical matters, so they can work with you to develop a treatment plan that meets your needs.

Questions to ask about treatment:
- Are there any risks associated with the treatment?
- How soon should treatment start? How long will it last?
- Are there other treatments available?
- How much will the treatment cost? Will my insurance cover it?
- Are there any research studies or clinical trials studying treatments for my condition?

LEARN ABOUT PREVENTION

Doctors and other health professionals may suggest you change your diet, activity level, or other aspects of your life to help you manage medical conditions. Research has shown that these changes, particularly getting more exercise and eating well, have positive effects on overall health.

Preventing disease is especially important for older adults. We know that it is never too late to stop smoking, improve your diet, or start exercising. Getting regular checkups and seeing other health professionals, such as dentists and eye specialists, help promote good health. Even people who have chronic diseases, such as arthritis or diabetes, can prevent further disability and, in some cases, control the progression of these diseases.

If a certain disease or health condition runs in your family, ask your doctor if there are steps you can take to:
- help prevent it
- manage it
- keep it from getting worse

Making Decisions with Your Doctor

If you want to discuss health and disease prevention with your doctor, say so when you make your next appointment. This lets the doctor plan to spend more time with you.

Questions to ask about prevention:
- Is there any way to prevent a condition that runs in my family?
- Are there ways to keep my condition from getting worse?
- How will making a change in my habits help me?
- Are there any risks in making this change?
- Are there support groups or community services that might help me?

It is just as important to talk with your doctor about lifestyle changes as it is to talk about medical treatment. For example: "I know that you have told me to eat more dairy products, but they really disagree with me. Is there something else I could eat instead?" or "Maybe an exercise class would help, but I have no way to get to the senior center. Is there something else you could suggest?"

As with treatments, consider all the alternatives, look at risks and benefits, and remember to consider your own point of view. Tell your doctor if you feel his or her suggestions would not work for you and explain why. Keep talking with your doctor to come up with a plan that works.

Talking about Exercise and Physical Activity

Exercise and physical activity are often just what the doctor ordered to:
- help you have more energy to do the things you want to do
- help maintain and improve your physical strength and fitness
- help improve mood and reduce feelings of depression
- help manage and prevent diseases such as heart disease, diabetes, some types of cancer, osteoporosis, and disabilities as you grow older
- help improve your balance and prevent falls

Many doctors now recommend that older adults try to make exercise and physical activity a part of everyday life. Add these to your list of things to talk about with your doctor. Ask how they would benefit you, if there are any activities you should avoid, and whether your doctor can recommend any specific kinds of exercise.[1]

---

[1] National Institute on Aging (NIA), "A Guide for Older Adults—Talking with Your Doctor," National Institutes of Health (NIH), March 2021. Available online. URL: https://order.nia.nih.gov/sites/default/files/2021-06/talking-with-your-doctor.pdf. Accessed February 16, 2024.

Chapter 18 | Seeking Out Information

"Evidence-based" information is based on a careful review of the latest scientific findings in medical journals and can help you make decisions about the best possible treatments for you.

Evidence-based information about treatments generally comes from two major types of scientific studies:
- **Clinical trials.** These trials are research studies on human volunteers to test new drugs or other treatments. Participants are randomly assigned to different treatment groups. Some get the research treatment, and others get a standard treatment or may be given a placebo (a medicine that has no effect) or no treatment. The results are compared to learn whether the new treatment is safe and effective.
- **Outcomes research.** This research looks at the effect of treatments and other health care on health outcomes (end results) for patients and populations. End results include effects that people care about, such as changes in their quality of life (QOL).

TAKE ADVANTAGE OF THE EVIDENCE-BASED INFORMATION THAT IS AVAILABLE

Health information is everywhere—in books, newspapers, and magazines and on the Internet, television, and radio. However, not all information is good information. Your best bets for sources of evidence-based information include the federal government, national nonprofit organizations, medical specialty groups, medical schools, and university medical centers. Some resources are listed subsequently, grouped by type of information.

Information
Information about your disease or condition and its treatment is available in the following sources:
- **Healthfinder®.** This site (https://health.gov/myhealthfinder)—sponsored by the U.S. Department of Health and Human Services (HHS)—offers carefully selected health information websites from government agencies, clearinghouses, nonprofit groups, and universities.
- **Health information resource database.** This database (www.health.gov/nhic/#Referrals)—sponsored by the National Health Information Center (NHIC)—includes 1,400 organizations and government offices that provide health information upon request. Information is also available over the telephone at 800-336-4797.
- **MedlinePlus®.** This site (www.nlm.nih.gov/medlineplus) has extensive information from the National Institutes of Health (NIH) and other trusted sources on over 650 diseases and conditions. The site includes many additional features.
- **National nonprofit groups.** Groups such as the American Heart Association (AHA), American Cancer Society (ACS), and American Diabetes Association (ADA) can be valuable sources of reliable information. Many have chapters nationwide. Check your phone book for a local chapter in your community. The Health Information Resource Database (www.health.gov/nhic/#Referrals) can help you find national offices of nonprofit groups.
- **Health or medical libraries.** Libraries that are run by the government, hospitals, professional groups, and other reliable organizations often welcome consumers. For a list of libraries in your area, use the MedlinePlus® "Find a Library" feature (www.nnlm.gov/membership/directory).

Seeking Out Information

Current Medical Research
You can find the latest medical research in medical journals at your local health or medical library and, in some cases, on the Internet. Here are two major online sources of medical articles:
- **Medline®/PubMed®**. This is the database of references of the National Library of Medicine (NLM) to more than 14 million articles published in 4,800 medical and scientific journals. All of the listings have information to help you find the articles at a health or medical library (https://pubmed.ncbi.nlm.nih.gov). Many listings also have short summaries of the article (abstracts), and some have links to the full article. The article might be free, or it might require a fee charged by the publisher.
- **PubMed Central® (PMC)**. This is the NLM's database of journal articles that are available free of charge to users (www.ncbi.nlm.nih.gov/pmc).

Clinical Trials
Perhaps you wonder whether there is a clinical trial that is right for you. Or you may want to learn about results from previous clinical trials that might be relevant to your situation. Here are two reliable resources:
- **ClinicalTrials.gov**. This site (https://clinicaltrials.gov) provides regularly updated information about federally and privately supported clinical research on people who volunteer to participate. The site has information about a trial's purpose, who may participate, locations, and phone numbers for more details. The site also describes the clinical trial process and includes news about recent clinical trial results.
- **Cochrane Collaboration**. This site (www.cochrane.org/search/site/reviews) writes summaries (reviews) about evidence from clinical trials to help people make informed decisions. You can search and read the review abstracts free of charge.

Outcomes Research

Outcomes research provides research about the benefits, risks, and outcomes (end results) of treatments so that patients and their doctors can make better-informed decisions. The U.S. Agency for Healthcare Research and Quality (AHRQ) supports improvements in health outcomes through research and sponsors products that result from research.

STEER CLEAR OF DECEPTIVE ADS AND INFORMATION

While searching for information either on or off the Internet, beware of "miracle" treatments and cures. They can cost you money and your health, especially if you delay or refuse proper treatment. Here are some tip-offs that a product truly is too good to be true:

- phrases such as "scientific breakthrough," "miraculous cure," "exclusive product," "secret formula," or "ancient ingredient"
- claims that the product treats a wide range of ailments
- using impressive-sounding medical terms (These often cover up a lack of good science behind the product.)
- case histories from consumers claiming "amazing" results
- claims that the product is available from only one source and for a limited time only
- claims of a "money-back guarantee"
- claims that others are trying to keep the product off the market
- ads that fail to list the company's name, address, or other contact information[1]

---

[1] Agency for Healthcare Research and Quality (AHRQ), "Next Steps after Your Diagnosis—Step 4: Seek Out Information," U.S. Department of Health and Human Services (HHS), November 2020. Available online. URL: www.ahrq.gov/questions/resources/diagnosis/step4.html. Accessed February 16, 2024.

Chapter 19 | **Getting a Second Opinion**

A second opinion is when another doctor examines your medical records and gives his or her views about your condition and how it should be treated.

You might want a second opinion to:
- be clear about what you have
- know all of your treatment choices
- have another doctor look at your choices with you

It is not pushy or rude to want a second opinion. Most doctors will understand that you need more information before making important decisions about your health.

Check to see whether your health plan covers a second opinion. In some cases, health plans require second opinions.

Here are some ways to find a doctor for a second opinion:
- Ask your doctor. Request someone who does not work in the same office because doctors who work together tend to share similar views.
- Contact your health plan or your local hospital, medical society, or medical school.
- Use the DoctorFinder online service of the American Medical Association (AMA; https://find-doctor.ama-assn.org).[1]

---

[1] Agency for Healthcare Research and Quality (AHRQ), "Next Steps after Your Diagnosis—Step 3: Talk with Your Doctor," U.S. Department of Health and Human Services (HHS), November 2020. Available online. URL: www.ahrq.gov/questions/resources/diagnosis/step3.html. Accessed February 16, 2024.

MEDICARE PART B AND SECOND OPINION

Medicare Part B (medical insurance) helps pay for a second opinion before surgery. When your doctor says you have a health problem that needs surgery, you have the right to:
- know and understand your treatment choices
- have another doctor look at those choices with you (second opinion)
- participate in treatment decisions by making your wishes known

WHEN SHOULD YOU GET A SECOND OPINION?

If your doctor says you need surgery to diagnose or treat a health problem that is not an emergency, consider getting a second opinion. It is up to you to decide when and if you will have surgery.

Medicare does not pay for surgeries or procedures that are not medically necessary, such as cosmetic surgery. This means that Medicare would also not pay for second opinions for surgeries or procedures that are not medically necessary.

Do not wait for a second opinion if you need emergency surgery. Some types of emergencies may require surgery right away, such as:
- acute appendicitis
- blood clots or aneurysms
- accidental injuries

Before you visit the second doctor:
- Ask the first doctor to send your medical records to the second doctor. That way, you may not have to repeat any tests you already had.
- Call the second doctor's office and make sure they have your records.
- Write down a list of questions to take with you to the appointment.
- Ask a family member or friend to go to the appointment with you.

Getting a Second Opinion

During your visit with the second doctor:
- Tell the doctor what surgery your first doctor recommended.
- Tell the doctor what tests you already had.
- Ask the questions on your list and encourage your family member or friend to ask any questions they have.

Note: *The second doctor may ask you to have additional tests as a result of the visit. Medicare will help pay for these tests, just as it helps pay for other services that are medically necessary.*

WHAT IF THE FIRST AND SECOND OPINIONS ARE DIFFERENT?
You may want to:
- talk more about your condition with your first doctor
- talk to a third doctor (Medicare helps pay for a third opinion if the first and second opinions are different.)

Getting a second or third opinion does not mean you have to change doctors. If you decide to have surgery, you will choose which doctor you want to do the surgery.

HOW MUCH DOES MEDICARE PAY FOR A SECOND OPINION?
Medicare Part B helps pay for a second (or third) opinion and related tests, just as it helps pay for other services that are medically necessary.

If you have Medicare Part B and original Medicare:
- Medicare pays 80 percent of the Medicare-approved amount
- you usually pay 20 percent of the Medicare-approved amount after you pay your yearly Medicare Part B deductible

DO MEDICARE ADVANTAGE PLANS COVER SECOND OPINIONS?
If you have a Medicare Advantage plan, you have the right to get a second opinion. If the first two opinions are different, your plan

will help pay for a third opinion. Even though you have the right to get a second opinion, keep the following things in mind:
- Some plans will only help pay for a second opinion if you have a referral from your primary care doctor.
- Some plans will only help pay for a second opinion from a doctor who is in your plan's provider network.[2]

---

[2] "Getting a Second Opinion before Surgery," Centers for Medicare & Medicaid Services (CMS), December 2021. Available online. URL: www.medicare.gov/Pubs/pdf/02173-Getting-a-Second-Opinion-Before-Surgery.pdf. Accessed February 16, 2024.

Chapter 20 | Selecting a Complementary and Alternative Medicine Practitioner

Millions of Americans use complementary health approaches. Like any decision concerning your health, decisions about whether to use complementary approaches are important.

WHAT DO "COMPLEMENTARY," ALTERNATIVE," AND "INTEGRATIVE" MEAN?

You may have seen the terms "complementary and alternative medicine" (CAM), "complementary medicine," "alternative medicine," and "integrative medicine" on the Internet and in marketing, but what do they really mean? While the terms are often used to mean the array of health-care approaches with a history of use or origins outside of mainstream medicine, they are actually hard to define and may mean different things to different people.

The terms complementary and integrative refer to the use of nonmainstream approaches together with conventional medical approaches.

Alternative health approaches refer to the use of nonmainstream products or practices in place of conventional medicine. The National Center for Complementary and Integrative Health (NCCIH) advises against using any product or practice that has not been proven safe and effective as a substitute for conventional medical treatment or as a reason to postpone seeing your health-care provider about any health problem. In some instances, stopping—or not starting—conventional treatment can have serious consequences. Before making a decision not to use a proven conventional treatment, talk to your health-care providers.

ARE COMPLEMENTARY HEALTH APPROACHES SAFE?

As with any medical product or treatment, there can be risks with complementary approaches. These risks depend on the specific product or practice. Each needs to be considered on its own. However, if you are considering a specific product or practice, the following general suggestions can help you think about safety and minimize risks:

- **Be aware that individuals respond differently to health products and practices, whether conventional or complementary.** How you might respond to one depends on many things, including your state of health, how you use it, or your belief in it.
- **Keep in mind that "natural" does not necessarily mean "safe."** Think of mushrooms that grow in the wild: Some are safe to eat, while others are not.
- **Learn about factors that affect safety.** For a practice that is administered by a practitioner, such as chiropractic, these factors include the training, skill, and experience of the practitioner. For a product such as a dietary supplement, the specific ingredients and the quality of the manufacturing process are important factors.
- **Choose practitioners wisely.** If you decide to use a practice provided by a complementary health practitioner, choose the practitioner as carefully as you would your primary health-care provider.
- **Supplement safety warning.** If you decide to use a dietary supplement, such as an herbal product, be aware that some products may interact in harmful ways with medications (prescription or over the counter (OTC)) or other dietary supplements, and some may have side effects on their own.

- **Tell all your health-care providers about any complementary or integrative health approaches you use.** Give them a full picture of what you do to manage your health. This will help ensure coordinated and safe care.

HOW CAN YOU GET RELIABLE INFORMATION ABOUT A COMPLEMENTARY HEALTH APPROACH?

It is important to learn what scientific studies have discovered about the complementary health approach you are considering. Evidence from research studies is stronger and more reliable than something you have seen in an advertisement or on a website or something someone told you about that worked for them.

Understanding a product's or practice's potential benefits, risks, and scientific evidence is critical to your health and safety. Scientific research on many complementary health approaches is relatively new, so this kind of information may not be available for each one. However, many studies are underway, including those that NCCIH supports, and knowledge and understanding of complementary approaches are increasing all the time. Here are some ways to find reliable information:

- **Talk with your health-care providers.** Tell them about the complementary health approach you are considering and ask any questions you may have about safety, effectiveness, or interactions with medications (prescription or nonprescription) or dietary supplements.
- **Visit the NCCIH website (www.nccih.nih.gov).** The "Health Information" page has an A–Z list of complementary health products and practices, which describes what the science says about them and links to other objective sources of online information. The website also has contact information for the NCCIH Clearinghouse, where information specialists are available to assist you in searching the scientific literature and to suggest useful NCCIH publications.

- **Visit your local library or a medical library.** Ask the reference librarian to help you find scientific journals and trustworthy books with information on the product or practice that interests you.

HOW CAN YOU DETERMINE WHETHER STATEMENTS MADE ABOUT THE EFFECTIVENESS OF A COMPLEMENTARY HEALTH APPROACH ARE TRUE?

Before you begin using a complementary health approach, it is a good idea to ask the following questions:
- Is there scientific evidence (not just personal stories) to back up the statements?
- What is the source? Statements that manufacturers or other promoters of some complementary health approaches may make about effectiveness and benefits can sound reasonable and promising. However, the statements may be based on a biased view of the available scientific evidence.
- Does the federal government have anything to report about the product or practice?
    - Visit the NCCIH website or contact the NCCIH Clearinghouse to see if the NCCIH has information about the product or practice.
    - Visit the U.S. Food and Drug Administration (FDA) online at www.fda.gov to see if there is any information available about the product or practice.
    - Information specifically about dietary supplements can be found on the FDA's website at www.fda.gov/Food/DietarySupplements and on the website of the National Institutes of Health (NIH) Office of Dietary Supplements (ODS) at https://ods.od.nih.gov.
    - Visit the FDA's web page on recalls and safety alerts at www.fda.gov/safety/recalls-market-withdrawals-safety-alerts. The FDA has a rapid public notification system to provide information about tainted dietary supplements.

- Check with the Federal Trade Commission (FTC) at www.ftc.gov to see if there are any enforcement actions for deceptive advertising regarding the therapy. Also, visit the site's Consumer Information section at www.consumer.ftc.gov.
- How does the provider or manufacturer describe the approach?
  - Beware of terms such as "scientific breakthrough," "miracle cure," "secret ingredient," or "ancient remedy."
  - If you encounter claims of a "quick fix" that depart from previous research, keep in mind that science usually advances over time by small steps, slowly building an evidence base.
  - Remember: if it sounds too good to be true—for example, claims that a product or practice can cure a disease or works for a variety of ailments—it usually is.

IS THE HEALTH WEBSITE TRUSTWORTHY?

If you are visiting a health website for the first time, the following five quick questions can help you decide whether the site is a helpful resource:
- **Who?** Who runs the website? Can you trust them?
- **What?** What does the site say? Do its claims seem too good to be true?
- **When?** When was the information posted or reviewed? Is it up-to-date?
- **Where?** Where did the information come from? Is it based on scientific research?
- **Why?** Why does the site exist? Is it selling something?

ARE COMPLEMENTARY HEALTH APPROACHES TESTED TO SEE IF THEY WORK?

While scientific evidence now exists regarding the effectiveness and safety of some complementary health approaches, there remain many yet-to-be-answered questions about whether others are safe, whether they work for the diseases or medical conditions for which they are promoted, and how those approaches with health benefits may work. As the federal government's lead agency for scientific research on health interventions, practices, products, and disciplines that originate from outside mainstream medicine, the NCCIH supports scientific research to answer these questions and determine who might benefit most from the use of specific approaches.[1]

HOW DO YOU GO ABOUT SELECTING A PRACTITIONER?

If you are looking for a complementary health practitioner to help treat a medical problem, it is important to be as careful and thorough in your search as you are when looking for conventional care.

Here are some tips to help you in your search:
- **If you need names of practitioners in your area, first check with your doctor or other health-care provider.** A nearby hospital or medical school, professional organizations, state regulatory agencies or licensing boards, or even your health insurance provider may be helpful. Unfortunately, the NCCIH cannot refer you to practitioners.
- **Find out as much as you can about any potential practitioner, including education, training, licensing, and certifications.** The credentials required for complementary health practitioners vary tremendously from state to state and from discipline to discipline.
- **Find out whether the practitioner is willing to work together with your conventional health-care providers.** For safe, coordinated care, it is important for all of the professionals involved in your health to communicate and cooperate.
- **Explain all of your health conditions to the practitioner and find out about the practitioner's**

---

[1] "Are You Considering a Complementary Health Approach?" National Center for Complementary and Integrative Health (NCCIH), September 2016. Available online. URL: www.nccih.nih.gov/health/are-you-considering-a-complementary-health-approach. Accessed February 16, 2024.

- **training and experience in working with people who have your conditions.** Choose a practitioner who understands how to work with people with your specific needs, even if general well-being is your goal. And remember that health conditions can affect the safety of complementary approaches; for example, if you have glaucoma, some yoga poses may not be safe for you.
- **Do not assume that your health insurance will cover the practitioner's services.** Contact your health insurance provider and ask. Insurance plans differ greatly in what complementary health approaches they cover, and even if they cover a particular approach, restrictions may apply.
- **Tell all your health-care providers about the complementary approaches you use and about all practitioners who are treating you.** Keeping your health-care providers fully informed helps you to stay in control and effectively manage your health.[2]

When patients tell their providers about their use of complementary health practices, they can better stay in control and more effectively manage their health. When providers ask their patients, they can ensure that they are fully informed and can help patients make wise health-care decisions.

Here are some tips to help you and your health-care providers start talking:

- **List the complementary health practices you use on your patient history form.** When completing the patient history form, be sure to include everything you use—from acupuncture to zinc. It is important to give health-care providers a full picture of what you do to manage your health.
- **At each visit, be sure to tell your providers about what complementary health approaches you are using.**

---

[2] "6 Things to Know When Selecting a Complementary Health Practitioner," National Center for Complementary and Integrative Health (NCCIH), August 26, 2013. Available online. URL: www.nccih.nih.gov/health/tips/things-to-know-when-selecting-a-complementary-health-practitioner. Accessed February 16, 2024.

Do not forget to include OTC and prescription medicines, as well as dietary and herbal supplements. Make a list in advance and take it with you. Some complementary health approaches can have an effect on conventional medicine, so your provider needs to know.
- **If you are considering a new complementary health practice, ask questions.** Ask your health-care providers about its safety, effectiveness, and possible interactions with medications (both prescription and nonprescription).
- **Do not wait for your providers to ask about any complementary health practice you are using.** Be proactive. Start the conversation.[3]

---

[3] "4 Tips: Start Talking with Your Health Care Providers about Complementary Health Approaches," National Center for Complementary and Integrative Health (NCCIH), March 14, 2012. Available online. URL: www.nccih.nih.gov/health/tips/tips-start-talking-with-your-health-care-providers-about-complementary-health-approaches. Accessed February 16, 2024.

Chapter 21 | Health-Care Quality Issues

Chapter Contents
Section 21.1—Understanding Health-Care Quality.................. 211
Section 21.2—Identifying Quality Laboratory Services............ 218
Section 21.3—Patient Safety in Ambulatory Care 224

Section 21.1 | Understanding Health-Care Quality

Getting quality health care can help you stay healthy and recover faster when you become sick. However, often people do not get high-quality care. Quality means different things to different people. Some people think that getting quality health care means seeing the doctor right away, being treated courteously by the doctor's staff, or having the doctor spend a lot of time with them.

While these things are important to all of us, clinical quality of care is even more important. Think of it like this: Getting quality health care is like taking your car to a mechanic. The people in the shop can be friendly and listen to your complaints, but the most important thing is whether they fix the problem with your car.

Health-care providers, the government, and many other groups are working hard to improve health-care quality. You also have a role to play to make sure you and your family members receive the best quality care possible.

BEING ACTIVE: TAKING CHARGE OF YOUR HEALTH CARE

The single, most important thing you can do to ensure you get high-quality health care is to find and use health information and take an active role in making decisions about your care.

Here are some steps you can take to improve your care:
- Work together with your doctor and other members of the health-care team to make decisions about your care.
- Be sure to ask questions.
- Ask your doctor what the scientific evidence has to say about your condition.
- Do your homework; go online or to the library to find out more information about your condition.
- Find and use quality information in making health-care choices; be sure the information comes from a reliable source.

TALKING WITH YOUR DOCTOR

Here are some examples of questions to ask your doctor. It is not a complete list. You will probably have many other questions. You should keep asking questions until you understand what is wrong with you and what you need to do to get better.

To understand your diagnosis, ask your doctor:
- What is wrong with me?
- What do I need to do to get better?
- Where can I get more information about my condition?

If you need a lab test, an x-ray, or another kind of test, ask your doctor:
- How will the test be done?
- How accurate will the results be?
- What are the benefits and risks of the test?
- When and how will I receive the results?
- What should I do if I do not receive the results?

If you receive a prescription for a new medicine, ask your doctor:
- What is the name of the medicine?
- What is it supposed to do?
- When should I take the medicine, and how much should I take?
- Does the medicine have any side effects?

If you need surgery, ask your doctor:
- What kind of operation do I need?
- Why do I need an operation?
- What are the benefits and risks of the operation?
- How long will it take to recover?
- What will happen if I do not have the operation?
- Are there any other treatments I could have instead of an operation?
- Where can I get a second opinion?

UNDERSTANDING HEALTH-CARE QUALITY
Research has shown that science-based measures can be used to assess quality for various conditions and for specific types of care. For example, quality health care is:
- doing the right thing (getting the health-care services you need)
- at the right time (when you need them)
- in the right way (using the appropriate test or procedure)
- to achieve the best possible results

Providing quality health care also means striking the right balance of services by:
- avoiding underuse (e.g., not screening a person for high blood pressure (HBP))
- avoiding overuse (e.g., performing tests that a patient does not need)
- eliminating misuse (e.g., providing medications that may have dangerous interactions)

It is usually believed that every doctor, nurse, pharmacist, hospital, and other provider gives high-quality care, but the fact is not always the case. Quality varies depending on where you live. Quality can vary from one state to another, and it can vary from one doctor's office across the street to another. Health-care quality varies widely and for many reasons.

IMPROVING HEALTH-CARE QUALITY
Improving health-care quality is a team effort, and it is ongoing on many levels. To succeed, every part of the health-care system must become involved, including government and private organizations, doctors, nurses, pharmacists, hospitals, other providers, and you, the patient.

One way to assess and track the quality of care is by using measures that are based on the latest scientific evidence. A health-care measure clearly defines which health-care services should be provided to patients who have or are at risk for certain conditions. Measures also set standards for screening, immunizations, and other preventive care.

Because measures are intended to set general standards for a broad population, they may or may not apply to you. Always check with your doctor about your level of risk for a particular condition and which types of screening and tests you should have.

Clinical Measures

Clinical measures can be used to assess the quality of care and patient satisfaction. Examples provided here are of measures that can be used to assess care quality for three of the most common conditions: diabetes, heart disease, and cancer.

DIABETES

More than 6 percent of all Americans have diabetes. Diabetes is the leading cause of blindness, leg amputation not resulting from trauma, and kidney disease. Diabetes increases the risk of complications in pregnant women, and it is a risk factor for heart disease and stroke. People who have diabetes are two to four times as likely to die from heart disease or stroke as those without diabetes.

The following five measures can be used to assess the quality of care for diabetes. If you have diabetes, you should receive the following tests and exams:

- regular hemoglobin A1C (blood glucose) testing
- regular cholesterol testing
- annual retinal eye exam
- annual foot exam
- flu shot each year

HEART DISEASE

Heart disease—or cardiovascular disease (CVD)—is a collection of diseases of the heart and blood vessels that includes heart attack, stroke, and heart failure.

Health-Care Quality Issues

Heart disease is the number one cause of death in the United States. Maintaining control of blood pressure and cholesterol can help you prevent heart attack and stroke.

The following are examples of measures that can be used to assess care for heart disease:
- For adults aged 18 and older:
  - blood pressure measurement
  - cholesterol testing
- In general:
  - if you smoke, being advised to stop smoking
  - if you suffer a heart attack, receiving aspirin within 24 hours of hospital admission and being prescribed beta-blocker therapy at hospital discharge

CANCER

In the United States, cancer is the second leading cause of death after heart disease. Each year, more than 1 million new cases of cancer are diagnosed. Four cancers—lung, colorectal, breast, and prostate—account for over half of the new cases reported each year.

Screening to permit early detection holds the most promise for successful cancer treatment. Talk to your doctor about screening tests for all of these cancers, especially if other members of your family have had these cancers or if you smoke.

The following are examples of quality measures for cancer screening:
- For breast and cervical cancer:
  - mammography exam for women aged 40 and older
  - Pap smear testing for women aged 18 and older
- For colorectal cancer:
  - fecal occult blood testing (FOBT; a test to detect blood in the stool) for men and women aged 50 and older
  - flexible sigmoidoscopy/colonoscopy exam for men and women aged 50 and older (Check with your doctor about how often you should have this screening.)

Finding Quality Information

A great deal of information about health-care quality, both online and in print, is available. New tools and resources for assessing and improving health-care quality are being developed.

REPORT CARDS

Report cards and other quality reports include consumer ratings, clinical performance measures, or both. They can help you select the right treatment and the right health-care provider based on what is most important to you. You may be able to get quality reports in the following ways:

- **Your employer.** Ask your personnel office for information on health plans.
- **Health plans.** Ask the plan's customer service office about quality reports.
- **Other health-care providers.** Hospitals, nursing homes, and community health clinics may have quality reports.

Several government agencies publish quality reports and other types of quality information. For example, the U.S. Department of Health and Human Services (HHS) has a quality tool that helps you compare the care provided by hospitals in your area. The website (www.medicare.gov/care-compare/?redirect=true&providerType=NursingHome) provided by the Centers for Medicare & Medicaid Services (CMS) has detailed information on the past performance of every Medicare- and Medicaid-certified nursing home in the country.

ACCREDITATION

Accreditation is another indicator that can be used to judge quality. Accreditation is a "seal of approval" given by a private, independent group. Health-care organizations—such as hospitals—must meet national standards, including clinical performance measures, in order to be accredited.

Health-Care Quality Issues

Accreditation reports present quality information on hospitals, nursing homes, and other health-care facilities. For example, the Joint Commission on Accreditation of Healthcare Organizations (JCAHO) prepares a performance report on each hospital that it surveys. Another group, the National Committee for Quality Assurance (NCQA), rates health plans such as health maintenance organizations (HMOs). The NCQA's Health Plan Report Card presents accreditation results for hundreds of health plans across the country.

If you need help in finding quality reports, accreditation reports, or other types of quality information, check with your local library or your local or state health department. You can find your state health department listed in the blue pages of your phone book.

CONSUMER RATINGS

Consumer ratings tell you what other people like you think about their health care. Some consumer ratings focus on health plans. For example, a survey called "Consumer Assessment of Healthcare Providers and Systems" (CAHPS®) asks people about the quality of care in their own health plans. Their answers can help you decide whether you want to join one of those plans. Hospital CAHPS (HCAHPS®) will ask patients about their experiences with hospital care.

CHOOSING QUALITY HEALTH CARE

Here are some tips for making quality a key factor in the health-care decisions you make about health plans, doctors, treatments, hospitals, and long-term care.

Look for a health plan that:
- has been given high ratings by its members on the things that are important to you
- has the doctors and hospitals you want or need
- provides the benefits (covered services) you need
- provides services where and when you need them
- has a documented history of doing a good job of preventing and treating illness

Look for a doctor who:
- has received high ratings for quality of care
- has the training and experience to meet your needs
- will work with you to make decisions about your health care

If you become ill, make sure you understand:
- your diagnosis
- how soon you need to be treated
- your treatment choices, including the benefits and risks of each treatment
- how much experience your doctor has in treating your condition

Look for a hospital that:
- is accredited by the JCAHO
- is rated highly by the state and by consumer groups or other organizations
- has a lot of experience and success in treating your condition
- monitors quality of care and works to improve quality

In choosing a nursing home or other long-term care facility, look for one that:
- has been found by state agencies and other groups to provide quality care
- provides a level of care, including staff and services, that will meet your needs[1]

Section 21.2 | Identifying Quality Laboratory Services

More than a billion laboratory tests that identify and measure chemicals, such as lead or cholesterol, are performed each year in the United States. The test results have a significant influence on medical decisions.

---

[1] Agency for Healthcare Research and Quality (AHRQ), "Guide to Health Care Quality: How to Know It When You See It," U.S. Department of Health and Human Services (HHS), September 2005. Available online. URL: https://archive.ahrq.gov/consumer/guidetoq/guidetoq.pdf. Accessed February 26, 2024.

Given the importance of laboratory test results, the National Center for Environmental Health (NCEH) of the Centers for Disease Control and Prevention (CDC) has programs to help assure the quality of these data, so patients and health-care providers (as well as researchers and public health officials) can be confident that laboratory test results they receive are accurate. These CDC programs focus specifically on laboratory tests that are related to chronic diseases, newborn screening disorders, nutritional status, and environmental exposures.

QUALITY ASSURANCE

Laboratory quality assurance (QA) encompasses a range of activities that enable laboratories to achieve and maintain high levels of accuracy and proficiency despite changes in test methods and the volume of specimens tested. A good QA system does the following four things:
- Establish standard operating procedures (SOPs) for each step of the laboratory testing process, ranging from specimen handling to instrument performance validation.
- Define administrative requirements, such as mandatory recordkeeping, data evaluation, and internal audits to monitor adherence to SOPs.
- Specify corrective actions, documentation, and the persons responsible for carrying out corrective actions when problems are identified.
- Sustain high-quality employee performance.

LABORATORY STANDARDIZATION

Laboratory standardization is achieved when test results have the same analytical accuracy and precision across measurement systems, laboratories, and over time. CDC's standardization programs consist of the following three main steps:
- **Reference system**. This system consists of reference methods and reference materials with target values assigned by the reference methods.

- **Traceability procedure.** In this procedure, participants use the reference materials created in the previous step to calibrate their tests or to verify the analytical accuracy and precision of their testing system.
- **Verification procedure.** In this procedure, the analytical accuracy and precision of the test calibrated in the previous step is being assessed under routine testing conditions.

Well-executed standardization programs greatly improve the quality of laboratory measurements that are used to detect signs of illnesses and to guide interventions to prevent or treat illnesses. Standardization also ensures the production of credible and comparable data across laboratories—a boon to epidemiologists and researchers who may need to pool data from multiple sources.

The CDC offers customized QA and standardization programs to help laboratories improve the quality and reliability of their measurement procedures. The following are the specific CDC services that are offered:
- reference materials
- proficiency testing
- training
- guidelines
- consultations

Each CDC laboratory QA and standardization program is voluntary, and most are free of charge.

CENTERS FOR DISEASE CONTROL AND PREVENTION'S LABORATORY QUALITY ASSURANCE PROGRAMS
Newborn Screening Quality Assurance Program

Newborn screening identifies conditions that can affect a child's long-term health or survival. The CDC's Newborn Screening and Molecular Biology Branch (NSMBB) manages the Newborn Screening Quality Assurance Program (NSQAP) to enhance and maintain the quality and accuracy of newborn screening results. The program provides training, consultation, proficiency testing, guidelines, and materials to state public health laboratories and other laboratories responsible for newborn screening in the United States and many other countries.

Lead and Multielement Proficiency Program
The CDC's Lead and Multielement Proficiency (LAMP) program is a voluntary laboratory standardization program that focuses on whole blood multianalyte QA. More than 100 laboratories, including 30 international labs, participate in the LAMP program. Each quarter, these laboratories are required to analyze a CDC-provided set of blood samples and return those results to the CDC. The CDC provides detailed reports to the labs about how well they performed these analyses. LAMP program results are not used for accreditation or certification; however, the program does improve the precision and accuracy of blood lead, cadmium, and mercury measurements. In the future, arsenic, selenium, and uranium measurements will be added to the program.

Ensuring the Quality of Urinary Iodine Procedures
Iodine deficiency disorders are thought to affect more than a billion people worldwide. Accurate laboratory tests can detect iodine deficiency. Urinary iodine (UI) analysis is the most common method used, worldwide, for assessing the iodine status of a population. Ensuring the Quality of Iodine Procedures (EQUIP) is a standardization program that addresses laboratory QA issues related to testing for iodine deficiency. The CDC's EQUIP program currently assists more than 126 iodine laboratories in more than 60 countries. The CDC provides each laboratory with quality control materials, analytical guidelines, and technical training and consultation so that these laboratories can accurately measure iodine levels in their national surveys. Three times a year, the CDC sends participating laboratories EQUIP samples for analysis.

Proficiency of Arsenic Speciation
The CDC established the Proficiency in Arsenic Speciation (PAsS) program to help laboratories worldwide assess the accuracy of their arsenic analysis and provide them with technical support.

Arsenic in drinking water has been recognized for many decades in some regions of the world. People in these areas use groundwater as their drinking water source. This water can become contaminated by naturally occurring sources of arsenic and/or human activities.

Accurate laboratory tests that can detect arsenic contamination are essential. Urinary arsenic analysis is the most common method used worldwide for assessing the arsenic contamination of a population. In 2009, the CDC established the PAsS program to help laboratories worldwide assess the accuracy of their arsenic analyses. The PAsS program is a standardization program that aids in the measurement of seven species of arsenic.

Vitamin A Laboratory-External Quality Assurance

The Vitamin A Laboratory-External Quality Assurance (VITAL-EQA) program is a standardization program designed to provide labs measuring nutritional markers in serum with an independent assessment of their analytical performance. The program assists labs in monitoring the degree of variability and bias in their assays. Information received from the program can then be used to:
- eliminate bias or precision problems in the assay system
- confirm the quality of analysis and increase the confidence level of the lab

Participation in the VITAL-EQA program is voluntary and free of charge. Results are not used for accreditation or certification.

Folate Performance Verification Program

The CDC's Nutritional Biomarkers Branch (NBB) established the folate performance verification program in 2019. The program provides an independent assessment of analytical performance for laboratories working to determine population folate status. The program complements a larger collaborative project between the CDC, the CDC Foundation, the Nutrition International Folate

Health-Care Quality Issues

Task Team, and the Bill and Melinda Gates Foundation to develop regional laboratory capacity for the measurement of blood folate levels.

The folate microbiologic assay used in the folate performance verification program was selected based on a World Health Organization (WHO) recommendation. It produces comparable data across laboratories when the laboratories use the same key reagents, such as the calibrator and microorganism. To facilitate the use of common key reagents, the CDC offers assay materials containing common key reagents for epidemiologic use in population surveys.

The performance verification program follows the Clinical Laboratory Standards Institute (CLSI) EP9-A2 guideline and provides 40 samples per matrix to allow a comprehensive method comparison to the microbiologic assay approved by the CDC Clinical Laboratory Improvement Amendments (CLIA). The program assesses the mean difference between the test and the CDC method, as well as the relationship between the two methods across the concentration range. It also provides eight quality control samples to assess multiday method imprecision. Some of the program materials are pooled serum, while others are single-donor materials.

The performance verification program is voluntary and nonregulatory and does not provide laboratory accreditation. Participation can be either on a onetime basis to assess method performance (e.g., upcoming survey) or on a continuous basis, where the 40 samples are analyzed over the course of one year (e.g., 10 samples per quarter). The program uses objective quality goals based on biologic variation to assess the acceptability of method performance.[2]

---

[2] "Laboratory Quality Assurance and Standardization Programs," Centers for Disease Control and Prevention (CDC), April 12, 2023. Available online. URL: www.cdc.gov/labstandards/index.html. Accessed February 26, 2024.

Section 21.3 | Patient Safety in Ambulatory Care

Despite the fact that the vast majority of health care takes place in the outpatient or ambulatory care setting, efforts to improve safety have mostly focused on the inpatient setting. However, a body of research dedicated to patient safety in ambulatory care has emerged over the past few years. These efforts have identified and characterized factors that influence safety in office practice, the types of errors commonly encountered in ambulatory care, and potential strategies for improving ambulatory safety.

FACTORS INFLUENCING SAFETY IN AMBULATORY CARE

Ensuring patient safety outside the hospital setting poses unique challenges for both providers and patients. A modified version of the original chronic care model (CCM) broadly encompasses the following three concepts that influence safety in ambulatory care:
- the role of patient and caregiver behaviors
- the role of provider-patient interactions
- the role of the community and health system

Specific types of errors can be linked to each of these three concepts.

TYPES OF SAFETY EVENTS IN AMBULATORY CARE

Since face-to-face interactions between providers and patients in the ambulatory setting are limited and occur weeks to months apart, patients must assume a much greater role in and responsibility for managing their own health. This elevates the importance of including the patient as a partner and ensuring that patients understand their illnesses and treatments. The need for outpatients to self-manage their own chronic diseases requires that they monitor their symptoms and, in some cases, adjust their own lifestyle or medications. For example, a patient with diabetes must measure his/her own blood sugars and perhaps adjust his/her insulin dose based on blood sugar values and dietary intake. A patient's inability or failure to perform such activities may compromise safety in the short term and clinical outcomes in the long term. Patients must also understand how and when to contact their caregivers outside routine appointments, and they must often play a role in ensuring their own care coordination (e.g., by keeping an updated list of medications).

The nature of interactions between patients and providers—and between different providers—may also be a source of adverse events. Patients consistently voice concerns about coordination of care, particularly when one patient sees multiple physicians, and indeed, communication between physicians in the outpatient setting is often suboptimal. Poorly handled care transitions (e.g., when a patient is discharged from the hospital or when care is transferred from one physician to another) also place patients at high risk for preventable adverse events. When a clinician is not immediately available—for example, after-hours—patients may have to rely on telephone advice for acute illnesses, an everyday practice that has its own inherent risks.

Underlying health system flaws have been documented to increase the risk for medical errors, particularly medication errors and diagnostic errors, issues that are certainly germane to ambulatory safety. Medication errors are very common in ambulatory care, with one landmark study finding that more than 4.5 million ambulatory care visits occur every year due to adverse drug events. Likewise, prescribing errors are startlingly common in ambulatory practice. Because the likelihood of a medication error is linked to a patient's understanding of the indication, dosage schedule, proper administration, and potential adverse effects, low health literacy and poor patient education contribute to elevated error risk.

The fragmentation of ambulatory care in outpatient settings increases the challenge of making a timely and accurate diagnosis. Indeed, a study estimated that 5 percent of adults in the United States experience a missed or delayed diagnosis each year. Data suggest that timely information availability and managing test results contribute to delayed and missed diagnoses in outpatient care. Although the use of electronic health records (EHRs) in the ambulatory setting is growing, many practices still lack reliable systems for following up on test results—a problem that has been implicated in missed and delayed diagnoses.

Finally, while an increasing amount of attention has been devoted to measuring and improving the culture of safety in acute care settings, less is known about safety culture in office practice. Burnout and work dissatisfaction, particularly among primary care physicians, may adversely affect the quality of care. The Medical Office Surveys on Patient Safety Culture (SOPS®) of the Agency for Healthcare Research and Quality (AHRQ) is designed to assess safety culture in ambulatory care, and its comparative database (which includes data from more than 900 participating practices) is freely available from the AHRQ.

IMPROVING SAFETY IN AMBULATORY CARE

Improving outpatient safety will require both structural reform of office practice functions as well as the engagement of patients in their own safety. While EHRs hold great promise for reducing medication errors and tracking test results, these systems have yet to reach their full potential. Coordinating care between different physicians remains a significant challenge, especially if the doctors do not work in the same office or share the same medical record system. Efforts are being made to increase the use of EHRs in ambulatory care, and physicians believe that the use of EHRs leads to higher quality and improved safety.

Patient engagement in outpatient safety involves the following two related concepts:
- educating patients about their illnesses and medications, using methods that require patients to demonstrate understanding (such as "teach-back")
- empowering patients and caregivers to act as a safety "double check" by providing access to advise and test results and encouraging patients to ask questions about their care

Success has been achieved in this area for patients taking high-risk medications, even in patients with low health literacy at baseline.

Health-Care Quality Issues

Although efforts to improve safety have largely focused on hospital care, the Joint Commission publishes the National Patient Safety Goals® (NPSGs) focused on ambulatory care. The AHRQ is also leading efforts to improve ambulatory quality and safety through programs and research funding. A 2016 systematic review commissioned by the World Health Organization (WHO) identified missed and delayed diagnoses and medication errors as the chief safety priorities in ambulatory care, and it highlighted the need to develop clear and consistent definitions for patient safety incidents in primary care.[3]

---

[3] Agency for Healthcare Research and Quality (AHRQ), "Ambulatory Care Safety," U.S. Department of Health and Human Services (HHS), September 7, 2019. Available online. URL: https://psnet.ahrq.gov/primer/ambulatory-care-safety. Accessed February 26, 2024.

Chapter 22 | Hospitalization

Chapter Contents
Section 22.1—Choosing a Hospital 231
Section 22.2—Medicare and Hospital Expenses 234
Section 22.3—Caregivers and Their Role during
 a Hospital Stay 238

Section 22.1 | Choosing a Hospital

When you are sick, you may go to the closest hospital or the hospital where your doctor practices. But which hospital is the best for your individual needs? Research shows that some hospitals do a better job taking care of patients with certain conditions than other hospitals. When you have a life-threatening emergency, always go to the nearest hospital. Understanding your choices will help you have a more informed discussion with your doctor or other health-care providers.

STEPS TO CHOOSING A HOSPITAL CHECKLIST
Step 1: Learn about the Care You Need and Your Hospital Choices

- Talk to your doctors or health-care providers:
  - Find out which hospitals they work with.
  - Ask which hospitals they think give the best care for your condition (e.g., have enough staffing, coordinate care, promote medication safety, and prevent infection).
  - Ask how well these hospitals check and improve their quality of care.
  - Ask if the hospitals participate in Medicare or in the network of your Medicare Advantage plan (such as a health maintenance organization (HMO) or preferred provider organization (PPO)) or other Medicare health plan if you have one.
- Based on your condition, ask the following questions to your doctors or health-care providers:
  - Should you consider a specialty hospital, teaching hospital (usually part of a university), community hospital, or one that does research or has clinical trials related to your condition?
  - If you need a surgeon or other type of specialist, what is their experience and success in treating your condition?
  - Who will be responsible for your overall care while you are in the hospital?

- Will you need care after leaving the hospital, and if so, what kind of care? Who will arrange this care?
- Are there any alternatives to hospital care?

Step 2: Think about Your Personal and Financial Needs
- Check your hospital insurance coverage:
  - Do you need permission from your Medicare health plan (such as a pre-authorization or a referral) before you are admitted for hospital care?
  - If you need care that is not emergency care, do you have to use only the network of your Medicare health plan? Do you have to use certain hospitals or see certain surgeons or specialists?
  - Do you have to pay more to use a hospital (surgeon or specialist) that does not participate in your Medicare health plan if you have one?
  - Do you need to meet certain requirements to get care after you leave the hospital?
- Think about your preferences:
  - Do you want a hospital located near family members or friends?
  - Does the hospital have convenient visiting hours and other rules that are important to you? (e.g., can a relative or someone helping with your care stay overnight in the room with you?)

Step 3: Find and Compare Hospitals Based on Your Condition and Needs
Visit Hospital Compare at www.medicare.gov/care-compare/?redirect=true&providerType=Hospital to:
- find hospitals by name, city, state, or zone improvement plan (ZIP) code
- check the results of patient surveys (what patients said about their hospital experience)
- compare the results of certain measures of quality that show how well these hospitals treat patients with certain conditions

Hospitalization

You can also call 800-MEDICARE (800-633-4227). Teletypewriter (TTY) users can call 877-486-2048.

Search online for other sources to compare the quality of the hospitals you are considering. Some states have laws that require hospitals to report data about the quality and cost of their care and post the data online.

Step 4: Discuss Your Hospital Options and Choose a Hospital
- Talk with family members or friends about the hospitals you are comparing.
- Talk to your doctor or health-care provider about how the hospital information you gathered applies to you.
- Considering all the previously mentioned factors, choose the hospital that is best for you.

HOSPITAL QUALITY QUICK CHECK
Here is a quick summary of what to look for when comparing hospitals. Look for a hospital that:
- has the best experience with your condition
- checks and improves the quality of its care
- performs well on measures of quality, including a national patient survey
- participates in Medicare
- meets your needs in terms of location and other factors, such as visiting hours
- is covered by your Medicare health plan[1]

---

[1] "Guide to Choosing a Hospital," Centers for Medicare & Medicaid Services (CMS), December 2017. Available online. URL: www.medicare.gov/Pubs/pdf/10181-Guide-Choosing-Hospital.pdf. Accessed February 28, 2024.

Section 22.2 | **Medicare and Hospital Expenses**

Did you know that even if you stay in a hospital overnight, you might still be considered an "outpatient?" Your hospital status (if the hospital considers you an "inpatient" or "outpatient") affects how much you pay for hospital services (such as x-rays, drugs, and lab tests) and may also affect whether Medicare will cover care you get in a skilled nursing facility (SNF) following your hospital stay:
- **Inpatient**. You are an inpatient starting when you are formally admitted to a hospital with a doctor's order. The day before you are discharged is your last inpatient day.
- **Outpatient**. You are an outpatient if you are getting emergency department services, observation services, outpatient surgery, lab tests, x-rays, or any other hospital services, and the doctor has not written an order to admit you to a hospital as an inpatient. In these cases, you are an outpatient even if you spend the night at the hospital.

Note: *Observation services are hospital outpatient services to help the doctor decide if you need to be admitted as an inpatient or can be discharged. You can get observation services in the emergency department or another area of the hospital.*

The decision for inpatient hospital admission is a complex medical decision based on your doctor's judgment and your need for medically necessary hospital care. An inpatient admission is generally appropriate for payment under Medicare Part A (hospital insurance) when you are expected to need two or more midnights of medically necessary hospital care. But, for you to become an inpatient, your doctor must order this admission, and the hospital must formally admit you.

WHAT DO YOU PAY AS AN INPATIENT?
Medicare Part A (hospital insurance) covers inpatient hospital services. Generally, this means you pay a onetime deductible for all of your hospital services for the first 60 days you are in a hospital.

Hospitalization

Medicare Part B (medical insurance) covers most of your doctor services when you are an inpatient. You pay 20 percent of the Medicare-approved amount for doctor services after paying the Part B deductible.

WHAT DO YOU PAY AS AN OUTPATIENT?

Part B covers outpatient hospital services. Generally, this means you pay a co-payment for each outpatient hospital service you get. This amount may vary by service.

Note: *The co-payment for a single outpatient hospital service cannot be more than the inpatient hospital deductible. However, your total co-payment for all outpatient services may be more than the inpatient hospital deductible.*

Generally, Part B does not cover prescription and over-the-counter (OTC) drugs you get in an outpatient setting (such as an emergency department), sometimes called "self-administered drugs." Also, for safety reasons, many hospitals have policies that do not allow patients to bring prescriptions or other drugs from home. If you have Medicare drug coverage (Part D), these drugs may be covered under certain circumstances. You will likely need to pay out of pocket for these drugs and submit a claim to your Medicare drug plan for a refund.

You can visit Medicare.gov website (www.medicare.gov) for detailed information, and you can also call 800-633-4227. Teletypewriter (TTY) users can call 877-486-2048.

Table 22.1 shows some common hospital situations and a description of how Medicare will pay. Remember, you pay deductibles, coinsurance, and co-payments.

HOW DOES YOUR HOSPITAL STATUS AFFECT THE WAY MEDICARE COVERS YOUR CARE IN A SKILLED NURSING FACILITY?

Medicare will only cover care you get in an SNF if you first have a qualifying inpatient hospital stay.

A qualifying inpatient hospital stay means you have been a hospital inpatient (you are formally admitted to the hospital after your doctor wrote an inpatient admission order) for at least three days in a row (counting the day you are admitted as an inpatient, but not counting the day of your discharge).

If you do not have a three-day inpatient hospital stay and you need care after your discharge from a hospital, ask if you can get care in other settings (such as home health care) or if any other programs (such as Medicaid or veterans' benefits) can cover your SNF care. Always ask your doctor or hospital staff if Medicare will cover your SNF stay.

HOW DO HOSPITAL OBSERVATION SERVICES AFFECT YOUR SKILLED NURSING FACILITY COVERAGE?

Your doctor may order "observation services" to help decide if you need to be admitted to a hospital as an inpatient or can be discharged. During the time you are getting observation services in a hospital, you are considered an outpatient. This means Medicare would not count this time toward the three-day inpatient hospital stay needed for Medicare to cover your SNF care.

If you have a Medicare Advantage plan, your costs and coverage may be different. Check with your plan. Visit the website www.medicare.gov/publications/10153-Medicare-Skilled-Nursing-Facility-Care.pdf for more information about how Medicare covers care in an SNF.

Table 22.2 shows some common hospital situations that may affect your SNF coverage.

WHAT ARE YOUR RIGHTS?

No matter what type of Medicare coverage you have, you have certain guaranteed rights, including the right to:
- get answers to your Medicare questions
- learn about all of your treatment choices and participate in treatment decisions
- get a decision about health-care payment or services or Medicare drug coverage
- appeal certain decisions about health-care payment, coverage of services, or drug coverage
- file complaints (sometimes called "grievances"), including complaints about the quality of your care

Hospitalization

Table 22.1. Medicare Payment on Common Hospital Situations

Situation	Inpatient or Outpatient	Medicare Part A Payment	Medicare Part B Payment
You are in the emergency department (also known as the "emergency room" (ER), and then you are formally admitted to the hospital with a doctor's order.	Outpatient until you are formally admitted as an inpatient based on your doctor's order. Inpatient after your admission.	Part A pays for your inpatient hospital stay and all related outpatient services provided during the three days before your admission date.	Part B pays for your doctor services.
You come to the ER with chest pain, and the hospital keeps you for two nights. One night is spent in observation, and the doctor writes an order for inpatient admission on the second day.	Outpatient until you are formally admitted as an inpatient based on your doctor's order. Inpatient after your admission.	Part A pays for your inpatient hospital stay and all related outpatient services provided during the day before your admission date.	Part B pays for your doctor services.
You go to a hospital for outpatient surgery, but they keep you overnight for high blood pressure (HBP). Your doctor does not write an order to admit you as an inpatient. You go home the next day.	Outpatient	Nothing	Part B pays for your doctor services and hospital outpatient services (such as surgery, lab tests, or intravenous medicines).
Your doctor writes an order for you to be admitted as an inpatient, and the hospital later tells you it is changing your hospital status to outpatient. Your doctor must agree, and the hospital must tell you in writing—while you are still a hospital patient before you are discharged—that your hospital status changed from inpatient to outpatient.	Outpatient	Nothing	Part B pays for your doctor services and hospital outpatient services.

Note: Even if you stay overnight in a regular hospital bed, you might be an outpatient. Ask your doctor or hospital.

Table 22.2. Skilled Nursing Facility Coverage on Common Hospital Situations

Situation	Is My Skilled Nursing Facility Stay Covered?
You come to the emergency room (ER) and are formally admitted to the hospital with a doctor's order. You spend three days in the hospital as an inpatient after admission. You are discharged on the fourth day.	Yes, if you meet all other coverage requirements. In this scenario, you meet the three-day inpatient hospital stay requirement for a covered skilled nursing facility (SNF) stay.
You come to the ER and spend one day getting observation services. Then, you are formally admitted to the hospital as an inpatient for two more days.	No, even though you spend a total of three days in the hospital, you are considered an outpatient while getting ER and observation services. These days do not count toward the three-day inpatient hospital stay requirement.

Note: Any days you spend in a hospital as an outpatient (before you are formally admitted as an inpatient based on the doctor's order) are not counted as inpatient days. An inpatient stay begins on the day you are formally admitted to a hospital as an inpatient with a doctor's order. That is your first inpatient day. The day of discharge does not count as an inpatient day.

Visit the website www.medicare.gov/media/publication/11534-medicare-rights-and-protections0.pdf for more information about your rights, the different levels of appeals, and Medicare notices.[2]

Section 22.3 | Caregivers and Their Role during a Hospital Stay

Hospital visits can be stressful for most people and their caregivers. Being prepared for an emergency and planned hospital visits can relieve some of that stress.

---

[2] "Are You a Hospital Inpatient or Outpatient?—If You Have Medicare—Ask!" Centers for Medicare & Medicaid Services (CMS), September 2021. Available online. URL: www.medicare.gov/publications/11435-Inpatient-or-Outpatient.pdf. Accessed February 28, 2024.

Hospitalization

HOSPITAL EMERGENCIES: WHAT YOU CAN DO
A trip to the emergency room (ER) can tire and frighten a person with a disease. Here are some ways to cope:
- Ask a friend or family member to go with you or meet you in the ER. He or she can stay with the person while you answer questions.
- Be ready to explain the symptoms and events leading up to the ER visit—possibly more than once to different staff members.
- Explain how best to talk with the person.
- Comfort the person. Stay calm and positive. How you are feeling will get absorbed by others.
- Be patient. It could be a long wait if the reason for your visit is not life-threatening.
- Recognize that results from the lab take time.
- Realize that just because you do not see staff at work does not mean they are not working.
- Be aware that ER staff may have limited training in a disease so try to help them better understand the person with the disease.
- Encourage hospital staff to see the person with the disease as an individual and not just another patient with a disease.
- Do not assume the person will be admitted to the hospital.
- If the person must stay overnight in the hospital, try to have a friend or family member stay with him or her.

Do not leave the ER without a plan. If you are sent home, make sure you understand all instructions for follow-up care.

WHAT TO PACK
An emergency bag with the following items, packed ahead of time, can make a visit to the ER go more smoothly:
- health insurance cards
- lists of current medical conditions, medicines being taken, and allergies

- health-care providers' names and phone numbers
- copies of health-care advance directives
- "personal information sheet" stating the person's preferred name and language; contact information of key family members and friends; the need for glasses, dentures, or hearing aids; behaviors of concern; how the person communicates needs and expresses emotions; and living situation
- snacks and bottles of water
- incontinence briefs if usually worn, moist wipes, and plastic bags
- comforting objects or music player with earphones
- a change of clothing, toiletries, and personal medications for yourself
- pain medicine, such as ibuprofen, acetaminophen, or aspirin (A trip to the ER may take longer than you think, and stress can lead to a headache or other symptoms.)
- a pad of paper and pen to write down information and directions given to you by hospital staff
- a small amount of cash
- a note on the outside of the emergency bag to remind you to take your cell phone and charger with you

By taking these steps in advance, you can reduce the stress and confusion that often accompany a hospital visit, particularly if the visit is an unplanned trip to the ER.

BEFORE A PLANNED HOSPITAL STAY

It is wise to accept that hospitalization is a "when" and not an "if" event. Due to the nature of any disease, it is very probable that, at some point, the person you are caring for may be hospitalized. Preparation can make all the difference. Here are some tips:
- **Think about and discuss hospitalization before it happens and as the disease progresses.** Hospitalization is a choice. Talk about when hospice may be a better and more appropriate alternative.

Hospitalization

- **Build a care team of family, friends, and/or professional caregivers to support the person during the hospital stay.** Do not try to do it all alone.
- **Ask the doctor if the procedure can be done during an outpatient visit.** If not, ask if tests can be done before admission to the hospital to shorten the hospital stay.
- **Ask questions about anesthesia, catheters, and intravenous (IV).** General anesthesia can have side effects so see if local anesthesia is an option.
- **Ask if regular medications can be continued during the hospital stay.**
- **Ask for a private room with a reclining chair or bed if insurance will cover it.** It will be calmer than a shared room.
- **Involve the person with the disease in the planning process as much as possible.**
- **Do not talk about the hospital stay in front of the person as if he or she is not there.** This can be upsetting and embarrassing.
- **Shortly before leaving home, tell the person with the disease that the two of you are going to spend a short time in the hospital.**

DURING THE HOSPITAL STAY
While the person with the disease is in the hospital, do the following:
- **Ask doctors to limit questions to the person, who may not be able to answer accurately.** Instead, talk with the doctor in private, outside the person's room.
- **Help hospital staff understand the person's normal functioning and behavior.** Ask them to avoid using physical restraints or medications to control behaviors.
- **Have a family member, trusted friend, or hired caregiver stay with the person at all times if possible—even during medical tests.** This may be hard to do, but it will help keep the person calm and less frightened, making the hospital stay easier.

- **Tell the doctor immediately if the person seems suddenly worse or different.** Medical problems, such as fever, infection, medication side effects, and dehydration, can cause delirium, a state of extreme confusion and disorientation.
- **Ask friends and family to make calls or use email or online tools to keep others informed about the person's progress.**
- **Help the person fill out menu requests.** Open food containers and remove trays. Assist with eating as needed.
- **Remind the person to drink fluids.** Offer fluids regularly and have him or her make frequent trips to the bathroom.
- **Assume the person will experience difficulty finding the bathroom and/or using a call button, bed adjustment buttons, or the phone.**
- **Communicate with the person in the way he or she will best understand and respond.**
- **Recognize that an unfamiliar place, medicines, invasive tests, and surgery will make a person with the disease more confused.** He or she will likely need more assistance with personal care.
- **Take deep breaths and schedule breaks for yourself.**

If anxiety or agitation occurs, try the following:
- Remove personal clothes from sight; they may remind the person of getting dressed and going home.
- Post reminders or cues, such as a sign labeling the bathroom door, if this comforts the person.
- Turn off the television, telephone ringer, and intercom. Minimize background noise to prevent overstimulation.
- Talk in a calm voice and offer reassurance. Repeat answers to questions when needed.
- Provide a comforting touch or distract the person with offers of snacks and beverages.

Hospitalization

- Consider "unexpressed pain" (i.e., furrowed brow, clenched teeth or fists, and kicking). Assume the person has pain if the condition or procedure is normally associated with pain. Ask for pain evaluation and treatment every four hours—especially if the person has labored breathing, loud moaning, crying, or grimacing or if you are unable to console or distract him or her.
- Listen to soothing music or try comforting rituals, such as reading, praying, singing, or reminiscing.
- Slow down; try not to rush the person.
- Avoid talking about subjects or events that may upset the person.

WORKING WITH HOSPITAL STAFF

Remember that not everyone in the hospital knows the same basic facts about a disease. You may need to help teach hospital staff what approach works best with the person, what distresses or upsets him or her, and ways to reduce this distress.

You can help the staff by providing them with a personal information sheet that includes the person's normal routine, how he or she prefers to be addressed, personal habits, likes and dislikes, possible behaviors (what might trigger them and how best to respond), and nonverbal signs of pain or discomfort.

Help staff understand what the person's "baseline" is (prior level of functioning). You should:
- place a copy of the personal information sheet with the chart in the hospital room and at the nurse's station
- with the hospital staff, decide who will do what for the person (e.g., you may want to be the one who helps with bathing, eating, or using the bathroom)
- inform the staff about any hearing difficulties and/or other communication problems and offer ideas for what works best in those instances
- make sure the person is safe (Tell the staff about any previous issues with wandering, getting lost, falls, and suspicious and/or delusional behavior.)

- not assume the staff knows the person's needs (Inform them in a polite and calm manner.)
- ask questions when you do not understand certain hospital procedures and tests or when you have any concerns (Do not be afraid to be an advocate.)
- plan early for discharge (Ask the hospital discharge planner about eligibility for home health services, equipment, or other long-term care options. Prepare for an increased level of caregiving.)
- realize that hospital staff are providing care for many people (Practice the art of patience.)[3]

---

[3] National Institute on Aging (NIA), "Going to the Hospital: Tips for Dementia Caregivers," National Institutes of Health (NIH), May 18, 2017. Available online. URL: www.nia.nih.gov/health/alzheimers-caregiving/going-hospital-tips-dementia-caregivers. Accessed February 28, 2024.

Chapter 23 | Surgery

Chapter Contents
Section 23.1—What You Need to Know about Surgery............247
Section 23.2—Anesthesia Basics..249
Section 23.3—Robotic Interventions...252
Section 23.4—Wrong-Site, Wrong-Procedure, and
                Wrong-Patient Surgery..257

Section 23.1 | What You Need to Know about Surgery

There are many reasons to have surgery. Some operations can relieve or prevent pain. Others can reduce a symptom of a problem or improve some body function. Some surgeries are done to find a problem. For example, a surgeon may do a biopsy, which involves removing a piece of tissue to examine under a microscope. Some surgeries, such as heart surgery, can save your life.

Some operations that once needed large incisions (cuts in the body) can now be done using much smaller cuts. This is called "laparoscopic surgery." Surgeons insert a thin tube with a camera to see and use small tools to do the surgery.

After surgery, there can be a risk of complications, including infection, too much bleeding, reaction to anesthesia, or accidental injury. There is almost always some pain with surgery.[1]

WHAT YOU SHOULD KNOW BEFORE YOUR SURGERY

Protect yourself and your loved ones from infections related to surgery. Having any type of surgery can be stressful. You might be asking yourself: What is the recovery process? How long will I be out of work? What do I do after leaving the hospital or surgery center?

An important question you might not have thought of is: How do I avoid getting a surgical site infection (SSI)?

An SSI is an infection patients can get during or after surgery. SSIs can happen on any part of the body where surgery takes place and can sometimes involve only the skin. Other SSIs are more serious and can involve tissues under the skin, organs, or implanted material.

These infections can make recovery from surgery more difficult because they can cause additional complications, stress, and medical cost. It is important that health-care providers, patients, and loved ones work together to prevent these infections.

---

[1] MedlinePlus, "Surgery," National Institutes of Health (NIH), October 31, 2016. Available online. URL: https://medlineplus.gov/surgery.html. Accessed February 28, 2024.

What Can Health-Care Providers Do to Ensure That the Surgical Site Is Clean?

To ensure the surgical site is clean, health-care providers can do the following:
- Clean their hands and arms up to the elbows with an antiseptic agent just before the surgery.
- Wear hair covers, masks, gowns, and gloves during surgery to keep the surgery area clean.
- Give you antibiotics before surgery starts when indicated.
- Clean the skin at the surgery site with a special soap that kills germs.

How Can You and Your Loved Ones Prevent Surgical Site Infections?

- **Before your surgery, discuss other health problems, such as diabetes, with your doctor**. These issues can affect your surgery and your treatment.
- **Quit smoking**. Patients who smoke get more infections.
- **Follow your doctor's instructions for cleaning your skin before your surgery**. For example, if your doctor recommends using a special soap before surgery, make sure you do so.
- **Avoid shaving near where you will have surgery**. Shaving with a razor can irritate your skin and make it easier to develop an infection. If someone tries to shave you before surgery, ask why this is necessary.

Protection against Surgical Site Infection

After surgery, be sure to follow the recommendations listed here to protect against SSI:
- Ask your provider to clean their hands before they examine you or check your wound.
- Do not allow visitors to touch the surgical wound or dressings.

Surgery

- Ask family and friends to clean their hands before and after visiting you.
- Make sure you understand how to care for your wound before you leave the medical facility.
- Always clean your hands before and after caring for your wound.
- Make sure you know who to contact if you have questions or problems after you get home.
- If you have any symptoms of an infection, such as redness and pain at the surgery site, drainage, or fever, call your doctor immediately.[2]

Section 23.2 | Anesthesia Basics

WHAT IS ANESTHESIA?

Anesthesia is a medical intervention that prevents patients from feeling pain during procedures such as surgery, certain screening and diagnostic tests, tissue sample removal (e.g., skin biopsies), and dental work. Anesthesiologists are doctors who have been specifically trained to give medicines used for anesthesia, which are called "anesthetics." Depending on the type of pain relief needed, anesthesiologists can deliver anesthetics through several methods:

- gas that the patient inhales through a mask covering the mouth and nose
- intravenous (IV) line with a needle inserted into a vein, giving direct access to the bloodstream
- catheter (thin tube) inserted into the space outside of the spinal cord or around peripheral nerves
- injection into a body part with a needle and syringe

---

[2] "What You Should Know before Your Surgery," Centers for Disease Control and Prevention (CDC), February 25, 2020. Available online. URL: www.cdc.gov/patientsafety/features/before-surgery.html. Accessed February 28, 2024.

- topical lotion or spray
- eye drops
- skin patch

Before the introduction of safe and effective anesthetics about 175 years ago, surgeries of any kind were rare, dangerous, and only used as a last resort. Patients who underwent surgeries at this time were fully conscious. Now, advances in anesthesia have allowed for lifesaving surgeries that would be impossible otherwise. Surgeries to treat cancer, organ transplants, and open heart surgery are only a few types of important techniques anesthesia has made possible. Modern anesthetics are typically very safe, but there are risks involved, including breathing problems, allergic reactions, and general confusion after surgery.

TYPES OF ANESTHESIA

There are four main types of anesthesia. Each has different effects on the body:

- **General anesthesia**. It affects the whole body, making patients unconscious and unable to move. Anesthesiologists will give general anesthesia for complex surgeries involving internal organs or other invasive or time-consuming procedures, such as back surgery. These anesthetics are given either through an IV line or as an inhaled gas.
- **Monitored sedation**. It is like general anesthesia in that it relaxes the body and may induce sleep. However, in monitored sedation, patients are still conscious and may even be able to talk, depending on the level of sedation needed. This form of anesthesia is often combined with pain relief for procedures such as a colonoscopy or complex dental work. These anesthetics are given through an IV line.
- **Regional anesthesia**. It numbs pain and sensation to only the part of the body that needs it, such as an arm, a leg, or everything below the waist. This type of anesthesia is used in hand and joint surgeries and

Surgery

C-section deliveries, as well as to ease the pain of childbirth. With regional anesthetics, patients stay conscious and comfortable. These medications are given through an injection or a catheter.
- **Local anesthesia**. It affects only a small part of the body. For example, this type of anesthetic is used to block pain in a single tooth during a dental procedure or in a part of the skin that needs stitches. As with regional anesthesia, patients who receive local anesthesia remain awake and comfortable. Local anesthetics are commonly given as an injection, topical lotion or spray, eye drops, or skin patch.

WHAT SCIENTISTS KNOW ABOUT HOW ANESTHESIA WORKS

Anesthesia prevents the feeling of pain by stopping nerves from passing signals to the brain. Scientists do not know exactly how all types of anesthetics work, but they do know that some anesthetics block pain by altering the following:
- **Neurotransmitter release**. Neurotransmitters are the chemical messengers that pass signals between nerve cells. They can cause signal transmission (excitatory) or block signal transmission (inhibitory). Certain general anesthetics cause the release of inhibitory neurotransmitters—while others block the release of excitatory neurotransmitters—to reduce the activation of nerve cells.
- **Activity of ion channel proteins**. Normally, ion channel proteins pass ions through nerve cell membranes to transmit signals. General and local anesthetics that work in this manner prevent ion passage to block signal transmission.[3]

---

[3] "Anesthesia," National Institute of General Medical Sciences (NIGMS), September 2023. Available online. URL: www.nigms.nih.gov/education/fact-sheets/Pages/anesthesia.aspx. Accessed February 28, 2024.

Section 23.3 | **Robotic Interventions**

WHAT ARE IMAGE-GUIDED ROBOTIC INTERVENTIONS?

Image-guided robotic interventions are medical procedures that integrate sophisticated robotic and imaging technologies, primarily to perform minimally invasive surgery. This integrated technology approach offers distinct advantages for both patients and physicians:

- **Imaging**. In image-guided procedures, the surgeon is guided by images from various techniques, including magnetic resonance (MR) and ultrasound. Images can also be obtained using tiny cameras attached to probes that are small enough to fit into a minimal incision. The camera allows the surgery to be performed using a much smaller incision than in traditional surgery.
- **Robotics**. The surgeon's hands and traditional surgical tools are too large for small incisions. Instead, thin, finger-like robotic tools are used to perform the surgery. As the surgeon watches the image on the screen, he or she uses a telemanipulator to transmit and direct hand and finger movements to a robot, which can be controlled by hydraulic, electronic, or mechanical means.

Robotic tools can also be controlled by computer. One advantage of a computerized system is that a surgeon could potentially perform the surgery from anywhere in the world.

WHAT ARE THE ADVANTAGES OF MINIMALLY INVASIVE PROCEDURES?

Minimally invasive surgery can reduce the damage to surrounding healthy tissues, thus decreasing the need for pain medication and reducing patients' recovery time. For surgeons, image-guided interventions using robots also have the advantage of reducing fatigue during long operations, allowing the surgeon to perform the procedure while seated.

WHAT ARE SOME EXAMPLES OF IMAGE-GUIDED ROBOTIC INTERVENTIONS, AND HOW ARE THEY USED?

- **Robotic prostatectomy.** Complete prostate removal is performed through a series of small incisions, compared with a single large incision of four to five inches in traditional surgery. The small incisions result in a shorter postoperative recovery, less scarring, and a faster return to normal activities.
- **Ablation techniques for early cancers.** Patients with early kidney cancer can be treated with minimally invasive procedures to destroy small tumors. Cryoablation uses cold energy to destroy the tumors. Doctors use computed tomography (CT) and ultrasound imaging to position a needle-like probe within each kidney tumor. Once in position, the tip of the probe is supercooled to encase the tumor in a ball of ice. Alternate freeze/thaw cycles kill the tumor cells. Other minimally invasive methods of destroying early kidney cancers include heating the tumor cells and surgical removal using a robotic device. Many patients can go home the same day and are able to perform regular activities in several days.
- **Orthopedics.** Image-guided robotic procedures are improving the precision and outcome of a number of orthopedic procedures. For example, partial knee resurfacing surgeries aim to target only the damaged sections of the knee joint. Orthopedic surgeons are combining the use of a robotic surgical arm and fiber-optic cameras in such procedures, which results in patients retaining more of their normal healthy tissue. Image-guided robotic procedures also improve total knee replacements, allowing precise alignment and positioning of knee implants. The result is more natural knee function, better range of motion, and improved balance for patients.

WHAT ARE NIBIB-FUNDED RESEARCHERS DEVELOPING IN THE AREA OF IMAGE-GUIDED ROBOTIC INTERVENTIONS TO IMPROVE MEDICAL CARE?

Portable Robot Uses Three-Dimensional Near-Infrared Imaging to Guide Needle Insertion into Veins

Drawing blood and inserting intravenous (IV) lines are the most commonly performed medical procedures in hospitals and clinics. However, for many patients, it can be difficult to find veins and accurately insert the needle, resulting in patient injury. Scientists funded by the National Institute of Biomedical Imaging and Bioengineering (NIBIB) are developing a portable, lightweight medical robot to help perform these procedures. The device uses three-dimensional (3D) near-infrared imaging to identify an appropriate vein for the robot to insert the needle. The goal is to integrate the imaging system and software into a miniaturized version of the prototype robot. The outcome will be a compact, low-cost system that will greatly improve the safety and accuracy of accessing veins.

Robot-Assisted Needle Guidance Aids Removal of Liver Tumors

Radiofrequency ablation (RFA) is a minimally invasive treatment that kills tumors with heat and can be a lifesaving option for patients who are not eligible for surgery. However, the broad use of RFA has been limited because the straight paths taken by the needles that carry tumor-killing electrodes may damage lungs or other sensitive organs. Also, large tumors require multiple needle insertions, which increase bleeding risk. To address the problem of tissue damage using straight needles, NIBIB-funded scientists are developing highly flexible needles that can be guided along controlled, curved paths through tissue, allowing the removal of tumors that are not accessible by a straight-line path. The technology combines needle flexibility with a 3D ultrasound guidance system that allows the doctor to correct the path of the needle to avoid unexpected obstacles as the needle advances toward the tumor. The device will ultimately increase the accuracy and reduce the damage to healthy tissue during tumor removal resulting in wider use of the technology for better patient outcomes.

Swallowable Capsule Identifies and Biopsies Abnormal Tissue in the Esophagus

Barrett esophagus is a precancerous condition that requires repeated biopsies to monitor abnormal tissue. NIBIB-funded researchers are developing a swallowable, pill-sized device to improve the management and treatment of this condition. The unsedated patient can easily swallow the pill, which is attached to a thin tether made of cable and optic fiber. The device detects microscopic areas of the esophagus that may show evidence of disease and uses a laser to collect samples from the suspicious tissue—a technology known as "laser capture microdissection." The physician then retrieves the device from the patient without discomfort and the collected microsamples are examined for visual evidence of disease, as well as genetic analysis. This minimally invasive device improves patient comfort and provides a precise molecular profile of the biopsied regions, which helps the physician better monitor and treat the disorder.[4]

RECOMMENDATIONS FOR PATIENTS AND HEALTH-CARE PROVIDERS ABOUT ROBOTICALLY ASSISTED SURGERY

Patients

Robotically assisted surgery (RAS) is an important treatment option but may not be appropriate in all situations. Talk to your physician about the risks and benefits of RASs, as well as the risks and benefits of other treatment options.

Patients who are considering treatment with RASs should discuss the options for these devices with their health-care provider and feel free to inquire about their surgeon's training and experience with these devices.

Health-Care Providers

RAS is safe and effective for performing certain procedures when used appropriately and with proper training. The U.S. Food and

---

[4] "Image-Guided Robotic Interventions," National Institute of Biomedical Imaging and Bioengineering (NIBIB), December 2019. Available online. URL: www.nibib.nih.gov/sites/default/files/2020-06/Image-Guided%20Robotic%20Interventions%20Fact%20Sheet_0.pdf. Accessed February 28, 2024.

Drug Administration (FDA) regulates devices to provide reasonable assurance of their safety and effectiveness for their intended uses. For RAS devices, this includes assuring manufacturers implement adequate training programs for both new and experienced users. The FDA does not supervise or provide accreditation for physician training nor does it oversee training and education related to legally marketed medical devices. Instead, the development and implementation of training is the responsibility of the manufacturer, physicians, and health-care facilities. In some cases, professional societies and specialty board certification organizations may also develop and support training for their specialty physicians. Specialty boards also maintain the certification status of their specialty physicians.

Physicians, hospitals, and facilities that use RAS devices should ensure surgeons are trained properly and have appropriate credentials to perform surgical procedures with these devices. Device users should ensure they maintain their credentialing. Hospitals and facilities should also ensure that other surgical staff who use these devices complete proper training.

Users of the device should realize there are several different models of RAS devices. Each model may operate differently and may not have the same functions. Users should know the differences between the models and make sure to get appropriate training on each model.

If you suspect a problem or complications associated with the use of RAS devices, the FDA encourages you to file a voluntary report through MedWatch: The FDA Safety Information and Adverse Event Reporting program (www.accessdata.fda.gov/scripts/medwatch). Health-care personnel employed by facilities that are subject to the FDA's user facility reporting requirements should follow the reporting procedures established by their facilities. Prompt reporting of adverse events can help the FDA identify and better understand the risks associated with medical devices.[5]

---

[5] "Computer-Assisted Surgical Systems," U.S. Food and Drug Administration (FDA), June 21, 2022. Available online. URL: www.fda.gov/medical-devices/surgery-devices/computer-assisted-surgical-systems. Accessed February 28, 2024.

Surgery

Section 23.4 | Wrong-Site, Wrong-Procedure, and Wrong-Patient Surgery

Few medical errors are as vivid and terrifying as those that involve patients who have undergone surgery on the wrong body part, undergone the incorrect procedure, or had a procedure intended for another patient. These "wrong-site, wrong-procedure, wrong-patient errors" (WSPEs) are rightly termed "never events"—errors that should never occur and indicate serious underlying safety problems.

Wrong-site surgery may involve operating on the wrong side, as in the case of a patient who had the right side of her vulva removed when the cancerous lesion was on the left, or on the incorrect body site. One example of surgery on the incorrect site is operating on the wrong level of the spine, a surprisingly common issue for neurosurgeons. A classic case of wrong-patient surgery involved a patient who underwent a cardiac procedure intended for another patient with a similar last name.

While much publicity has been given to these high-profile cases of WSPEs, these errors are in fact relatively rare. One study using the U.S. Department of Veterans Affairs (VA) data found that fully half of WSPEs occurred during procedures outside the operating room.

PREVENTING WRONG-SITE, WRONG-PROCEDURE, AND WRONG-PATIENT SURGERY

Early efforts to prevent WSPEs focused on developing redundant mechanisms for identifying the correct site, procedure, and patient, such as "sign your site" initiatives, that instructed surgeons to mark the operative site in an unambiguous fashion. However, it soon became clear that even this seemingly simple intervention was problematic. An analysis of the efforts of the United Kingdom (UK) to prevent WSPEs found that, although dissemination of a site-marking protocol did increase the use of preoperative site marking, implementation and adherence to the protocol differed significantly across surgical specialties and hospitals, and many clinicians voiced concerns about unintended consequences of the protocol. In some cases, there was even confusion over whether the marked site indicates the area to be operated on or the area to be avoided. Site marking remains a core component of the Joint Commission's Universal Protocol to prevent WSPEs.

Root cause analyses of WSPEs consistently reveal communication issues as a prominent underlying factor. The concept of the surgical time-out—a planned pause before beginning the procedure in order to review important aspects of the procedure with all involved personnel—was developed to improve communication in the operating room and prevent WSPEs. The Universal Protocol also specifies the use of a time-out prior to all procedures. Although initially designed for operating room procedures, time-outs are now required before any invasive procedure. Comprehensive efforts to improve surgical safety have incorporated time-out principles into surgical safety checklists; while these checklists have been proven to improve surgical and postoperative safety, the low baseline incidence of WSPEs makes it difficult to establish that a single intervention can reduce or eliminate WSPEs.

It is worth noting, however, that many cases of WSPEs would still occur despite full adherence to the Universal Protocol. Errors may happen well before the patient reaches the operating room; a time-out may be rushed or otherwise ineffective; and production pressures may contribute to errors during the procedure itself. Ultimately, preventing WSPEs depends on the combination of system solutions, strong teamwork and safety culture, and individual vigilance.

CURRENT CONTEXT

Wrong-patient, wrong-site, and wrong-procedure errors are all considered never events by the National Quality Forum (NQF) and are considered sentinel events by the Joint Commission. In February 2009, the Centers for Medicare & Medicaid Services (CMS) announced that hospitals will not be reimbursed for any costs associated with WSPEs. (CMS has not reimbursed hospitals for additional costs associated with many preventable errors since 2007.)[6]

---

[6] Agency for Healthcare Research and Quality (AHRQ), "Wrong-Site, Wrong-Procedure, and Wrong-Patient Surgery," U.S. Department of Health and Human Services (HHS), September 7, 2019. Available online. URL: https://psnet.ahrq.gov/primer/wrong-site-wrong-procedure-and-wrong-patient-surgery. Accessed February 28, 2024.

Part 4 | Health Literacy and Making Informed Health Decisions

Chapter 24 | Understanding Health Literacy

WHAT IS HEALTH LITERACY?
The definition of health literacy was updated in August 2020 with the release of the U.S. government's Healthy People 2030 initiative. The update addresses personal health literacy and organizational health literacy and provides the following definitions:
- **Personal health literacy.** It is the degree to which individuals have the ability to find, understand, and use information and services to inform health-related decisions and actions for themselves and others.
- **Organizational health literacy.** It is the degree to which organizations equitably enable individuals to find, understand, and use information and services to inform health-related decisions and actions for themselves and others.

These definitions are a change from the health literacy definition used in Healthy People 2010 and Healthy People 2020: "the degree to which individuals have the capacity to obtain, process, and understand basic health information and services needed to make appropriate health decisions."

The following are the new definitions:
- Emphasize people's ability to use health information rather than just understand it.
- Focus on the ability to make "well-informed" decisions rather than "appropriate" ones.

- Acknowledge that organizations have a responsibility to address health literacy.
- Incorporate a public health perspective.

From a public health perspective, the organizational definition acknowledges that health literacy is connected to health equity. Health equity is the attainment of the highest level of health for all people. We will achieve health equity when everyone has the opportunity to be as healthy as possible.

Is Health Literacy Important for Everyone?

Yes, health literacy is important for everyone because, at some point in our lives, we all need to be able to find, understand, and use health information and services.

Taking care of our health is part of everyday life, not just when we visit a doctor, clinic, or hospital. Health literacy can help us prevent health problems, protect our health, and better manage health problems when they arise.

Even people who read well and are comfortable using numbers can face health literacy issues when:
- they are not familiar with medical terms or how their bodies work
- they have to interpret statistics and evaluate risks and benefits that affect their health and safety
- they are diagnosed with a serious illness and are scared and confused
- they have health conditions that require complicated self-care
- they are voting on an issue affecting the community's health and relying on unfamiliar technical information

Why Do We Have a Health Literacy Problem?

When organizations or people create and give others health information that is too difficult for them to understand, we create a health literacy problem. When we expect them to figure out health services with many unfamiliar, confusing, or even conflicting steps, we also create a health literacy problem.

How Can We Help People Now?
We can help people use the health literacy skills they have, by doing the following:
- Create and provide information and services people can understand and use most effectively with the skills they have.
- Work with educators and others to help people become more familiar with health information and services and build their health literacy skills over time.
- Build our own skills as communicators of health information.
- Work with trusted messengers to share your information.
- Build health-literate organizations.
- Consider the cultural and linguistic norms, environment, and history of your intended audience when developing your information and messages.
- Use certified translators and interpreters who can adapt to your intended audience's language preferences, communication expectations, and health literacy skills.

WHAT ARE ADULT LITERACY AND NUMERACY?
The U.S. Department of Education (ED) defines adult literacy and numeracy in terms of skills that help people accomplish tasks and realize their purposes. Researchers can measure literacy and numeracy skills, but skills are not static. People can build their skills, and even adults with limited skills can get better results when their environments accommodate the skills they have.
- **Literacy**. It is understanding, evaluating, using, and engaging with written text to participate in society, achieve one's goals, and develop one's knowledge and potential.
- **Numeracy**. It is the ability to access, use, interpret, and communicate mathematical information and ideas, to engage in and manage the mathematical demands of a range of situations in adult life.

WHAT ARE THE POPULATION MEASURES OF LITERACY, NUMERACY, HEALTH LITERACY, AND TECHNOLOGY SKILLS?

Adult Health Literacy Skills

Literacy and health literacy are not the same, but they are related. The ED collects and reports data on adult literacy and numeracy skills. In 2006, they published the only national data on health literacy skills. The study found that adults who self-report the worst health also have the most limited literacy, numeracy, and health literacy skills.

Adult Literacy and Numeracy Skills

The most current adult literacy data comes from the Program for the International Assessment of Adult Competencies (PIACC). The PIACC is a comparative study among participating countries. It assesses adults' proficiency in three domains: literacy, numeracy, and problem-solving in technology-rich environments.

In each of these domains, adults perform tasks with different levels of complexity. Their skills with these tasks are quantified and categorized into proficiency levels. The National Center for Education Statistics (NCES) posts the most current results (https://nces.ed.gov/surveys/piaac/national_results.asp).

Youth Literacy Skills

The ED also collects and reports data on school-aged children and youth. Elementary school children with weak literacy and numeracy skills often struggle academically through the middle and high school years. Research shows that academic success, risky behaviors, and health status are linked.[1]

---

[1] "Health Literacy Basics," Centers for Disease Control and Prevention (CDC), March 30, 2021. Available online. URL: www.cdc.gov/healthliteracy/basics.html. Accessed February 13, 2024.

Chapter 25 | eHealth Literacy

These days it seems as if everyone has a smartphone. Health services are increasingly being delivered through web-based and mobile resources. Examples of electronic health (eHealth) services include:
- electronic communication between patients and health-care providers
- electronic medical records (EMRs)
- patient portals
- personal health records

Mobile health (mHealth), a subcategory of eHealth, includes using tablets and phones to access apps and wearable tracking devices.[1]

NEED FOR EHEALTH LITERACY
Searching online for health information is an easy and affordable way for Americans to learn more about their health, self-diagnose an illness, and manage a health condition. Approximately 6 in 10 American adults search online for health information, and the trend is expected to increase as ownership of mobile devices grows and access to high-speed Internet expands.[2]

---

[1] "Tackling eHealth Literacy," Centers for Disease Control and Prevention (CDC), March 5, 2018. Available online. URL: https://blogs.cdc.gov/publichealthmatters/2018/03/tackling-ehealth-literacy. Accessed February 16, 2024.
[2] "eHealth Literacy, Online Help-Seeking Behavior, and Willingness to Participate in mHealth Chronic Disease Research among African Americans, Florida, 2014–2015," Centers for Disease Control and Prevention (CDC), November 17, 2016. Available online. URL: www.cdc.gov/pcd/issues/2016/16_0210.htm. Accessed February 16, 2024.

WHAT IS AN ELECTRONIC HEALTH RECORD?

An electronic health record (EHR) is a digital version of a patient's paper chart. EHRs are real-time, patient-centered records that make information available instantly and securely to authorized users. While an EHR does contain the medical and treatment histories of patients, an EHR system is built to go beyond standard clinical data collected in a provider's office and can be inclusive of a broader view of a patient's care. EHRs are a vital part of health information technology (IT) and can:

- contain a patient's medical history, diagnoses, medications, treatment plans, immunization dates, allergies, radiology images, and laboratory and test results
- allow access to evidence-based tools that providers can use to make decisions about a patient's care
- automate and streamline provider workflow

One of the key features of an EHR is that health information can be created and managed by authorized providers in a digital format capable of being shared with other providers across more than one health-care organization. EHRs are built to share information with other health-care providers and organizations—such as laboratories, specialists, medical imaging facilities, pharmacies, emergency facilities, and school and workplace clinics—so they contain information from all clinicians involved in a patient's care.[3]

ELECTRONIC HEALTH RECORDS FOSTER PATIENT PARTICIPATION

Providers and patients who share access to electronic health information can collaborate in informed decision-making. Patient participation is especially important in managing and treating chronic conditions such as asthma, diabetes, and obesity.

EHRs can help health-care providers by:
- **Ensuring high-quality care**. With EHRs, health-care providers can give patients full and accurate

---

[3] HealthIT.gov, "What Is an Electronic Health Record (EHR)?" Office of the National Coordinator for Health Information Technology (ONC), September 10, 2019. Available online. URL: www.healthit.gov/faq/what-electronic-health-record-ehr. Accessed February 16, 2024.

eHealth Literacy

information about all of their medical evaluations. They can also offer follow-up information, such as self-care instructions, reminders for other follow-up care, and links to web resources, after an office visit or a hospital stay.
- **Creating an avenue for communication with their patients.** With EHRs, health-care providers can manage appointment schedules electronically and exchange emails with their patients. Quick and easy communication between patients and health-care providers may help the latter identify symptoms earlier. And it can position providers to be more proactive by reaching out to patients. Health-care providers can also provide information to their patients through patient portals tied into their EHR system.[4]

KEEPING YOUR ELECTRONIC HEALTH INFORMATION SECURE

Most of us feel that our health information is private and should be protected. The federal government put in place the Health Insurance Portability and Accountability Act (HIPAA) of 1996 Privacy Rule to ensure you have rights over your own health information, no matter what form it is in. The government also created the HIPAA Security Rule to require specific protections to be in place in order to safeguard your electronic health information. A few possible measures that can be built into EHR systems include:
- **Access control tools.** These tools, such as passwords and personal identification numbers (PINs), help limit access to your information to authorized individuals.
- **Encrypting your stored information.** This means your health information cannot be read or understood except by those using a system that can "decrypt" it with a "key."
- **Audit trail.** This feature records who accessed your information, what changes were made, and when.

---

[4] HealthIT.gov, "Increase Patient Participation in Their Care," Office of the National Coordinator for Health Information Technology (ONC), September 26, 2018. Available online. URL: www.healthit.gov/topic/health-it-and-health-information-exchange-basics/increase-patient-participation-their-care. Accessed February 16, 2024.

Finally, federal law requires doctors, hospitals, and other health-care providers to notify you of a security "breach." The law also requires the health-care provider to notify the Secretary of the U.S. Department of Health and Human Services (HHS). If a security breach affects more than 500 residents of a state or jurisdiction, the health-care provider must also notify prominent media outlets serving the state or jurisdiction. This requirement helps patients know if something has gone wrong with the protection of their information and helps keep providers accountable for EHR protection.[5]

---

[5] "Privacy, Security, and Electronic Health Records," U.S. Department of Health and Human Services (HHS), March 17, 2013. Available online. URL: www.hhs.gov/sites/default/files/ocr/privacy/hipaa/understanding/consumers/privacy-security-electronic-records.pdf. Accessed February 16, 2024.

Chapter 26 | Health Communication and Technology

All people have some ability to manage their health and the health of those they care for. However, with the increasing complexity of health information and health-care settings, most people need additional information, skills, and supportive relationships to meet their health needs.

Disparities in access to health information, services, and technology can result in lower usage rates of preventive services, less knowledge of chronic disease management, higher rates of hospitalization, and poorer reported health status.

Both public and private institutions are increasingly using the Internet and other technologies to streamline the delivery of health information and services. This results in an even greater need for health professionals to develop additional skills in the understanding and use of consumer health information.

The increase in online health information and services challenges users with limited literacy skills or limited experience using the Internet. For many of these users, the Internet is stressful and overwhelming—even inaccessible. Much of this stress can be reduced through the application of evidence-based best practices in user-centered design.

In addition, despite increased access to technology, other forms of communication are essential to ensuring that everyone, including nonweb users, is able to obtain, process, and understand health information to make good health decisions. These include printed materials, media campaigns, community outreach, and interpersonal communication.

Ideas about health and behaviors are shaped by the communication, information, and technology that people interact with every day. Health communication and health information technology (IT) are central to health care, public health, and the way our society views health. These processes make up the ways and the context in which professionals and the public search for, understand, and use health information, significantly affecting their health decisions and actions.

The objectives in this topic area describe many ways health communication and health IT can have a positive effect on health, health care, and health equity. They include:
- supporting shared decision-making between patients and providers
- providing personalized self-management tools and resources
- building social support networks
- delivering accurate, accessible, and actionable health information that is targeted or tailored
- facilitating the meaningful use of health IT and the exchange of health information among health-care and public health professionals
- enabling quick and informed responses to health risks and public health emergencies
- increasing health literacy skills
- providing new opportunities to connect with culturally diverse and hard-to-reach populations
- providing sound principles in the design of programs and interventions that result in healthier behaviors
- increasing Internet and mobile access

IMPORTANCE OF HEALTH COMMUNICATION AND HEALTH INFORMATION TECHNOLOGY

Effective use of communication and technology by health-care and public health professionals can bring about an age of patient- and public-centered health information and services. By strategically

combining health IT tools and effective health communication processes, there is the potential to:
- improve health-care quality and safety
- increase the efficiency of health-care and public health service delivery
- improve the public health information infrastructure
- support care in the community and at home
- facilitate clinical and consumer decision-making
- build health skills and knowledge

EMERGING ISSUES IN HEALTH COMMUNICATION AND HEALTH INFORMATION TECHNOLOGY

During the coming decade, the speed, scope, and scale of adoption of health IT will only increase. Social media and emerging technologies promise to blur the line between expert and peer health information. Monitoring and assessing the effect of these new media, including mobile health, on public health will be challenging.

Equally challenging will be helping health professionals and the public adapt to the changes in health-care quality and efficiency due to the creative use of health communication and health IT. Continual feedback, productive interactions, and access to evidence on the effectiveness of treatments and interventions will likely transform the traditional patient-provider relationship. It will also change the way people receive, process, and evaluate health information. Capturing the scope and effect of these changes—and the role of health communication and health IT in facilitating them—will require multidisciplinary models and data systems.

Such systems will be critical to expanding the collection of data to better understand the effects of health communication and health IT on population health outcomes, health-care quality, and health disparities.[1]

---

[1] Office of Disease Prevention and Health Promotion (ODPHP), "Health Communication and Health Information Technology," U.S. Department of Health and Human Services (HHS), February 6, 2022. Available online. URL: www.healthypeople.gov/2020/topics-objectives/topic/health-communication-and-health-information-technology. Accessed February 14, 2024.

NATIONAL ACTION PLAN TO IMPROVE HEALTH LITERACY

The National Action Plan to Improve Health Literacy seeks to engage organizations, professionals, policymakers, communities, individuals, and families in a linked, multisector effort to improve health literacy. The action plan is based on two core principles:
- All people have the right to health information that helps them make informed decisions.
- Health services should be delivered in ways that are easy to understand and that improve health, longevity, and quality of life (QOL).

The Action Plan contains the following seven goals that will improve health literacy and strategies for achieving them:
- Develop and disseminate health and safety information that is accurate, accessible, and actionable.
- Promote changes in the health-care system that improve health information, communication, informed decision-making, and access to health services.
- Incorporate accurate, standards-based, and developmentally appropriate health and science information and curricula in childcare and education through the university level.
- Support and expand local efforts to provide adult education, English language instruction, and culturally and linguistically appropriate health information services in the community.
- Build partnerships, develop guidance, and change policies.
- Increase basic research and the development, implementation, and evaluation of practices and interventions to improve health literacy.
- Increase the dissemination and use of evidence-based health literacy practices and interventions.

Many strategies highlight the actions that particular organizations or professions can take to further these goals. It will take everyone working together in a linked and coordinated manner

Health Communication and Technology

to improve access to accurate and actionable health information and usable health services. By focusing on health literacy issues and working together, we can improve the accessibility, quality, and safety of health care; reduce costs; and improve the health and QOL of millions of people in the United States.[2]

---

[2] Office of Disease Prevention and Health Promotion (ODPHP), "National Action Plan to Improve Health Literacy," U.S. Department of Health and Human Services (HHS), August 24, 2021. Available online. URL: https://health.gov/our-work/national-health-initiatives/health-literacy/national-action-plan-improve-health-literacy. Accessed February 14, 2024.

Chapter 27 | Patient Rights and Responsibilities

Chapter Contents
Section 27.1—Health-Care Rights and Responsibilities 277
Section 27.2—Health Information Privacy Rights 281
Section 27.3—How to Keep Your Health Information
              Private and Secure 287

Section 27.1 | Health-Care Rights and Responsibilities

WHAT ARE YOUR HEALTH-CARE RIGHTS AND RESPONSIBILITIES?

As a patient, you have certain rights. Some are guaranteed by federal law, such as the right to get a copy of your medical records and keep them private. Many states have additional laws protecting patients, and health-care facilities often have a patient bill of rights.

An important patient right is informed consent. This means that if you need a treatment, your health-care provider must give you the information you need to make a decision.

Many hospitals have patient advocates who can help you if you have problems. Many states have an ombudsman office for problems with long-term care. Your state's department of health may also be able to help.[1]

HEALTH INSURANCE RIGHTS AND PROTECTIONS

The health-care law offers rights and protections that make coverage more fair and easy to understand. Some rights and protections apply to plans in the Health Insurance Marketplace® or other individual insurance, some apply to job-based plans, and some apply to all health coverage. The protections outlined subsequently may not apply to grandfathered health insurance plans.

The health-care law protects you by:
- requiring insurance plans to cover people with preexisting health conditions, including pregnancy, without charging more
- providing free preventive care
- giving young adults more coverage options
- ending lifetime and yearly dollar limits on coverage of essential health benefits
- helping you understand the coverage you are getting
- holding insurance companies accountable for rate increases

---

[1] MedlinePlus, "Patient Rights," National Institutes of Health (NIH), August 31, 2016. Available online. URL: https://medlineplus.gov/patientrights.html. Accessed February 16, 2024.

- making it illegal for health insurance companies to cancel your health insurance just because you get sick
- protecting your choice of doctors
- protecting you from employer retaliation

Additional rights and benefits include:
- breast-feeding equipment and support
- birth control methods and counseling
- mental health and substance abuse services
- the right to appeal a health plan decision
- the right to choose an individual Marketplace plan rather than the one your employer offers you[2]

FREQUENTLY ASKED QUESTIONS ABOUT HEALTH INFORMATION RIGHTS
Do I Have the Right to See and Get a Copy of My Health Records?

The Health Insurance Portability and Accountability Act (HIPAA) Privacy Rule gives you the right to inspect, review, and receive a copy of your health and billing records that are held by health plans and health-care providers covered under the HIPAA.
- In a few special cases, you may not be able to get all of your information. For example, your doctor may decide that something in your file could physically endanger you or someone else and may not have to give this information to you.
- In most cases, your copies must be given to you within 30 days. However, if your health information is not maintained or accessible on-site, your health-care provider or health plan can take up to 60 days to respond to your request. If, for some reason, they cannot take action by these deadlines, your provider or plan may extend the deadline by another 30 days if they

---

[2] "Health Insurance Rights & Protections," Centers for Medicare & Medicaid Services (CMS), June 22, 2013. Available online. URL: www.healthcare.gov/health-care-law-protections/rights-and-protections. Accessed February 16, 2024.

Patient Rights and Responsibilities

give you a reason for the delay in writing and tell you when to expect your copies.
- The provider cannot charge a fee for searching for or retrieving your information, but you may have to pay for the cost of copying and mailing.

Your state may also have laws that give you the right to see and copy your medical records. If there is a difference between state and federal law, your provider must follow the law that gives you the most rights.

Do I Have a Right to Know When My Health-Care Provider Has Shared My Health Information with People Outside of His or Her Practice?

You have a right to receive an "accounting of disclosures," which is a list of certain instances when your health-care provider or health plan has shared your health information with another person or organization. There are some major exceptions to this right. As of now, an accounting of disclosures does not include information about when your health-care provider or health plan shares your information with another person or organization for treatment, payment, or health-care operations.

Can I Ask to Correct the Information in My Health Records?

You can ask your health-care provider or health plan to correct your health record by adding information to make it more accurate or complete. This is called the "right to amend." For example, if you and your hospital agree that your record has the wrong result for a test, the hospital must change it. If you and your health provider or health plan do not agree that an amendment is necessary, you still have the right to have your disagreement noted in your record. In most cases, your record should be changed within 60 days, but the provider can take an extra 30 days if they provide a reason.

Do I Have the Right to Receive a Notice That Tells Me How My Health Information Is Being Used and Shared?

You can learn how your health information is used and shared by your provider or health insurer. They must give you a notice that tells you how they legally may use and share your health information and how you can exercise your rights. In most cases, you should get this notice on your first visit to a provider or in the mail from your health plan, and you can ask for a copy at any time. This is the document that providers often ask for you to sign to indicate that you have received it.

Who Has to Follow the Parts of the HIPAA Privacy Rule That Give Me Rights with Respect to My Health Information?

- most doctors, nurses, pharmacies, hospitals, clinics, nursing homes, and many other health-care providers
- health insurance companies, health maintenance organizations (HMOs), and most employer group health plans
- certain government programs that pay for health care, such as Medicare and Medicaid

Do I Have the Right to File a Complaint?

If you believe your information was used or shared in a way that is not allowed under the HIPAA Privacy Rule, or if you were not able to exercise your health information rights, you can file a complaint with your provider or health insurer. The privacy notice you receive from them will tell you how to file a complaint. You can also file a complaint with the U.S. Department of Health and Human Services' (HHS) Office for Civil Rights (OCR) or your state's Attorneys General Office.

Are State Governments Involved in Protecting Privacy Rights?

The HIPAA Privacy Rule sets a federal "floor" of privacy protections—a minimum level of privacy that health-care providers and health plans must meet. Many states have health information

Patient Rights and Responsibilities

privacy laws that have additional protections that are above this floor. In addition, even though the HIPAA is a federal law, state Attorneys General have been given the authority to enforce the HIPAA.[3]

Section 27.2 | Health Information Privacy Rights

Most of us believe that our medical and other health information is private and should be protected, and we want to know who has this information. The Privacy Rule, a federal law, gives you rights over your health information and sets rules and limits on who can look at and receive your health information. The Privacy Rule applies to all forms of individuals' protected health information, whether electronic, written, or oral. The Security Rule is a federal law that requires security for health information in electronic form.

Who Must Follow These Laws?

We call the entities that must follow the HIPAA regulations "covered entities."

Covered entities include the following:
- **Health plans**. This includes health insurance companies, health maintenance organizations (HMOs), company health plans, and certain government programs that pay for health care, such as Medicare and Medicaid.
- **Health-care providers**. Most health-care providers conduct certain business electronically, such as electronically billing your health insurance, including most doctors, clinics, hospitals, psychologists, chiropractors, nursing homes, pharmacies, and dentists.

---

[3] HealthIT.gov, "Your Health Information Rights," Office of the National Coordinator for Health Information Technology (ONC), September 7, 2017. Available online. URL: www.healthit.gov/topic/privacy-security-and-hipaa/your-health-information-rights. Accessed February 16, 2024.

- **Health-care clearinghouses.** These include entities that process nonstandard health information they receive from another entity into a standard (i.e., standard electronic format or data content), or vice versa.

In addition, business associates of covered entities must follow parts of the HIPAA regulations.

Often, contractors, subcontractors, and other outside persons and companies that are not employees of a covered entity will need to have access to your health information when providing services to the covered entity. We call these entities "business associates." Examples of business associates include:
- companies that help your doctors get paid for providing health care, including billing companies and companies that process your health-care claims
- companies that help administer health plans
- people such as outside lawyers, accountants, and information technology (IT) specialists
- companies that store or destroy medical records

Covered entities must have contracts in place with their business associates, ensuring that they use and disclose your health information properly and safeguard it appropriately. Business associates must also have similar contracts with subcontractors. Business associates (including subcontractors) must follow the use and disclosure provisions of their contracts, the Privacy Rule, and the safeguard requirements of the Security Rule.

Who Is Not Required to Follow These Laws?

Many organizations that have health information about you do not have to follow these laws.

Examples of organizations that do not have to follow the Privacy and Security Rules include:
- life insurers
- employers
- workers compensation carriers
- most schools and school districts

Patient Rights and Responsibilities

- many state agencies such as child protective service agencies
- most law enforcement agencies
- many municipal offices

What Information Is Protected
- information your doctors, nurses, and other health-care providers put in your medical record
- conversations your doctor has about your care or treatment with nurses and others
- information about you in your health insurer's computer system
- billing information about you at your clinic
- most other health information about you held by those who must follow these laws

How This Information Is Protected
- Covered entities must put in place safeguards to protect your health information and ensure they do not use or disclose your health information improperly.
- Covered entities must reasonably limit uses and disclosures to the minimum necessary to accomplish their intended purpose.
- Covered entities must have procedures in place to limit who can view and access your health information as well as implement training programs for employees about how to protect your health information.
- Business associates must also put in place safeguards to protect your health information and ensure they do not use or disclose your health information improperly.

What Rights Does the Privacy Rule Give You Over Your Health Information?
Health insurers and providers who are covered entities must comply with your right to:
- ask to see and get a copy of your health records
- have corrections added to your health information

- receive a notice that tells you how your health information may be used and shared
- decide if you want to give your permission before your health information can be used or shared for certain purposes, such as marketing
- request that a covered entity restrict how it uses or discloses your health information
- get a report on when and why your health information was shared for certain purposes
- if you believe your rights are being denied or your health information is not being protected, you can:
  - file a complaint with your provider or health insurer
  - file a complaint with the HHS

You should get to know these important rights, which help you protect your health information.

You can ask your provider or health insurer questions about your rights.

Who Can Look at and Receive Your Health Information?

The Privacy Rule sets rules and limits on who can look at and receive your health information.

To make sure that your health information is protected in a way that does not interfere with your health care, your information can be used and shared:
- for your treatment and care coordination
- to pay doctors and hospitals for your health care and to help run their businesses
- with your family, relatives, friends, or others you identify who are involved with your health care or your health-care bills, unless you object
- to make sure doctors give good care and nursing homes are clean and safe
- to protect the public's health, such as by reporting when the flu is in your area
- to make required reports to the police, such as reporting gunshot wounds

Patient Rights and Responsibilities

Your health information cannot be used or shared without your written permission unless this law allows it. For example, without your authorization, your provider generally cannot:
- give your information to your employer
- use or share your information for marketing or advertising purposes or sell your information[4]

SHARING HEALTH INFORMATION WITH FAMILY MEMBERS AND FRIENDS

The Health Insurance Portability and Accountability Act (HIPAA) requires most doctors, nurses, hospitals, nursing homes, and other health-care providers to protect the privacy of your health information. However, if you do not object, a health-care provider or health plan may share relevant information with family members or friends involved in your health care or payment for your health care in certain circumstances.

When Your Health Information Can be Shared

Under the HIPAA, your health-care provider may share your information face-to-face, over the phone, or in writing. A health-care provider or health plan may share relevant information if:
- you give your provider or plan permission to share the information
- you are present and do not object to sharing the information
- you are not present, and the provider determines based on professional judgment that it is in your best interest

EXAMPLES
- An emergency room doctor may discuss your treatment in front of your friend when you ask your friend to come into the treatment room.

---

[4] "Your Rights under HIPAA," U.S. Department of Health and Human Services (HHS), January 19, 2022. Available online. URL: www.hhs.gov/hipaa/for-individuals/guidance-materials-for-consumers/index.html. Accessed February 16, 2024.

- Your hospital may discuss your bill with your daughter who is with you and has a question about the charges, if you do not object.
- Your doctor may discuss the drugs you need to take with your health aide who has come with you to your appointment.
- Your nurse may not discuss your condition with your brother if you tell her not to.
- The HIPAA also allows health-care providers to give prescription drugs, medical supplies, x-rays, and other health-care items to a family member, friend, or other person you send to pick them up.
- A health-care provider or health plan may also share relevant information if you are not around or cannot give permission when a health-care provider or plan representative believes, based on professional judgment, that sharing the information is in your best interest.
- You had emergency surgery and are still unconscious. Your surgeon may tell your spouse about your condition, either in person or by phone while you are unconscious.
- Your doctor may discuss your drugs with your caregiver who calls your doctor with a question about the right dosage.
- A doctor may not tell your friend about a past medical problem that is unrelated to your current condition.[5]

---

[5] "Sharing Health Information with Family Members and Friends," U.S. Department of Health and Human Services (HHS), August 7, 2016. Available online. URL: www.hhs.gov/sites/default/files/ocr/privacy/hipaa/understanding/consumers/sharing-family-friends.pdf. Accessed February 16, 2024.

Patient Rights and Responsibilities

Section 27.3 | **How to Keep Your Health Information Private and Secure**

PROTECTING THE PRIVACY AND SECURITY OF YOUR HEALTH INFORMATION

The privacy and security of patient health information is a top priority for patients and their families, health-care providers and professionals, and the government. Federal laws require many of the key persons and organizations that handle health information to have policies and security safeguards in place to protect your health information—whether it is stored on paper or electronically.

The Health Insurance Portability and Accountability Act of 1996 (HIPAA) Privacy, Security, and Breach Notification Rules are the main federal laws that protect your health information. The Privacy Rule gives you rights with respect to your health information. The Privacy Rule also sets limits on how your health information can be used and shared with others. The Security Rule sets rules for how your health information must be kept secure with administrative, technical, and physical safeguards.

You may have additional protections and health information rights under your state's laws. There are also federal laws that protect specific types of health information, such as information related to federally funded alcohol and substance abuse treatment.

Your Privacy Rights

If you believe your health information privacy has been violated, the U.S. Department of Health and Human Services (HHS) has a division, the Office for Civil Rights (OCR), to educate you about your privacy rights, enforce the rules, and help you file a complaint.

Security

Health-care providers and other key persons and organizations that handle your health information must protect it with passwords, encryption, and other technical safeguards. These are designed to make sure that only the right people have access to your information.

Be Responsible
While federal law can protect your health information, you should also use common sense to make sure that private information does not become public. If you access your health records online, make sure you use a strong password and keep it a secret. Keep in mind that if you post information online in a public forum, you cannot assume it is private or secure.[6]

HEALTH IT: HOW TO KEEP YOUR HEALTH INFORMATION PRIVATE AND SECURE
There are laws that protect the privacy of your health information held by those who provide you health-care services. But, as it becomes easier to get and share your own health information online, you need to take steps to protect it. This applies whether you are downloading a copy of your health information via Blue Button, emailing your doctor, taking an online health survey, or using a variety of digital apps or devices to monitor your health.

DOES THE HEALTH INSURANCE PORTABILITY AND ACCOUNTABILITY ACT PROTECT ALL HEALTH INFORMATION?
You may have heard about the HIPPA, Privacy and Security Rules. These are federal laws that set national standards for protecting the privacy and security of health information. Health information that is kept by health-care providers, health plans and organizations acting on their behalf is protected by these federal laws. However, you should know that there are many organizations that do not have to follow these laws. Some examples of health information that is not covered by the HIPAA include health information that patients:
- store in a mobile app or on a mobile device, such as a smartphone or tablet

---

[6] HealthIT.gov, "Protecting Your Privacy & Security," Office of the National Coordinator for Health Information Technology (ONC), December 17, 2018. Available online. URL: www.healthit.gov/topic/protecting-your-privacy-security. Accessed February 16, 2024.

Patient Rights and Responsibilities

- share over social media websites or health-related online communities, such as message boards
- store in a personal health record (PHR) that is not offered through a health provider or health plan covered by the HIPAA

KEEP YOUR ELECTRONIC HEALTH INFORMATION SECURE

There are a number of ways you can help protect your electronic health information. Here are some tips to ensure your personal health information is private and secure when accessing it electronically.

When Creating a Password
- Use a password or other function on your home computer or mobile device so that you are the only one who can access your information.
- Use a strong password and update it often.
- Do not share your password with anyone.

When Using Social Media
- Think carefully before you post anything on the Internet that you do not want to be made public—do not assume that an online public forum is private or secure.
- If you decide to post health information on a social media platform, consider using the privacy setting to limit others' access.
- Be aware that information posted on the web may remain permanently.

When Using Mobile Devices
- Research mobile apps—software programs that perform one or more specific functions—before you download and install any of them. Be sure to use known app websites or trusted sources.

- Read the terms of service and privacy notice of the mobile app to verify that the app will perform only the functions you approve.
- Consider installing or using encryption software for your device. Encryption software is now widely available and increasingly affordable.
- Install and activate remote wiping and/or remote disabling on your mobile devices. The remote wipe feature allows you to permanently delete data stored on a lost or stolen mobile device. Remote disabling enables you to lock data stored on a lost or stolen mobile device, and unlock the data if the device is recovered.[7]

---

[7] HealthIT.gov, "Health IT: How to Keep Your Health Information Private and Secure," Office of the National Coordinator for Health Information Technology (ONC), September 17, 2013. Available online. URL: www.healthit.gov/sites/default/files/how_to_keep_your_health_information_private_and_secure.pdf. Accessed February 16, 2024.

Chapter 28 | Personal Health Records and Patient Portals

WHAT IS A PERSONAL HEALTH RECORD?
A personal health record (PHR) is an electronic application through which patients can maintain and manage their health information (and that of others for whom they are authorized) in a private, secure, and confidential environment.[1]

ARE THERE DIFFERENT TYPES OF PERSONAL HEALTH RECORDS?
There are two main kinds of PHRs:
- **Standalone PHRs.** With a standalone PHR, patients fill in information from their own records, and the information is stored on patients' computers or the Internet. In some cases, a standalone PHR can also accept data from external sources, including providers and laboratories. With a standalone PHR, patients could add diet or exercise information to track progress over time. Patients can decide whether to share the information with providers, family members, or anyone else involved in their care.
- **Tethered/connected PHRs.** A tethered or connected PHR is linked to a specific health-care organization's

---

[1] HealthIT.gov, "What Is a Personal Health Record?" Office of the National Coordinator for Health Information Technology (ONC), May 2, 2016. Available online. URL: www.healthit.gov/faq/what-personal-health-record. Accessed February 23, 2024.

electronic health record (EHR) system or to a health plan's information system. With a tethered PHR, patients can access their own records through a secure portal and see, for example, the trend of their lab results over the last year, their immunization history, or due dates for screenings.[2]

WHAT IS A PATIENT PORTAL?

A patient portal is a secure online website that gives patients convenient, 24-hour access to personal health information from anywhere with an Internet connection. Using a secure username and password, patients can view health information such as:
- recent doctor visits
- discharge summaries
- medications
- immunizations
- allergies
- lab results

Some patient portals also allow you to:
- securely message your doctor
- request prescription refills
- schedule nonurgent appointments
- check benefits and coverage
- update contact information
- make payments
- download and complete forms
- view educational materials

With your patient portal, you can be in control of your health and care. Patient portals can also save your time, help you communicate with your doctor, and support care between visits.[3]

---

[2] HealthIT.gov, "Are There Different Types of Personal Health Records (PHRs)?" Office of the National Coordinator for Health Information Technology (ONC), July 30, 2019. Available online. URL: www.healthit.gov/faq/are-there-different-types-personal-health-records-phrs. Accessed February 23, 2024.

[3] HealthIT.gov, "What Is a Patient Portal?" Office of the National Coordinator for Health Information Technology (ONC), September 29, 2017. Available online. URL: www.healthit.gov/faq/what-patient-portal. Accessed February 23, 2024.

Chapter 29 | Making Sense of Internet Health Information

Many older adults share a common concern: "Can I trust the health information I find online?" There are thousands of medical websites. Some provide up-to-date medical news and reliable health information, and some do not. Choosing trustworthy websites is an important step in gathering reliable health information.

WHERE CAN YOU FIND RELIABLE HEALTH INFORMATION ONLINE?
The National Institutes of Health (NIH) website (www.nih.gov) is a good place to start for reliable health information. The Centers for Disease Control and Prevention (CDC) website (www.cdc.gov) is another.

As a rule, health websites sponsored by federal government agencies are accurate sources of information. You can reach all federal websites by visiting www.usa.gov. Medical and health-care organizations, hospitals, and academic medical institutions may also be reliable sources of health information.

Your health-care provider can also suggest ideal sources of online information. If your doctor's office has a website, it may include a list of recommended links.

QUESTIONS TO ASK BEFORE TRUSTING A WEBSITE
If you search, you will likely find websites for multiple health organizations, including many you may not recognize. The following questions can help determine which ones are trustworthy.

What Is the Purpose of the Website, and Who Owns or Sponsors It?

Why was the site created? Is the purpose of the site to inform or explain, or is it trying to sell a product or service? Understanding the motive of the website can help you better judge its content. The goal of any trustworthy health information website is to provide accurate, recent, and useful information versus trying to make a sale.

Knowing who pays for a website may provide you with insight into the mission or goal of the site. For example, if a business pays for the site, the health information may favor that business and its products. Sometimes the website address (called a "URL") is helpful for identifying the type of agency or organization that owns the site, for example:

- .gov identifies a U.S. government agency
- .edu identifies an educational institution, such as a school, college, or university
- .org usually identifies nonprofit organizations, such as medical or research societies and advocacy groups
- .com identifies commercial websites, such as businesses and pharmaceutical companies

While many commercial websites do provide accurate, useful health information, it can be hard to distinguish this content from marketing and promotional materials in some cases. Any advertisements on a site should be clearly marked as such. Watch out for ads designed to look like neutral health information.

Who Wrote the Information? Who Reviewed It?

Website pages often, but not always, identify the authors and contributors. If the author is listed, are they an expert in the field? Look for health-care professionals or scientific researchers with in-depth knowledge of the topic. Does the author work for an organization and, if so, what are the goals of that organization? A contributor's connection to the website, and any financial stake they have regarding the information on the website, should be made clear.

Making Sense of Internet Health Information

If the material is not authored by an expert, has the information been reviewed by a health-care professional or other credentialed specialist? Dependable health information websites will share sources and citations.

Trustworthy websites will also have contact information—an email address, phone number, and/or mailing address—that you can use to reach the site's sponsor.

Be cautious about testimonials, individual blogs, and posts on discussion boards. Personal stories may be helpful and comforting, but not everyone experiences health problems the same way. Also, there is a big difference between information written by a single person interested in a topic and a website developed by professionals using researched and peer-reviewed scientific evidence.

No online information, even if it is accurate and trustworthy, should replace seeing a health-care professional who can thoroughly evaluate your unique situation and provide specific advice.

When Was the Information Written and Updated?

Look for websites that stay current with their health information. You do not want to make decisions about your care based on out-of-date content. Often, the date the information was created and reviewed or updated will appear at the bottom of the page. Pages on the same site may be updated at different times, and some may be updated more often than others. Older information is not useless, but using the most recent, evidence-based information is ideal.

Is Your Privacy Protected? Does the Website Clearly State a Privacy Policy?

Read the website's privacy policy. It is usually at the bottom of the page or on a separate page titled "Privacy Policy" or "Our Policies." If a website says it uses "cookies," your information may not be private. Cookies are small text files that enable a website to collect and remember information about your visit. While cookies may enhance your web experience, they can also compromise your online privacy, so it is important to read about the information the website collects and how the organization will use it. Many websites will ask you ahead of time if you want to accept cookies, but others may not. If you are concerned about the potential use of information gathered by cookies, you can choose to disable the use of cookies through your Internet browser settings.

How Can You Protect Your Health Information?

If you are asked to share personal information, be sure to find out how the information will be used. Secure websites that collect personal information responsibly have an "s" after "http" in the start of their website addresses (https://) and often require that you create a username and password.

Be careful about sharing your Social Security number (SSN). Find out why your number is needed, how it will be used, and what will happen if you do not share this information. Only enter your SSN on secure websites. You might consider calling your doctor's office or health insurance company to give this information over the phone rather than providing it online.

Taking the following precautions may help protect your information:

- **Beware of health fraud scams and pay attention when browsing the Internet.** Do not open unexpected links. Hover your mouse over a link to confirm that clicking it will take you to a reputable website.
- **Always use a strong password.** Include a variation of numbers, letters, and symbols. Some websites may allow you to use a phrase as well. Create a unique password for each website and change it frequently.
- **Use two-factor authentication when you can.** This security feature requires the use of two different types of personal information to log into your mobile devices or accounts.
- **Do not enter sensitive information over public Wi-Fi.**
- **Be careful about the information you share through social media sites.** For example, do not share personal information, such as where you live or your contact information, on a public channel.

Making Sense of Internet Health Information

Does the Website Offer Quick and Easy Solutions to Your Health Problems? Does It Promise Miracle Cures?

Be cautious about websites claiming any single remedy will cure many different illnesses. Also, be wary of sites suggesting simple or unproven treatments for a disease. Question dramatic writing or promises of cures that seem too good to be true and look for other websites with the same information. Even if a website links to a trustworthy source, it does not mean that the site has the other organization's endorsement or support.

HEALTH AND MEDICAL APPS

Mobile medical applications ("apps") are a type of software you can install and run on your smartphone. Medical apps can support your health in many ways. For example, they can help track your eating habits or physical activity, access test results from a lab, or monitor a health condition. They can also provide helpful reminders to exercise or take medications. But anyone can develop a health app—for any reason—and apps may include inaccurate or misleading information. Before you download or use an app, make sure you know who produced it.

When you download an app, it may ask for your location, your email, or other personal information. Apps may also collect data about you as you use them. Ensure the information collected is relevant to the app, you know how the information will be used, and you feel comfortable sharing this information. Responsible app developers will make this information readily available before you download it.

SOCIAL MEDIA, HEALTH NEWS, AND HEALTH BOOKS

Social media websites and apps are online communities through which people can connect with friends, family, and strangers. Social media is one way people share health information and news stories with each other. Some of this information may be true, but too often, some of it is not. Recognize that just because a post is from a friend or colleague, it does not necessarily mean that the information is accurate, complete, or applicable to your health. Check the source of the information, and make sure the original author is credible. Fact-checking websites can also help you determine if a story is reliable.

Evaluating health information in books is similar to finding reliable information on websites or social media. Make sure to check who wrote the book, how recent the information is, and where the content came from. When in doubt, ask your health-care provider about what you read.

TRUST YOURSELF AND TALK WITH YOUR DOCTOR

Use your good judgment when gathering health information online. There are websites on nearly every health topic, and many have no rules for overseeing the quality of the information provided. Use the information you find online as one tool to become more informed. Do not count on any one website and check your sources. Discuss what you find with your doctor before making any changes to your health care.[1]

---

[1] National Institute on Aging (NIA), "How to Find Reliable Health Information Online," National Institutes of Health (NIH), January 12, 2023. Available online. URL: www.nia.nih.gov/health/healthy-aging/how-find-reliable-health-information-online. Accessed February 14, 2024.

Chapter 30 | Informed Consent

Informed consent is an essential process through which the research team explains the trial to you before you decide whether to take part.

The research team explains the trial's purpose, procedures, and possible risks and benefits. You have the right to ask questions and learn about all that is involved in the trial, including all your treatment options, details about treatment, tests, and possible risks and benefits.

They will also discuss other rights, including your rights to decide to take part in and to leave the study at any time. You have the right to both hear and read the information in a language you can understand.

After discussing the study with you, the research team will give you an informed consent form to read. The form includes written details about the information that was discussed with you and describes the privacy of your medical records. If you agree to take part in the study, you sign the form.

But even after you sign the consent form, you can leave the study at any time. You can always ask questions. And as new information becomes available, the research team will inform you.[1]

TIPS ON INFORMED CONSENT

The process of obtaining informed consent must comply with the requirements of 45 CFR 46.116. The documentation of informed

---

[1] "Are Clinical Trials Safe?" National Cancer Institute (NCI), September 18, 2023. Available online. URL: www.cancer.gov/research/participate/clinical-trials/safety. Accessed February 14, 2024.

consent must comply with 45 CFR 46.117. The following comments may help in the development of an approach and proposed language by investigators for obtaining consent and its approval by Institutional Review Boards (IRBs):

- **Informed consent is a process, not just a form.** Information must be presented to enable persons to voluntarily decide whether or not to participate as a research subject. It is a fundamental mechanism to ensure respect for persons through the provision of thoughtful consent for a voluntary act. The procedures used in obtaining informed consent should be designed to educate the subject population in terms that they can understand. Therefore, informed consent language and its documentation (especially an explanation of the study's purpose, duration, experimental procedures, alternatives, risks, and benefits) must be written in "lay language," (i.e., understandable to the people being asked to participate). The written presentation of information is used to document the basis for consent and for the subjects' future reference. The consent document should be revised when deficiencies are noted or when additional information will improve the consent process.
- **Use of the first person.** For example, "I understand that …" can be interpreted as suggestive, may be relied upon as a substitute for sufficient factual information, and can constitute coercive influence over a subject. The use of scientific jargon and legalese is not appropriate. Think of the document primarily as a teaching tool not as a legal instrument.
- **Describe the overall experience that will be encountered.** Explain the research activity, and how it is experimental (e.g., a new drug, extra tests, separate research records, or nonstandard means of management, such as flipping a coin for random assignment or other design issues). Inform the human subjects of the reasonably foreseeable harms,

discomforts, inconveniences, and risks that are associated with the research activity. If additional risks are identified during the course of the research, the consent process and documentation will require revisions to inform subjects as they are recontacted or newly contacted.
- **Describe the benefits that subjects may reasonably expect to encounter.** There may be none other than a sense of helping the public at large. If payment is given to defray the incurred expense for participation, it must not be coercive in amount or method of distribution.
- **Describe any alternatives to participating in the research project.** For example, in drug studies, the medication(s) may be available through their family doctor or clinic without the need to volunteer for the research activity.
- **The regulations insist that the subjects be told the extent to which their personally identifiable private information will be held in confidence.** For example, some studies require disclosure of information to other parties. Some studies inherently are in need of a Certificate of Confidentiality (CoC) which protects the investigator from involuntary release (e.g., subpoena) of the names or other identifying characteristics of research subjects. The IRB will determine the level of adequate requirements for confidentiality in light of its mandate to ensure the minimization of risk and determination that the residual risks warrant the involvement of subjects.
- **If research-related injury (i.e., physical, psychological, social, financial, or otherwise) is possible in research that is more than minimal risk, an explanation must be given of whatever voluntary compensation and treatment will be provided.** Note that the regulations do not limit injury to physical injury. This is a common misinterpretation.

- **The regulations prohibit waiving or appearing to waive any legal rights of subjects.** Therefore, for example, consent language must be carefully selected that deals with what the institution is voluntarily willing to do under circumstances, such as providing for compensation beyond the provision of immediate or therapeutic intervention in response to a research-related injury. In short, subjects should not be given the impression that they have agreed to and are without recourse to seek satisfaction beyond the institution's voluntarily chosen limits.
- **The regulations provide for the identification of contact persons who would be knowledgeable to answer questions of subjects about the research, rights as a research subject, and research-related injuries.** These three areas must be explicitly stated and addressed in the consent process and documentation. Furthermore, a single person is not likely to be appropriate to answer questions in all areas. This is because of potential conflicts of interest or the appearance of such. Questions about the research are frequently best answered by the investigator(s). However, questions about the rights of research subjects or research-related injuries (where applicable) may best be referred to those not on the research team. These questions could be addressed to the IRB, an ombudsman, an ethics committee, or other informed administrative body. Therefore, each consent document can be expected to have at least two names with local telephone numbers for contacts to answer questions in these specified areas.
- **The statement regarding voluntary participation and the right to withdraw at any time can be taken almost verbatim from the regulations (45 CFR 46.116 [a][8]).** It is important not to overlook the need to point out that no penalty or loss of benefits will occur as a result of not participating or withdrawing at any time. It is equally

Informed Consent

important to alert potential subjects to any foreseeable consequences to them should they unilaterally withdraw while dependent on some intervention to maintain normal function.

- **Do not forget to ensure provision for appropriate additional requirements that concern consent.** Some of these requirements can be found in sections 46.116(b), 46.205 (a)(2), 46.207(b), 46.208 (b), 46.209(d), 46.305 (a)(5-6), 46.408(c), and 46.409 (b). The IRB may impose additional requirements that are not specifically listed in the regulations to ensure that adequate information is presented in accordance with institutional policy and local law.[2]

---

[2] "Informed Consent Tips (1993)," U.S. Department of Health and Human Services (HHS), March 18, 2016. Available online. URL: www.hhs.gov/ohrp/regulations-and-policy/guidance/informed-consent-tips/index.html. Accessed February 14, 2024.

Chapter 31 | **Preventing Medical Errors**

Medical errors can occur anywhere in the health-care system: hospitals, clinics, surgery centers, doctors' offices, nursing homes, pharmacies, and patients' homes. Errors can involve medicines, surgery, diagnosis, equipment, or lab reports.

One in seven Medicare patients in hospitals experience a medical error. They can happen during even the most routine tasks, such as when a hospital patient on a salt-free diet is given a high-salt meal.

Most errors result from problems created by today's complex health-care system. But errors also happen when doctors and patients have problems communicating. The tips here tell what you can do to get safer care.

WHAT YOU CAN DO TO STAY SAFE
The best way you can help prevent errors is to be an active member of your health-care team. That means taking part in every decision about your health care. Research shows that patients who are more involved with their care tend to get better results.

Medicines
- **Make sure that all of your doctors know about every medicine you are taking.** This includes prescription and over-the-counter (OTC) medicines and dietary supplements, such as vitamins and herbs.
- **Bring all of your medicines and supplements to your doctor visits.** "Brown bagging" your medicines can help

you and your doctor talk about them and find out if there are any problems. It can also help your doctor keep your records up-to-date and help you get better quality care.
- **Make sure your doctor knows about any allergies and adverse reactions you have had to medicines.** This can help you to avoid getting medicines that could harm you.
- **When your doctor writes a prescription for you, make sure you can read it.** If you cannot read your doctor's handwriting, your pharmacist might not be able to either.
- **Ask for information about your medicines in terms you can understand—both when your medicines are prescribed and when you get them:**
  - What is the medicine for?
  - How am I supposed to take it and for how long?
  - What side effects are likely? What do I do if they occur?
  - Is this medicine safe to take with other medicines or dietary supplements I am taking?
  - What food, drink, or activities should I avoid while taking this medicine?
- **Ask when you pick up your medicine from the pharmacy.** Is this the medicine that my doctor prescribed?
- **Ask if you have any questions about the directions on your medicine labels.** Medicine labels can be hard to understand. For example, ask if "four times daily" means taking a dose every six hours around the clock or just during regular waking hours.
- **Ask your pharmacist for the best device to measure your liquid medicine.** For example, many people use household teaspoons, which often do not hold a true teaspoon of liquid. Special devices, such as marked syringes, help people measure the right dose.
- **Ask for written information about the side effects your medicine could cause.** If you know what might happen, you will be better prepared if it does or if something unexpected happens.

Hospital Stays
- **If you are in a hospital, consider asking all health-care workers who will touch you whether they have washed their hands.** Handwashing can prevent the spread of infections in hospitals.
- **When you are being discharged from the hospital, ask your doctor to explain the treatment plan you will follow at home.** This includes learning about your new medicines, making sure you know when to schedule follow-up appointments, and finding out when you can get back to your regular activities. It is important to know whether or not you should keep taking the medicines you were taking before your hospital stay. Getting clear instructions may help prevent an unexpected return trip to the hospital.

Surgery
- **If you are having surgery, make sure that you, your doctor, and your surgeon all agree on exactly what will be done.** Having surgery at the wrong site (e.g., operating on the left knee instead of the right) is rare. But even once is too often. The good news is that wrong-site surgery is 100 percent preventable. Surgeons are expected to sign their initials directly on the site to be operated on before the surgery.
- **If you have a choice, choose a hospital where many patients have had the procedure or surgery you need.** Research shows that patients tend to have better results when they are treated in hospitals that have a great deal of experience with their condition.

Other Steps
- **Speak up if you have questions or concerns.** You have a right to question anyone who is involved with your care.
- **Make sure that someone, such as your primary care doctor, coordinates your care.** This is especially

important if you have many health problems or are in the hospital.
- **Make sure that all your doctors have your important health information.** Do not assume that everyone has all the information they need.
- **Ask a family member or friend to go to appointments with you.** Even if you do not need help now, you might need it later.
- **Know that more is not always better.** It is a good idea to find out why a test or treatment is needed and how it can help you. You could be better off without it.
- **If you have a test, do not assume that no news is good news.** Ask how and when you will get the results.
- **Learn about your condition and treatments by asking your doctor and nurse and by using other reliable sources.** For example, treatment options based on the latest scientific evidence are available from the Effective Health Care (EHC) Program, Agency for Healthcare Research and Quality (AHRQ) website (https://effectivehealthcare.ahrq.gov/products). Ask your doctor if your treatment is based on the latest evidence.[1]

---

[1] Agency for Healthcare Research and Quality (AHRQ), "20 Tips to Help Prevent Medical Errors: Patient Fact Sheet," U.S. Department of Health and Human Services (HHS), November 2020. Available online. URL: www.ahrq.gov/questions/resources/20-tips.html. Accessed February 14, 2024.

Chapter 32 | Health-Care Fraud Scams

A PERVASIVE PROBLEM

Fraudulent products cannot deliver on their baseless promises and could cause serious injury or even death. Besides wasting money and delaying potentially life-saving diagnoses and scientifically tested and proven treatments, fraudulent products sometimes contain hidden drug ingredients that can be harmful when unknowingly taken by consumers.

For example, in recent years, U.S. Food and Drug Administration (FDA) laboratories have found hundreds of weight-loss products, illegally marketed as dietary supplements, that contained sibutramine, a Schedule IV controlled substance and the active ingredient in a prescription weight-loss drug. This prescription drug was later withdrawn from the U.S. market after studies showed that it was associated with an increased risk of heart attack and stroke. Furthermore, fraudulent products may be manufactured by unregistered facilities under unknown, unclean, or dangerous conditions.

Health fraud scams can involve a variety of FDA-regulated products. For example, the FDA found an expensive laser device being sold with fraudulent cure-all claims to treat cancer, human immunodeficiency virus/acquired immunodeficiency syndrome (HIV/AIDS), and diabetes. Three individuals were sentenced to prison for their involvement in the $16.6 million fraudulent scheme to distribute misbranded devices.

TIPS TO PROTECT YOURSELF FROM HEALTH-CARE FRAUD SCAMS

Here are six tip-offs to help you identify rip-offs:

- **One product does it all.** Be suspicious of products that claim to cure a wide range of diseases. The agency continues to send warning letters and take enforcement action as appropriate against companies marketing fake cure-all products. These miracle cures do not exist—they are bogus—and the only thing these companies are selling is false hope.
- **Personal success testimonials.** Success stories, such as "It cured my diabetes" or "It immediately stopped my coronavirus disease (COVID-19) infection," are easy to make up and are not a substitute for scientific evidence. Reviews found on popular online marketplaces and social media can be fake.
- **Quick fixes.** Few diseases or conditions can be treated quickly, even with legitimate products. Beware of language such as, "Lose 30 pounds in 30 days," "protects from viral infections," or "eliminates skin cancer in days."
- **All-natural cure or treatment.** Do not be fooled by descriptions such as "all-natural cure." Such phrases are often used in health fraud as an attention-grabber to suggest that a product is safer than conventional treatments. These terms do not necessarily equate to safety. Some plants found in nature (such as poisonous mushrooms) can be harmful or even kill when consumed. Moreover, the FDA has found numerous products promoted as all-natural cures or treatments that contain hidden and dangerously high doses of prescription drug ingredients or other active pharmaceutical ingredients.
- **Miracle cure.** Alarms should go off when you see this claim or others like it such as "new discovery," "guaranteed results," or "secret ingredient." If a real cure for a serious disease were FDA-approved, it would be widely reported through the media and prescribed

Health-Care Fraud Scams

by licensed health professionals—not plastered on advertisements in social media and messaging apps, or buried in websites, print ads, and TV infomercials.
- **Conspiracy theories**. Claims such as "This is the cure our government or Big Pharma does not want you to know about" are used to distract consumers from the obvious, common sense questions about the so-called miracle cure.

Even with these tips, fraudulent health products are not always easy to spot. If consumers are tempted to buy an unproven product or one with questionable claims, they should check with their doctor or other health-care professional first.[1]

---

[1] "6 Tip-Offs to Rip-Offs: Don't Fall for Health Fraud Scams," U.S. Food and Drug Administration (FDA), March 4, 2021. Available online. URL: www.fda.gov/consumers/consumer-updates/6-tip-offs-rip-offs-dont-fall-health-fraud-scams. Accessed February 15, 2024.

Chapter 33 | Medical Identity Theft

WHAT IS MEDICAL IDENTITY THEFT?
Medical identity theft is when someone uses your personal information—such as your name, Social Security number (SSN), health insurance account number, or Medicare number—to see a doctor, get prescription drugs, buy medical devices, submit claims with your insurance provider, or get other medical care.

If the thief's health information is mixed with yours, it could affect the medical care you are able to get or the health insurance benefits you are able to use. It could also hurt your credit.

HOW TO PROTECT YOUR MEDICAL INFORMATION FROM THEFT
Here is what you can do to protect your medical information.

Protect Documents That Contain Your Medical Information
Keep your medical records, health insurance records, and any other documents with medical information in a safe place. These may include:
- health insurance enrollment forms
- health insurance cards
- prescriptions
- prescription bottles
- billing statements from your doctor or other medical provider
- explanation of benefits (EOB) statements from your health insurance company

When you decide to get rid of those documents, shred them before you throw them away. If you do not have a shredder, look for a local shred day. If it is something that is hard to shred—such as a prescription bottle—use a marker to block out any medical and personal information.

If you get statements with medical information in the mail, take your mail out of the mailbox as soon as you can.

To limit the amount of medical information you get by mail, consider getting your medical bills or EOB statements online.

Ask Questions before You Give Out Your Medical Information
Some doctor's offices might ask for your SSN to identify you. Ask if they can use a different identifier or just the last four digits of your SSN.

If another organization asks for information such as your health insurance account number or Medicare number, or for details about your health, ask the following questions first:
- Why do you need it?
- How will you protect it?
- Will you share it? If so, with whom?

Protect Your Medical Information from Scammers Online and on Your Phone
Do not give your medical information to someone who calls, emails, or texts you unexpectedly. It could be a scammer trying to steal your information.

Instead, log in to your online medical account from a website you know is real. Or contact the company or provider using a phone number you know is real.

HOW TO KNOW IF SOMEONE IS USING YOUR MEDICAL INFORMATION
Besides taking steps to protect your medical information, it pays to know how to tell if someone is using your medical information. Some warning signs are as follows:
- You get a bill from your doctor for services you did not get.

Medical Identity Theft

- You notice errors in your EOB statement such as services you did not get or prescription medications you do not take.
- You get a call from a debt collector about a medical debt you do not owe.
- You review your credit report and see medical debt collection notices that you do not recognize.
- You get a notice from your health insurance company saying you reached your benefit limit.
- You are denied insurance coverage because your medical records show a preexisting condition you do not have.

WHAT TO DO IF SOMEONE IS USING YOUR MEDICAL INFORMATION

If you think someone is using your personal information to see a doctor, get prescription drugs, buy medical devices, submit claims with your insurance provider, or get other medical care, taking these steps will help you limit the damage.

Review Your Medical Records and Report Errors

- **Get your medical records.** Contact each doctor, clinic, hospital, pharmacy, laboratory, and health insurance company where the thief may have used your information. Explain the situation and ask for copies of these medical records. You may have to submit records request forms and pay fees to get copies of your records. If the provider refuses to give you copies of the records to protect the identity thief's privacy rights, you can appeal. Contact the person listed in your provider's Notice of Privacy Practices (NPP), the patient representative, or the ombudsman. Explain the situation to that person and ask for your medical records.
- **Review your medical records.** Look for any errors, such as visits you did not make and services you did not get.
- **Report errors.** Report any errors to your health-care provider in writing. Include a copy of the medical record

showing the incorrect information and explain why it is incorrect. Send the letter in a way that lets you track it and confirm that someone received it, such as a certified mail.

Your health-care provider must respond to your request within 30 days and must notify other health-care providers who may have the same mistake in their records.

Review Your Credit Reports and Report Medical Billing Errors
- **Get your credit reports.** Get your free credit reports from the three credit bureaus at https://consumer.ftc.gov/articles/free-credit-reports.
- **Review your credit reports.** Look for medical billing errors, such as medical debt collection notices, that you do not recognize.
- **Report errors.** Report any medical billing errors to all three credit bureaus by following the "What To Do Next" steps on IdentityTheft.gov (www.identitytheft.gov/#/Steps).

Create a Personal Recovery Plan
A thief who uses your personal information to see a doctor, get prescription drugs, buy medical devices, submit claims with your insurance provider, or get other medical care may also use it in other situations. Go to IdentityTheft.gov website (www.identity-theft.gov) to create a personal recovery plan.[1]

---

[1] "What to Know about Medical Identity Theft," Federal Trade Commission (FTC), May 2021. Available online. URL: https://consumer.ftc.gov/articles/what-know-about-medical-identity-theft. Accessed February 15, 2024.

Part 5 | Prescription and Over-the-Counter Medications

Chapter 34 | Understanding Medications

Chapter Contents
Section 34.1—About Medication and Their Categories............321
Section 34.2—Medicine's Life inside the Body........................327
Section 34.3—Pharmacogenomics..329
Section 34.4—As You Age: You and Your Medications.............333

Section 34.1 | About Medication and Their Categories

Medicines can treat diseases and improve your health. If you are like most people, you need to take medicine at some point in your life. You may need to take medicine every day, or you may only need to take medicine once in a while. Either way, you want to make sure that your medicines are safe and that they will help you get better. In the United States, the U.S. Food and Drug Administration (FDA) is in charge of ensuring that your prescription and over-the-counter (OTC) medicines are safe and effective.

There are always risks associated with taking medicines. It is important to think about these risks before you take a medicine. Even safe medicines can cause unwanted side effects or interactions with food, alcohol, or other medicines you may be taking. Some medicines may not be safe during pregnancy. To reduce the risk of reactions and make sure that you get better, it is important for you to take your medicines correctly. You should also be careful when giving medicines to children, since they can be more vulnerable to the effects of medicines.[1]

WHAT ARE PRESCRIPTION DRUGS?
Prescription drugs are:
- prescribed by a doctor
- bought at a pharmacy
- prescribed for and intended to be used by one person
- regulated by the FDA through the New Drug Application (NDA) process (This is the formal step a drug sponsor takes to ask that the FDA considers approving a new drug for marketing in the United States. An NDA includes all animal and human data and analyses of the data, as well as information about how the drug behaves in the body and how it is manufactured.)

---

[1] MedlinePlus, "Medicines," National Institutes of Health (NIH), May 20, 2021. Available online. URL: https://medlineplus.gov/medicines.html. Accessed February 20, 2024.

WHAT ARE OVER-THE-COUNTER DRUGS?
Over-the-counter drugs are:
- drugs that do not require a doctor's prescription
- bought off-the-shelf in stores
- regulated by the FDA through OTC drug monographs (OTC drug monographs are a kind of "recipe book" covering acceptable ingredients, doses, formulations, and labeling. Monographs will continually be updated adding additional ingredients and labeling as needed. Products conforming to a monograph may be marketed without further FDA clearance, while those that do not, must undergo separate review and approval through the "New Drug Approval System.")[2]

HOW ARE THE MEDICATIONS CATEGORIZED?
The medications are categorized as follows:
- **Analgesics.** Drugs that relieve pain. There are two main types: nonnarcotic analgesics for mild pain and narcotic analgesics for severe pain.
- **Antacids.** Drugs that relieve indigestion and heartburn by neutralizing stomach acid.
- **Antianxiety drugs.** Drugs that suppress anxiety and relax muscles (sometimes called "anxiolytics," "sedatives," or "minor tranquilizers").
- **Antiarrhythmics.** Drugs used to control irregularities of a heartbeat.
- **Antibacterials.** Drugs used to treat infections.
- **Antibiotics.** Drugs made from naturally occurring and synthetic substances that combat bacterial infection. Some antibiotics are effective only against limited types of bacteria. Others, known as "broad-spectrum antibiotics," are effective against a wide range of bacteria.

---

[2] "Prescription Drugs and Over-the-Counter (OTC) Drugs: Questions and Answers," U.S. Food and Drug Administration (FDA), November 13, 2017. Available online. URL: www.fda.gov/drugs/frequently-asked-questions-popular-topics/prescription-drugs-and-over-counter-otc-drugs-questions-and-answers. Accessed February 20, 2024.

Understanding Medications

- **Anticoagulants and thrombolytics.** Anticoagulants prevent blood from clotting. Thrombolytics help dissolve and disperse blood clots and may be prescribed for patients with recent arterial or venous thrombosis.
- **Anticonvulsants.** Drugs that prevent epileptic seizures.
- **Antidepressants.** There are three main groups of mood-lifting antidepressants: tricyclics, monoamine oxidase inhibitors (MAOIs), and selective serotonin reuptake inhibitors (SSRIs).
- **Antidiarrheals.** Drugs used for the relief of diarrhea. Two main types of antidiarrheal preparations are simple adsorbent substances and drugs that slow down the contractions of the bowel muscles so that the contents are propelled more slowly.
- **Antiemetics.** Drugs used to treat nausea and vomiting.
- **Antifungals.** Drugs used to treat fungal infections, the most common of which affect the hair, skin, nails, or mucous membranes.
- **Antihistamines.** Drugs used primarily to counteract the effects of histamine, one of the chemicals involved in allergic reactions.
- **Antihypertensives.** Drugs that lower blood pressure. The types of antihypertensives marketed include diuretics, beta-blockers, calcium channel blockers, angiotensin-converting enzyme (ACE) inhibitors, and centrally acting antihypertensives and sympatholytics.
- **Antiinflammatories.** Drugs used to reduce inflammation—the redness, heat, swelling, and increased blood flow found in infections and in many chronic noninfective diseases such as rheumatoid arthritis (RA) and gout.
- **Antineoplastics.** Drugs used to treat cancer.
- **Antipsychotics.** Drugs used to treat symptoms of severe psychiatric disorders. These drugs are sometimes called "major tranquilizers."
- **Antipyretics.** Drugs that reduce fever.

- **Antivirals**. Drugs used to treat viral infections or to provide temporary protection against infections such as influenza.
- **Beta-blockers**. Beta-adrenergic blocking agents, or beta-blockers for short, reduce the oxygen needs of the heart by reducing the heartbeat rate.
- **Bronchodilators**. Drugs that open up the bronchial tubes within the lungs when the tubes have become narrowed by muscle spasm. Bronchodilators ease breathing in diseases such as asthma.
- **Cold cures**. Although there is no drug that can cure a cold, aches, pains, and fever that accompany a cold can be relieved by aspirin or acetaminophen often accompanied by a decongestant, antihistamine, and, sometimes, caffeine.
- **Corticosteroids**. These hormonal preparations are used primarily as antiinflammatories in arthritis or asthma or as immunosuppressives, but they are also useful for treating some malignancies or compensating for a deficiency of natural hormones in disorders such as Addison disease.
- **Cough suppressants**. Simple cough medicines, which contain substances, such as honey, glycerin, or menthol, soothe throat irritation but do not actually suppress coughing. They are most soothing when taken as lozenges and dissolved in the mouth. As liquids, they are probably swallowed too quickly to be effective. A few drugs are actually cough suppressants. There are two groups of cough suppressants:
    - those that alter the consistency or production of phlegm such as mucolytics and expectorants
    - those that suppress the coughing reflex such as codeine (narcotic cough suppressants), antihistamines, dextromethorphan, and isoproterenol (nonnarcotic cough suppressants)
- **Cytotoxins**. Drugs that kill or damage cells. Cytotoxins are used as antineoplastics (drugs used to treat cancer) and also as immunosuppressives.

Understanding Medications

- **Decongestants**. Drugs that reduce swelling of the mucous membranes that line the nose by constricting blood vessels, thus relieving nasal stuffiness.
- **Diuretics**. Drugs that increase the quantity of urine produced by the kidneys and passed out of the body, thus ridding the body of excess fluid. Diuretics reduce waterlogging of the tissues caused by fluid retention in disorders of the heart, kidneys, and liver. They are useful in treating mild cases of high blood pressure (HBP).
- **Expectorant**. A drug that stimulates the flow of saliva and promotes coughing to eliminate phlegm from the respiratory tract.
- **Hormones**. Chemicals produced naturally by the endocrine glands (thyroid, adrenal, ovary, testis, pancreas, and parathyroid). In some disorders, for example, diabetes mellitus, in which too little of a particular hormone is produced, synthetic equivalents or natural hormone extracts are prescribed to restore the deficiency. Such treatment is known as "hormone replacement therapy" (HRT).
- **Hypoglycemics (oral)**. Drugs that lower the level of glucose in the blood. Oral hypoglycemic drugs are used in diabetes mellitus if it cannot be controlled by diet alone but does require treatment with injections of insulin.
- **Immunosuppressives**. Drugs that prevent or reduce the body's normal reaction to invasion by disease or by foreign tissues. Immunosuppressives are used to treat autoimmune diseases (in which the body's defenses work abnormally and attack its own tissues) and to help prevent rejection of organ transplants.
- **Laxatives**. Drugs that increase the frequency and ease of bowel movements, either by stimulating the bowel wall (stimulant laxative), by increasing the bulk of bowel contents (bulk laxative), or by lubricating them (stool-softeners, or bowel movement-softeners). Laxatives may be taken by mouth or directly into the

lower bowel as suppositories or enemas. If laxatives are taken regularly, the bowels may ultimately become unable to work properly without them.
- **Muscle relaxants**. Drugs that relieve muscle spasm in disorders such as backache. Antianxiety drugs (minor tranquilizers) that also have a muscle-relaxant action are used most commonly.
- **Sex hormones (female)**. There are two groups of these hormones (estrogens and progesterone), which are responsible for development of female secondary sexual characteristics. Small quantities are also produced in males. As drugs, female sex hormones are used to treat menstrual and menopausal disorders and are also used as oral contraceptives. Estrogen may be used to treat cancer of the breast or prostate; progestins, a synthetic progesterone, are used to treat endometriosis.
- **Sex hormones (male)**. Androgenic hormones, of which the most powerful is testosterone, are responsible for development of male secondary sexual characteristics. Small quantities are also produced in females. As drugs, male sex hormones are given to compensate for hormonal deficiency in hypopituitarism or disorders of the testes. They may be used to treat breast cancer in women, but either synthetic derivatives called "anabolic steroids," which have less marked side effects, or specific antiestrogens are often preferred. Anabolic steroids also have a bodybuilding effect that has led to their (usually nonsanctioned) use in competitive sports, for both men and women.
- **Sleeping drugs**. The two main groups of drugs that are used to induce sleep are benzodiazepines and barbiturates. All such drugs have a sedative effect in low doses and are effective sleeping medications in higher doses. Benzodiazepine drugs are used more widely than barbiturates because they are safer, the side effects are less marked, and there is less risk of eventual physical dependence.

Understanding Medications

- **Tranquilizer.** This is a term commonly used to describe any drug that has a calming or sedative effect. However, the drugs that are sometimes called "minor tranquilizers" should be called "antianxiety drugs," and the drugs that are sometimes called "major tranquilizers" should be called "antipsychotics."
- **Vitamins.** Chemicals essential in small quantities for good health. Some vitamins are not manufactured by the body, but adequate quantities are present in a normal diet. People whose diets are inadequate or who have digestive tract or liver disorders may need to take supplementary vitamins.[3]

Section 34.2 | Medicine's Life inside the Body

Pharmacology is the scientific field that studies how the body reacts to medicines and how medicines affect the body. Scientists funded by the National Institutes of Health (NIH) are interested in many aspects of pharmacology, including one called "pharmacokinetics," which deals with understanding the entire cycle of a medicine's life inside the body.

Knowing more about each of the four main stages of pharmacokinetics—absorption, distribution, metabolism, and excretion—aids the design of medicines that are more effective and that produce fewer side effects.[4]

- **Absorption.** The body absorbs the medicine from its administration point into the bloodstream. The amount absorbed varies depending on the route of administration and the medicine's molecular properties.

---

[3] "General Drug Categories," U.S. Food and Drug Administration (FDA), December 7, 2015. Available online. URL: www.fda.gov/drugs/investigational-new-drug-ind-application/general-drug-categories. Accessed February 20, 2024.

[4] "A Medicine's Life inside the Body," National Institute of General Medical Sciences (NIGMS), May 2, 2014. Available online. URL: https://biobeat.nigms.nih.gov/2014/05/a-medicines-life-inside-the-body. Accessed February 20, 2024.

Pharmacologists determine the bioavailability of a medicine, or the percentage of the administered dose that gets into the blood. The lower the bioavailability, the less medicine enters the blood, and thus, it eventually reaches the therapeutic target, than was administered.

- **Distribution**. Once the medicine is in the bloodstream, the blood distributes it throughout the body. Blood permeates all the body's organs, so the medicine reaches all of them—but that is not always ideal for a medicine that needs to act only in a specific site. Sometimes pharmacologists can alter the chemical makeup of a molecule to make it more likely to reach the therapeutic target, whether that is a specific protein, tissue, or organ.
- **Metabolism**. The body sees medicines as foreign substances that need to be removed, and to help with that process, it can metabolize—or change the chemical structure of—the medicine. Most metabolism occurs via enzymes in the liver that make the medicine more water-soluble, but it can also occur in the intestines, skin, kidneys, lungs, or blood. Metabolism usually inactivates a medicine, so pharmacologists try to block that from happening to keep the active medicine around longer. Alternatively, they can exploit these enzymes by designing drugs to be administered in an inactive form that the metabolic enzymes will then activate.
- **Excretion**. Most medicines leave the body through the kidneys filtering them and their metabolites out of blood and into urine. Some are excreted into other bodily fluids such as bile, sweat, saliva, or milk. Pharmacologists study how the body eliminates medicines through a combination of metabolism and excretion, a process called "clearance." Understanding what organs are responsible for clearing a medicine is especially important when doctors are prescribing medications to patients with kidney or liver dysfunction.

Understanding Medications

Pharmacologists determine how the body acts on medicines under a variety of conditions before clinicians ever prescribe them to patients. Data from pharmacologists allow clinicians to choose the appropriate medicine, dose, and route of administration for their patients.[5]

Section 34.3 | Pharmacogenomics

WHAT IS PHARMACOGENOMICS?

Pharmacogenomics is an important example of the field of precision medicine, which aims to tailor medical treatment to each person or to a group of people. Pharmacogenomics looks at how your deoxyribonucleic acid (DNA) affects the way you respond to drugs. In some cases, your DNA can affect whether you have a bad reaction to a drug or whether a drug helps you or has no effect. Pharmacogenomics can improve your health by helping you know ahead of time whether a drug is likely to benefit you and be safe for you to take. Knowing this information can help your doctor find medicine that will work best for you.

HOW DOES PHARMACOGENOMICS WORK?

Drugs interact with your body in numerous ways, depending both on how you take the drug and where the drug acts in your body. After you take a drug, your body needs to break it down and get it to the intended area. Your DNA can affect multiple steps in this process to influence how you respond to the drug. Some examples of these interactions are as follows:
- **Drug receptors.** Some drugs need to attach to proteins on the surface of cells called "receptors" in order to

---

[5] "What Happens to Medicine in Your Body?" National Institute of General Medical Sciences (NIGMS), September 11, 2023. Available online. URL: https://biobeat.nigms.nih.gov/2023/09/what-happens-to-medicine-in-your-body. Accessed February 20, 2024.

work properly. Your DNA determines what type of receptors you have and how many, which can affect your response to the drug. You might need a higher or lower amount of the drug than most people or a different drug (see Figure 34.1).

- **Example: Breast cancer and trastuzumab emtansine (T-DM1).** Some breast cancers make too much human epidermal growth factor receptor 2 (HER2), and this extra HER2 helps cancer develop and spread. The drug T-DM1 can be used to treat this type of breast cancer and works by attaching to HER2 on cancerous cells and killing them. If you have breast cancer, your doctor may test a sample of your tumor to determine if T-DM1 is the right treatment for you. If your tumor has a high amount of HER2 (HER2-positive), your doctor may prescribe T-DM1. If your tumor does not have enough HER2 (HER2-negative), T-DM1 will not work for you.

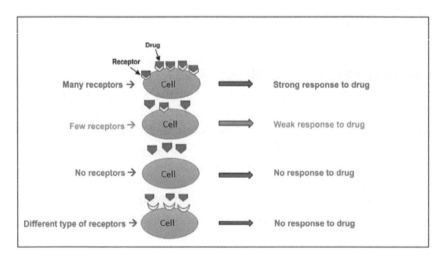

Figure 34.1. Drug Receptors

Centers for Disease Control and Prevention (CDC)

Understanding Medications

- **Drug uptake.** Some drugs need to be actively taken into the tissues and cells in which they act. Your DNA can affect uptake of certain drugs. Decreased uptake can mean that the drug does not work as well and can cause it to build up in other parts of your body, which can cause problems. Your DNA can also affect how quickly some drugs are removed from the cells in which they act. If drugs are removed from the cell too quickly, they might not have time to act (see Figure 34.2).
  - **Example: Statins and muscle problems.** Statins are a type of drug that act in the liver to help lower cholesterol. In order for statins to work correctly, they must first be taken into the liver. Statins are transported into the liver by a protein made by the *SLCO1B1* gene. Some people have a specific change in this gene that causes less of a statin called "simvastatin" to be taken into the liver. When taken at high doses, simvastatin can build up in the blood, causing muscle problems, including weakness and pain. Before prescribing simvastatin, your doctor may recommend genetic testing for the *SLCO1B1* gene to check if simvastatin is the best statin for you or to determine what dose would work best.

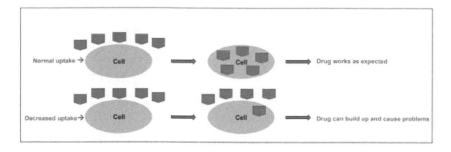

Figure 34.2. Drug Uptake

Centers for Disease Control and Prevention (CDC)

- **Drug breakdown.** Your DNA can affect how quickly your body breaks down a drug. If you break the drug down more quickly than most people, your body gets rid of the drug faster, and you might need more of the drug or a different drug. If your body breaks the drug down more slowly, you might need less of the drug (see Figure 34.3).
  - **Example: Depression and amitriptyline.** The breakdown of the antidepressant drug amitriptyline is influenced by two genes called "*CYP2D6*" and "*CYP2C19*." If your doctor prescribes amitriptyline, he or she might recommend genetic testing for the *CYP2D6* and *CYP2C19* genes to help decide what dose of the drug you need. If you break down amitriptyline too fast, you will need a higher dose for it to work, or you may need to use a different drug. If you break down amitriptyline very slowly, you will need to take a smaller dose or will need to take a different drug to avoid a bad reaction.

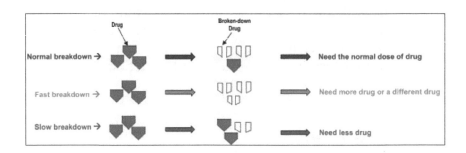

Figure 34.3. Drug Breakdown
Centers for Disease Control and Prevention (CDC)

- **Targeted drug development.** Pharmacogenomic approaches to drug development target the underlying problem rather than just treating symptoms. Some diseases are caused by specific changes (mutations) in a gene. The same gene can have different types of mutations, which have different effects. Some mutations may result in a protein that does not work correctly, while others may mean that the protein is not made at all. Drugs can be created based on how the mutation affects the protein, and these drugs will only work for a specific type of mutation.

- **Example: Cystic fibrosis (CF) and ivacaftor.** CF is caused by mutations in the *CFTR* gene, which affect the CFTR protein. The CFTR protein forms a channel, which acts as a passageway to move particles across the cells in your body. For most people, the protein is made correctly, and the channel can open and close. Some mutations that cause CF result in a channel that is closed. The drug ivacaftor acts on this type of mutation by forcing the channel open. Ivacaftor would not be expected to work for people with CF whose mutations cause the channel not to be made at all.

WHAT DOES THIS MEAN FOR YOUR HEALTH?

While pharmacogenomic testing is currently used for only a few drugs, the field is growing very quickly. Improved understanding of how pharmacogenomics can protect your health and improve your treatment will be increasingly important. Talk to your health-care provider about what pharmacogenomics might mean for your health.[6]

Section 34.4 | As You Age: You and Your Medications

As you get older, you may be faced with more health conditions that you need to treat on a regular basis. It is important to be aware that more use of medicines and normal body changes caused by

---

[6] "Pharmacogenomics: What Does It Mean for Your Health?" Centers for Disease Control and Prevention (CDC), May 20, 2022. Available online. URL: www.cdc.gov/genomics/disease/pharma.htm. Accessed February 20, 2024.

aging can increase the chance of unwanted or maybe even harmful drug interactions. The more you know about your medicines and the more you talk with your health-care professionals, the easier it is to avoid problems with medicines.

As you get older, body changes can affect the way medicines are absorbed and used. For example, changes in the digestive system can affect how fast medicines enter the bloodstream. Changes in body weight can influence the amount of medicine you need to take and how long it stays in your body. The circulatory system may slow down, which can affect how fast drugs get to the liver and kidneys. The liver and kidneys may also work more slowly, affecting the way a drug breaks down and is removed from the body.

DRUG INTERACTIONS

Because of these body changes, there is also a bigger risk of drug interactions among older adults. Therefore, it is important to know about drug interactions.

- **Drug-drug interactions**. These can happen when two or more medicines react with each other to cause unwanted effects. This kind of interaction can also cause one medicine to not work as well or even make one medicine stronger than it should be. For example, you should not take aspirin if you are taking a prescription blood thinner, such as warfarin, unless your health-care professional tells you to.
- **Drug-condition interactions**. These can happen when a medical condition you already have makes certain drugs potentially harmful. For example, if you have high blood pressure (HBP) or asthma, you could have an unwanted reaction if you take a nasal decongestant.
- **Drug-food interactions**. These result from drugs reacting with foods or drinks. In some cases, food in the digestive tract can affect how a drug is absorbed. Some medicines may also affect the way nutrients are absorbed or used in the body.
- **Drug-alcohol interactions**. These can happen when the medicine you take reacts with an alcoholic drink.

Understanding Medications

For instance, mixing alcohol with some medicines may cause you to feel tired and slow your reactions.

It is important to know that many medicines do not mix well with alcohol. As you grow older, your body may react differently to alcohol, as well as to the mix of alcohol and medicines. Keep in mind that some problems you might think are medicine-related, such as loss of coordination, memory loss, or irritability, could be the result of a mix between your medicine and alcohol.

What Side Effects Mean

Side effects are unplanned symptoms or feelings you have when taking a medicine. Most side effects are not serious and go away on their own; others can be more bothersome and even serious. To help prevent possible problems with medicines, seniors must know about the medicine they take and how it makes them feel.

Keep track of side effects to help your doctor know how your body is responding to a medicine. New symptoms or mood changes may not be a result of getting older but could be from the medicine you are taking or another factor, such as a change in diet or routine. If you have an unwanted side effect, call your doctor right away.

TALK TO YOUR TEAM OF HEALTH-CARE PROFESSIONALS

It is important to go to all your medical appointments and to talk to your team of health-care professionals (doctors, pharmacists, nurses, or physician assistants) about your medical conditions, the medicines you take, and any health concerns you have. Making a list of comments, questions, or concerns before your visit or call to a health-care professional may help. Also, think about having a close friend or relative come to your appointment with you if you are unsure about talking to your health-care professional or would prefer someone to help you understand and remember answers to your questions. Here are some other things to keep in mind:

- **All medicines count**. Tell your team of health-care professionals about all the medicines you take, including prescription and over-the-counter (OTC)

medicines, such as pain relievers, antacids, cold medicines, and laxatives. Do not forget to include eye drops, dietary supplements, vitamins, herbals, and topical medicines, such as creams and ointments.
- **Keep in touch with your doctors**. If you regularly take prescription medicine, ask your doctor to check how well it is working. Check to see whether you still need to take it and, if so, whether there is anything you can do to cut back. Do not stop taking the medicine on your own without first talking with your doctor.
- **Medical history**. Tell your health-care professional about your medical history. The doctor will want to know whether you have any food, medicine, or other allergies. He or she will also want to know about other conditions you have or had and how you are being treated or were treated for them by other doctors. It is helpful to keep a written list of your health conditions that you can easily share with your doctors. Your primary care doctor should also know about any specialist doctors you may see on a regular basis.
- **Eating habits**. Mention your eating habits. If you follow or have recently changed to a special diet (a very low-fat diet, for instance, or a high-calcium diet), talk to your doctor about this. Tell your doctor about how much coffee, tea, or alcohol you drink each day and whether you smoke. These things may make a difference in the way your medicine works.
- **Recognizing and remembering to take your medicines**. Let your health-care professional know whether you have trouble telling your medicines apart. The doctor can help you find better ways to recognize your medicines. Also, tell your doctor if you have problems remembering when to take your medicines or how much to take. Your doctor may have some ideas to help, such as a calendar or pillbox.
- **Swallowing tablets**. If you have trouble swallowing tablets, ask your doctor, nurse, or pharmacist for ideas. Maybe there is a liquid medicine you could use or

Understanding Medications

maybe you can crush your tablets. Do not break, crush, or chew tablets without first asking your health-care professional.
- **Your lifestyle**. If you want to make your medicine schedule more simple, talk about it with your doctor. He or she may have another medicine or other ideas. For example, if taking medicine four times a day is a problem for you, maybe the doctor can give you medicine you only need to take once or twice a day.
- **Put it in writing**. Ask your health-care professional to write out a complete medicine schedule, with directions on exactly when and how to take your medicines. Find out from your primary care doctor how your medicine schedule should be changed if you see more than one doctor.
- **Keep a record of your medicines**. List all prescription and OTC medicines, dietary supplements, vitamins, and herbals you take.

YOUR PHARMACIST CAN HELP, TOO

One of the most important services a pharmacist can offer is to talk to you about your medicines. A pharmacist can help you understand how and when to take your medicines, what side effects you might expect, or what interactions may occur. A pharmacist can answer your questions privately in the pharmacy or over the telephone.

Here are some other ways your pharmacist can help:
- Many pharmacists keep track of medicines on their computers. If you buy your medicines at one store and tell your pharmacist all the OTC and prescription medicines or dietary supplements you take, your pharmacist can help make sure your medicines do not interact harmfully with one another.
- Ask your pharmacist to place your prescription medicines in easy-to-open containers if you have a hard time taking off childproof caps and do not have young children living in or visiting your home. Remember to keep all medicines out of sight and reach of children.

- Your pharmacist may be able to print labels on prescription medicine containers in larger type if reading the medicine label is hard for you.
- Your pharmacist may be able to give you written information to help you learn more about your medicines.

WHAT TO ASK YOUR DOCTOR OR PHARMACIST
- What is the name of the medicine, and what is it supposed to do? Is there a less expensive alternative?
- How and when do I take the medicine and for how long?
- Should it be taken with water, food, or with a special medicine, or at the same time as other medicines?
- What do I do if I miss or forget a dose?
- Should it be taken before, during, or after meals?
- What is the proper dose? For example, does "four times a day" means you have to take it in the middle of the night?
- What does your doctor mean by "as needed"?
- Are there any other special instructions to follow?
- What foods, drinks, other medicines, dietary supplements, or activities should I avoid while taking this medicine?
- Will any tests or monitoring be required while I am taking this medicine? Do I need to report back to the doctor?
- What are the possible side effects, and what do I do if they occur?
- When should I expect the medicine to start working, and how will I know if it is working?
- Will this new prescription work safely with the other prescription and OTC medicines or dietary supplements I am taking?
- Do you have a patient profile form for me to fill out? Does it include space for my OTC drugs and any dietary supplements?
- Is there written information about my medicine? Ask the pharmacist to review the most important information with you. (Ask if it is available in large print or in a language other than English if you need it.)

Understanding Medications

- What is the most important thing I should know about this medicine? Ask the pharmacist any questions that may not have been answered by your doctor.
- Can I get a refill? If so, when?
- How and where should I store this medicine?

CUTTING MEDICINE COSTS

Medicines are an important part of treating an illness because they often allow people to remain active and independent. But medicine can be expensive. Here are some ideas to help lower costs:

- **Tell your doctor if you are worried about the cost of your medicine.** Your doctor may not know how much your prescription costs but may be able to tell you about another less expensive medicine, such as a generic drug or OTC product.
- **Ask for discount.** Ask for a discount if you are a senior citizen.
- **Shop around.** Look at prices at different stores or pharmacies. Lower medicine prices may not be a bargain if you need other services, such as home delivery, patient medication profiles, or pharmacist consultation, or if you cannot get a senior citizen discount.
- **Ask for medicine samples.** If your doctor gives you a prescription for a new medicine, ask your doctor for samples you can try before filling the prescription.
- **Buy bulk.** If you need to take medicine for a long period of time and your medicine does not expire quickly, you may be able to buy a larger amount of medicine for less money.
- **Try mail order.** Mail-order pharmacies can provide medications at lower prices. However, it is a good idea to talk with your doctor before using such a service. Make sure to find a backup pharmacy in case there is a problem with the mail service.[7]

---

[7] "As You Age: You and Your Medicines," U.S. Food and Drug Administration (FDA), February 19, 2019. Available online. URL: www.fda.gov/drugs/information-consumers-and-patients-drugs/you-age-you-and-your-medicines. Accessed February 20, 2024.

Chapter 35 | Using Medications Safely

For many people, taking medication is a regular part of their daily routine, and these medicines are relied upon to treat disease and improve health. Although medicines can make you feel better and help you get well, it is important to know that all medicines, both prescription and over the counter (OTC), have risks as well as benefits.

The benefits of medicines are the helpful effects you get when you use them, such as lowering blood pressure, curing infection, or relieving pain. The risks of medicines are the chances that something unwanted or unexpected could happen to you when you use them. Risks could be less serious things, such as an upset stomach, or more serious things, such as liver damage. Here are some tips from the U.S. Food and Drug Administration (FDA) and some of its public health partners to help you weigh the risks and benefits when you make decisions about the medicines you use.

When a medicine's benefits outweigh its known risks, the FDA considers it safe enough to approve. But before using any medicine—as with many things that you do every day—you should think through the benefits and the risks in order to make the best choice for you.

There are several types of risks from medicine use:
- the possibility of a harmful interaction between the medicine and a food, beverage, dietary supplement (including vitamins and herbals), or another medicine (Combinations of any of these products could increase the chance that there may be interactions.)
- the chance that the medicine may not work as expected
- the possibility that the medicine may cause additional problems

WAYS TO LOWER THE RISKS OF MEDICINES

Here are some specific ways to lower the risks and obtain the full benefits of medicines:

Talk with Your Doctor, Pharmacist, or Other Health-Care Professionals

- Keep an up-to-date, written list of all the medicines (prescription and OTC) and dietary supplements, including vitamins and herbals, that you use—even those you only use occasionally.
- Share this list with all of your health-care professionals.
- Tell them about any allergies or sensitivities that you may have.
- Tell them about anything that could affect your ability to take medicines, such as difficulty swallowing or remembering to take them.
- Tell them if you are or might become pregnant or if you are nursing a baby.
- Always ask your health-care professional questions about any concerns or thoughts that you may have.

Know Your Medicines: Prescription and Over the Counter

- the brand and generic names
- what they look like
- how to store them properly
- when, how, and how long to use them
- how and under what conditions you should stop using them
- what to do if you miss a dose
- what they are supposed to do and when to expect results
- side effects and interactions
- whether you need any tests or monitoring
- written information to take with you

Read the Label and Follow Directions

- Make sure you understand the directions; ask if you have questions or concerns.

Using Medications Safely

- Always double-check that you have the right medicine.
- Keep medicines in their original labeled containers, whenever possible.
- Never combine different medicines in the same bottle.
- Read and follow the directions on the label and the directions from your doctor, pharmacist, or other health-care professional. If you stop the medicine or want to use the medicine differently than directed, consult with your health-care professional.

Avoid Interactions

- Ask whether there are interactions with any other medicines or dietary supplements (including vitamins or herbal supplements), beverages, or foods.
- Use the same pharmacy for all of your medicine needs, whenever possible.
- Before starting any new medicine or dietary supplement (including vitamins or herbal supplements), ask again whether there are possible interactions with what you are currently using.

Monitor the Effects of Your Medicines and Other Products That You Use

- Ask whether there is anything you can do to minimize side effects, such as eating before you take a medicine to reduce stomach upset.
- Pay attention to how you are feeling; note any changes. Write down the changes so that you can remember to tell your doctor, pharmacist, or other health-care professional.
- Know what to do if you experience side effects and when to notify your doctor.
- Know when you should notice an improvement and when to report back.

Weighing the Risks, Making the Choice

The benefit-risk decision is sometimes difficult to make. The best choice depends on your particular situation.

You must decide what risks you can and will accept in order to get the benefits you want. For example, if facing a life-threatening illness, you might choose to accept more risk in the hope of getting the benefits of a cure or living a longer life. On the other hand, if you are facing a minor illness, you might decide that you want to take very little risk. In many situations, the expert advice of your doctor, pharmacist, or other health-care professionals can help you make the decision.[1]

TIPS FOR TALKING WITH YOUR PHARMACIST

Your pharmacist can help you learn how to use your prescription and OTC medicines safely and effectively. You can also use these tips when talking with your other health-care providers.

Tell Your Pharmacist

- every medicine you use, especially if you use multiple pharmacies, even if it is the same pharmacy chain:
  - Keep a record and give it to your pharmacist. List all the prescription and OTC medicines, vitamins, herbals, and other supplements you use. Tell your pharmacist exactly how you are taking the medicine.
  - Do not forget to tell your pharmacist about any changes to your medicines. This includes anything you have stopped taking.
- if you have had any allergic reactions or problems with medicines, dietary supplements, food, medical devices, or other medical treatments
  - What kind of reaction did you have? Did your throat swell up? Did you get a rash? Or was it a stomach ache or diarrhea?
- any medical conditions you have or have had, including any abnormal lab results

---

[1] "Think It Through: Managing the Benefits and Risks of Medicines," U.S. Food and Drug Administration (FDA), June 18, 2018. Available online. URL: www.fda.gov/drugs/information-consumers-and-patients-drugs/think-it-through-managing-benefits-and-risks-medicines. Accessed February 16, 2024.

Using Medications Safely

- anything that could affect your use of medicine, such as trouble with swallowing, reading small labels, understanding English, remembering to take your medicine, distinguishing the look of one medicine from another, paying for medicines, or transportation to the pharmacy (Your pharmacist may be able to help, so just ask!)
- if you plan to start or have started something new such as a new medicine, supplement, diet, or exercise regime (Your pharmacist can help you avoid medicines, supplements, foods, and other things that do not mix well with your medicines.)
- if you are pregnant, plan to become pregnant, are breastfeeding, or plan to breastfeed
- the best phone number to reach you and your present address (This is in case the pharmacist has any questions for you or if there are any issues. If you prefer to receive text messages instead of phone calls, let your pharmacy know! Many pharmacies have the ability to text.)
- if there have been any changes to your insurance plan/policy/card

Ask Your Pharmacist
- What is the most important information I should know about this medicine?
- How do I pronounce the name of my medicine? Does it go by any other name(s)? What are the brand and generic (nonbrand) names?
- Are there any cheaper options? Is a generic available? Are there any co-pay assistance coupons?
- How does this medicine work, and what is it used for?
- How and when should I use it? How much do I use? Should I take it with food or without food, before a meal or after a meal? What time of the day should I use it? How many times a day is it used? Is there a limit on how often I should use it?
- How long should I use it? Can I stop using the medicine or use less if I feel better? In what circumstances should I stop taking this medicine?

- What should I do if I ...miss a dose? ....throw up shortly after taking a dose? ....use too much? ....lose the medicine?
- Will this take the place of anything else I am taking?
- When will the medicine start working? How should I expect to feel?
- Are there any special directions for using this?
- Should I avoid any other medicines, dietary supplements, drinks, foods, activities, or other things? Do I have to space this medicine out from any other medicines or food?
- Does this medicine contain any ingredients I am allergic to?
- Is there anything I should watch for, such as allergic reactions or side effects? What are the serious side effects? What do I do if I get any?
- Will I need any tests to check the medicine's effects (blood tests, x-rays, and other)? When will I need those?
- How and where should I store this medicine? Is it stored at room temperature or refrigerated or frozen? What should I do if I left it in a hot car?
- When should I throw out this medicine? When does it expire?
- Is there a medication guide or other patient information for this medicine?
- Where and how can I get more written information?
- When should I contact my doctor about this medicine? In what situation should I call 911?

Before You Leave the Pharmacy after Picking Up Your Prescription

- **Look to be sure you have the right medicine.** If you have bought the medicine before, make sure this medicine has the same shape, color, size, markings, and packaging. Anything different? Do not hesitate to ask your pharmacist. If it seems different when you use it, tell your pharmacist, doctor, or other health-care professional.
- **Be sure you know the right dose for the medicine, and you know how to use it.** Unsure about anything? Ask your pharmacist.

Using Medications Safely

- **For liquid medicines, make sure there is a measuring spoon, cup, or syringe.** If the medicine does not come with a special measuring tool, ask your pharmacist for one. (Spoons used for eating and cooking may give the wrong dose. Do not use them.)
- **Be sure you have any information the pharmacist can give you about the medicine.** Read it and save it.
- **Get the pharmacy's phone number and hours, so you can call back for any questions or refills.**[2]

---

[2] "Stop - Learn - Go: Tips for Talking with Your Pharmacist to Learn How to Use Medicines Safely," U.S. Food and Drug Administration (FDA), October 15, 2019. Available online. URL: www.fda.gov/drugs/resources-drugs/stop-learn-go-tips-talking-your-pharmacist-learn-how-use-medicines-safely. Accessed February 16, 2024.

Chapter 36 | Over-the-Counter Medicines

Over-the-counter (OTC) medicines are drugs you can buy without a prescription. American medicine cabinets contain a growing choice of nonprescription, OTC medicines to treat an expanding range of ailments. OTC medicines often do more than relieve aches, pains, and itches. Some can prevent diseases such as tooth decay, cure diseases such as athlete's foot, and, with a doctor's guidance, help manage recurring conditions such as vaginal yeast infection, migraine, and minor pain in arthritis.

The U.S. Food and Drug Administration (FDA) determines whether medicines are prescription or nonprescription. The term "prescription" (Rx) refers to medicines that are safe and effective when used under a doctor's care. Nonprescription or OTC drugs are medicines the FDA decides are safe and effective for use without a doctor's prescription.

The FDA also has the authority to decide when a prescription drug is safe enough to be sold directly to consumers over the counter. This regulatory process allowing Americans to take a more active role in their health care is known as the "Rx-to-OTC switch." As a result of this process, more than 700 products sold over the counter today use ingredients or dosage strengths available only by prescription 30 years ago.

Increased access to OTC medicines is especially important for our maturing population. Two out of three older Americans rate their health as excellent to good, but four out of five report at least one chronic condition.

Fact is, the OTC medicines offer greater opportunity to treat more of the aches and illnesses most likely to appear in our later years. As we live longer, work longer, and take a more active role in our own health care, the need grows to become better informed about self-care.

The best way to become better informed—for young and old alike—is to read and understand the information on OTC labels. Next to the medicine itself, label comprehension is the most important part of self-care with OTC medicines.

With new opportunities in self-medication come new responsibilities and an increased need for knowledge. The FDA and the Consumer Healthcare Products Association (CHPA) have prepared the following information to help Americans take advantage of self-care opportunities.

OVER-THE-COUNTER MEDICINES KNOW-HOW: IT IS ON THE LABEL

You would not ignore your doctor's instructions for using a prescription drug so do not ignore the label when taking an OTC medicine. Here is what to look for:

- **Product name**. The brand name or generic name of the product.
- **Active ingredients**. Therapeutic substances in medicine.
- **Purpose**. Product category such as antihistamine, antacid, or cough suppressant.
- **Uses**. Symptoms or diseases the product will treat or prevent.
- **Warnings**. When not to use the product, when to stop taking it, when to see a doctor, and possible side effects.
- **Directions**. How much to take, how to take it, and how long to take it.
- **Other information**. Such as storage information.
- **Inactive ingredients**. Substances such as binders, colors, or flavoring.

You can help yourself read the label too.

Always remember to look for the statement describing the tamper-evident feature(s) before you buy the product and when you use it.

When it comes to medicines, more does not necessarily mean better. You should never misuse OTC medicines by taking them

Over-the-Counter Medicines

longer or in higher doses than the label recommends. Symptoms that persist are a clear signal it is time to see a doctor.

Be sure to read the label each time you purchase a product. Just because two or more products are from the same brand family does not mean they are meant to treat the same conditions or contain the same ingredients.

Remember, if you read the label and still have questions, talk to a doctor, nurse, or pharmacist.

DRUG INTERACTIONS: A WORD TO THE WISE

Although mild and relatively uncommon, interactions involving OTC drugs can produce unwanted results or make medicines less effective. It is especially important to know about drug interactions if you are taking prescription and OTC drugs at the same time.

Some drugs can also interact with foods and beverages, as well as with health conditions such as diabetes, kidney disease, and high blood pressure (HBP).

Here are a few drug interaction cautions for some common OTC ingredients:

- Avoid alcohol if you are taking antihistamines, cough-cold products with the ingredient dextromethorphan, or drugs that treat sleeplessness.
- Do not use drugs that treat sleeplessness if you are taking prescription sedatives or tranquilizers.
- Check with your doctor before taking products containing aspirin if you are taking a prescription blood thinner or if you have diabetes or gout.
- Do not use laxatives when you have stomach pain, nausea, or vomiting.
- Unless directed by a doctor, do not use a nasal decongestant if you are taking a prescription drug for HBP or depression, or if you have heart or thyroid disease, diabetes, or prostate problems.

This is not a complete list. Read the label! Drug labels change as new information becomes available. That is why it is important to read the label each time you take medicine.

TIME FOR A MEDICINE CABINET CHECKUP
- Be sure to look through your medicine supply at least once a year.
- Always store medicines in a cool, dry place or as stated on the label.
- Throw away any medicines that are past the expiration date.
- To make sure no one takes the wrong medicine, keep all medicines in their original containers.

PREGNANCY AND BREASTFEEDING
Drugs can pass from a pregnant woman to her unborn baby. A safe amount of medicine for the mother may be too much for the unborn baby. If you are pregnant, always talk with your doctor before taking any drugs, prescription or OTC.

Although most drugs pass into breast milk in concentrations too low to have any unwanted effects on the baby, breastfeeding mothers still need to be careful. Always ask your doctor or pharmacist before taking any medicine while breastfeeding. A doctor or pharmacist can tell you how to adjust the timing and dosing of most medicines so that the baby is exposed to the lowest amount possible, or whether the drugs should be avoided altogether.

OVER-THE-COUNTER DRUGS FOR KIDS
Over-the-counter drugs rarely come in one-size-fits-all. Here are some tips about giving OTC medicines to children:
- Children are not just small adults so do not estimate the dose based on their size.
- Read the label. Follow all directions.
- Follow any age limits on the label.
- Some OTC products come in different strengths. Be aware!
- Know the difference between a tablespoon (tbsp.) and a teaspoon (tsp.). They are very different doses.
- Be careful about converting dose instructions. If the label says two teaspoons, it is best to use a measuring

Over-the-Counter Medicines

spoon or a dosing cup marked in teaspoons, not a common kitchen spoon.
- Do not play doctor. Do not double the dose just because your child seems sicker than last time.
- Before you give your child two medicines at the same time, talk to your doctor or pharmacist.
- Never let children take medicine by themselves.
- Never call medicine candy to get your kids to take it. If they come across the medicine on their own, they are likely to remember that you called it "candy."

CHILD-RESISTANT PACKAGING

Child-resistant closures are designed for repeated use to make it difficult for children to open. Remember, if you do not relock the closure after each use, the child-resistant device cannot do its job—keeping children out!

It is best to store all medicines and dietary supplements where children can neither see nor reach them. Containers of pills should not be left on the kitchen counter as a reminder. Purses and briefcases are among the worst places to hide medicines from curious kids. And, since children are natural mimics, it is a good idea not to take medicine in front of them. They may be tempted to "play house" with your medicine later on.

PROTECT YOURSELF AGAINST TAMPERING

Makers of OTC medicines seal most products in tamper-evident packaging (TEP) to help protect against criminal tampering. TEP works by providing visible evidence if the package has been disturbed. But OTC packaging cannot be 100 percent tamper-proof. Here is how to help protect yourself:
- Be alert to the tamper-evident features on the package before you open it. These features are described on the label.
- Inspect the outer packaging before you buy it. When you get home, inspect the medicine inside.
- Do not buy an OTC product if the packaging is damaged.

- Do not use any medicine that looks discolored or different in any way.
- If anything looks suspicious, be suspicious. Contact the store where you bought the product. Take it back!
- Never take medicines in the dark.[1]

---

[1] "Over-the-Counter Medicines: What Is Right for You?" U.S. Food and Drug Administration (FDA), September 3, 2013. Available online. URL: www.fda.gov/drugs/choosing-right-over-counter-medicine-otcs/over-counter-medicines-whats-right-you. Accessed February 16, 2024.

Chapter 37 | Buying Prescription Drugs

Chapter Contents

Section 37.1—Using Your Health Insurance Coverage
          for Getting Prescription Medications................ 357
Section 37.2—Cost May Result in Underuse of
          Medications.. 359
Section 37.3—E-prescribing 361
Section 37.4—Safely Purchase Prescription
          Medicine Online 362
Section 37.5—Truth in Advertising: Advertisements for
          Prescription Drugs.. 364
Section 37.6—Imported Drugs Raise Safety Concerns............ 367

Section 37.1 | **Using Your Health Insurance Coverage for Getting Prescription Medications**

Health plans will help pay the cost of certain prescription medications. You may be able to buy other medications, but medications on your plan's formulary (approved list) usually will be less expensive for you.

DOES YOUR NEW INSURANCE PLAN COVER YOUR PRESCRIPTION?

To find out which prescriptions are covered through your new Marketplace plan, do the following:
- Visit your insurer's website to review a list of prescriptions your plan covers.
- See your Summary of Benefits and Coverage (SBC), which you can get directly from your insurance company or by using a link that appears in the detailed description of your plan in your Marketplace account.
- Call your insurer directly to find out what is covered. Have your plan information available. The number is available on your insurance card, the insurer's website, or the detailed plan description in your Marketplace account.
- Review any coverage materials that your plan mailed to you.

WHAT DO YOU DO IF YOU ARE AT THE PHARMACY TO PICK UP YOUR PRESCRIPTION AND THEY SAY YOUR PLAN NO LONGER COVERS IT?

Some insurance companies may provide a onetime refill for your medication after you first enroll. Ask your insurance company if they offer a onetime refill until you can discuss next steps with your doctor.

If you cannot get a onetime refill, you have the right to follow your insurance company's drug exceptions process, which allows you to get a prescribed drug that is not normally covered by your health plan. Because the details of every plan's exceptions process are different, you should contact your insurance company for more information.

Generally, to get your drug covered through the exceptions process, your doctor must confirm to your health plan (orally or in writing) that the drug is appropriate for your medical condition based on one or more of the following:

- All other drugs covered by the plan have not been or would not be as effective as the drug you are asking for.
- Any alternative drug covered by your plan has caused or is likely to cause side effects that may be harmful to you.
- If there is a limit on the number of doses you are allowed:
  - that the allowed dosage has not worked for your condition
  - the drug likely would not work for you based on your physical or mental makeup (e.g., Based on your body weight, you may need to take more doses than what is allowed by your plan.)

If you get the exception:

- your health plan generally will treat the drug as covered and charge you the co-payment that applies to the most expensive drugs already covered on the plan (e.g., a nonpreferred brand drug)
- any amount you pay for the drug generally will count toward your deductible and/or maximum out-of-pocket limits

CAN YOU GET THE NONCOVERED DRUG DURING THE EXCEPTIONS PROCESS?

While you are in the exceptions process, your plan may give you access to the requested drug until a decision is made.

YOUR INSURER DENIED YOUR REQUEST FOR AN EXCEPTION. NOW WHAT DO YOU DO?

If your health insurance company will not pay for your prescription, you have the right to appeal the decision and have it reviewed by an independent third party.

Buying Prescription Drugs

CAN YOU GO TO YOUR REGULAR PHARMACY TO GET YOUR MEDICATION?

Just like different health plans cover different medications, different health plans allow you to get your medications from different pharmacies (called "in-network pharmacies"). Call your insurance company or visit their website to find out whether your regular pharmacy is in-network under your new plan and, if not, what pharmacies in your area are in-network. You can also learn if you can get your prescription delivered in the mail.[1]

Section 37.2 | Cost May Result in Underuse of Medications

Little is known about the role of positive financial behaviors (behaviors that allow maintenance of financial stability with financial resources) in mitigating cost-related nonadherence (CRN) to health regimens.

One in four Americans reports financial difficulty in paying medical bills; this difficulty has significant public health implications, especially for the 50 percent of the population that is managing chronic illness. Seven systematic reviews concluded that several factors influence adherence to treatment, but the cost to the patient is one that demonstrates a consistent negative effect. Nearly 18 percent of chronically ill Americans report underusing medications and delaying or not fulfilling therapeutic recommendations because of cost, which is referred to as "CRN" and varies by therapeutic class across chronic therapies. Nearly 56 percent of American adults with common chronic diseases self-report non-fulfillment of medication as a result of financial hardship.

Health insurance coverage is a strong predictor of financial burden. Nearly half of Americans have literacy challenges with health insurance and pay more for health care out of pocket because of

---

[1] "Getting Prescription Medications," Centers for Medicare & Medicaid Services (CMS), October 4, 2014. Available online. URL: www.healthcare.gov/using-marketplace-coverage/prescription-medications. Accessed February 16, 2024.

these challenges, despite improvements as a result of the Affordable Care Act (ACA).

Although health literacy and health insurance literacy are commonly discussed as integral for individuals to have the capacity to obtain, process, and understand basic health information or services and health insurance, financial literacy in the context of health has received little attention. Financial literacy is a set of skills and knowledge that allows individuals to make informed decisions with their financial resources, and it is associated with more frequent engagement in health-promoting behaviors. Studies show that social determinants of health that contribute to financial burden correlate with CRN. Therefore, financial burden may be experienced in the context of a growing concern for financial insecurity and may not be exclusively health related. Given the role that cost to the patient plays in adherence to therapeutic regimens, improving financial literacy to influence positive financial behaviors (behaviors that allow individuals to maintain financial stability with their financial resources) may have implications for CRN and may be a necessary adjunct to policy reforms.

Few interventions have aimed to mitigate CRN beyond reducing out-of-pocket costs, which have shown modest improvements in health status. Whether positive financial behavior is protective of CRN has not been explored and may have implications for behavioral interventions to promote financial literacy, especially among people who have chronic illnesses.

An intervention strategy focused on improving financial literacy may be relevant for high-risk groups who report high levels of financial stress.[2]

---

[2] "Effect of Financial Stress and Positive Financial Behaviors on Cost-Related Nonadherence to Health Regimens among Adults in a Community-Based Setting," Centers for Disease Control and Prevention (CDC), April 7, 2016. Available online. URL: www.cdc.gov/pcd/issues/2016/16_0005.htm. Accessed February 16, 2024.

Section 37.3 | E-prescribing

Electronic prescribing (e-prescribing) enables a prescriber to electronically send an accurate, error-free, and understandable prescription directly to a pharmacy from the point of care and is an important element in improving the quality of patient care. The inclusion of e-prescribing in the Medicare Modernization Act (MMA) of 2003 gave momentum to the movement, and the July 2006 Institute of Medicine (IOM) report on the role of e-prescribing in reducing medication errors received widespread publicity, helping build awareness of e-prescribing's role in enhancing patient safety. Adopting the standards to facilitate e-prescribing is one of the key action items in the federal government's plan to expedite the adoption of electronic medical records and build a national electronic health information infrastructure in the United States.[3]

THE BENEFITS OF E-PRESCRIBING

e-Prescribing allows health-care providers to enter prescription information into a computer device—such as tablet, laptop, or desktop computer—and securely transmit the prescription to pharmacies using a special software program and connectivity to a transmission network. When a pharmacy receives a request, it can begin filling the medication right away.

e-prescribing can:
- help improve health-care quality and patient safety by reducing medication errors and checking for drug interactions
- make care more convenient by allowing providers to electronically request prescription refills

e-Prescribing is more convenient, cheaper, and safer for doctors, pharmacies, and patients.[4]

---

[3] "E-Prescribing," Centers for Medicare & Medicaid Services (CMS), February 22, 2024. Available online. URL: www.cms.gov/medicare/regulations-guidance/electronic-prescribing. Accessed February 16, 2024.
[4] HealthIT.gov, "What Is Electronic Prescribing?" Office of the National Coordinator for Health Information Technology (ONC), September 10, 2019. Available online. URL: www.healthit.gov/faq/what-electronic-prescribing. Accessed February 16, 2024.

Section 37.4 | Safely Purchase Prescription Medicine Online

Protect yourself and your family by being cautious when buying medicine online. Some pharmacy websites operate legally and offer convenience, privacy, cost savings, and safeguards for purchasing medicines.

Not all websites are the same. The U.S. Food and Drug Administration (FDA) warns that there are many unsafe online pharmacies that claim to sell prescription drugs at deeply discounted prices, often without requiring a prescription. These Internet-based pharmacies often sell unapproved, counterfeit or otherwise unsafe medicines outside the safeguards followed by licensed pharmacies.

Many unsafe online pharmacies use fake "storefronts" to mimic licensed pharmacies or to make you think their medicines come from countries with high safety standards. But the medicines they sell could have been made anywhere, with little care or concern for safety and effectiveness. Also, these drugs could be fake, expired, or otherwise unsafe for you and your family.

How can you tell if an online pharmacy is operating legally? The FDA's BeSafeRx page (www.fda.gov/drugs/quick-tips-buying-medicines-over-internet/besaferx-your-source-online-pharmacy-information) has resources and tools to help you make safer and more informed decisions when buying prescription medicines online.

WARNING SIGNS OF AN UNSAFE ONLINE PHARMACY

Beware of online pharmacies that:
- do not require a doctor's prescription
- are not licensed in the United States and by your state board of pharmacy
- do not have a licensed pharmacist on staff to answer your questions
- send medicine that looks different from what you receive at your usual pharmacy or arrives in packaging that is broken, is damaged, is in a foreign language, has no expiration date, or is expired

- offer deep discounts or prices that seem too good to be true
- charge you for products you never ordered or received
- do not provide clear written protections of your personal and financial information
- sell your information to other websites

These pharmacies often sell medicines that can be dangerous because they may:
- have too much or too little of the active ingredient you need to treat your disease or condition
- not contain the right active ingredient
- contain the wrong ingredients or other harmful substances

The active ingredient of an approved drug product is what makes the medicine effective for the illness or condition it is intended to treat. If a medicine has unknown active ingredients, it could fail to have the intended effect, could have an unexpected interaction with other medicines you are taking, could cause dangerous side effects, or could cause other serious health problems, such as serious allergic reactions.

Also, these drugs may not have been stored properly, such as in a warehouse without necessary temperature controls, which may cause the medicine to be ineffective in treating your condition.

KNOW THE SIGNS OF A SAFE ONLINE PHARMACY

There are ways you can identify a safe online pharmacy. These pharmacies:
- always require a doctor's prescription
- provide a physical address and telephone number in the United States
- have a licensed pharmacist on staff to answer your questions
- are licensed with a state board of pharmacy

Another way to help ensure you are using a safe and legal online pharmacy is to check the pharmacy's license in the state's board of pharmacy license database by using the location tool (www.fda.gov/drugs/besaferx-your-source-online-pharmacy-information/locate-state-licensed-online-pharmacy) on the FDA's BeSafeRx website. If your online pharmacy is not listed, do not use that pharmacy.[5]

Section 37.5 | Truth in Advertising: Advertisements for Prescription Drugs

Your health-care provider is the best source of information about the right medicines for you. Prescription drug advertisements can provide useful information for consumers to work with their health-care providers to make wise decisions about treatment. The following are the correct versions of different types of drug ads.

If you think a prescription drug ad violates the law, contact (www.fda.gov/about-fda/center-drug-evaluation-and-research-cder/office-prescription-drug-promotion-opdp) the U.S. Food and Drug Administration's (FDA) Office of Prescription Drug Promotion (OPDP).

CORRECT PRODUCT CLAIM AD

A product claim ad names a drug, says what condition it treats, and talks about both its benefits and its risks. An ad must present the benefits and risks of a prescription drug in a balanced fashion. Balance depends on both the information in the ad itself and how the information is presented.

- **Identifying drug brands.** Product claim ads must identify the drug's brand and generic names.
- **Product claim ads must accurately state an FDA-approved use for the drug.** In addition, the ad may

---

[5] "How to Buy Medicines Safely from an Online Pharmacy," U.S. Food and Drug Administration (FDA), November 16, 2022. Available online. URL: www.fda.gov/consumers/consumer-updates/how-buy-medicines-safely-online-pharmacy. Accessed February 16, 2024.

not make a claim that is not supported by substantial evidence or substantial clinical experience.
- **Prescription requirement**. Product claim ads should say that the drug is given by prescription only.
- **The ad should provide the required fair balance of information about the risks and benefits of the drug.** The ad as a whole should not put more emphasis on the drug's benefits than its risks.
- **If a person is pictured in an ad, he or she should be in the approved age range for users of the drug.**
- **As required by the Food and Drug Administration Amendments Act (FDAAA) of 2007, print ads must include the statement "You are encouraged to report negative side effects of prescription drugs to the FDA."**
- **Print ads must include a "brief summary" of all the risks listed in the drug's FDA-approved prescribing information**. The brief summary contains one or more pages of important information about a drug's risks. The brief summary usually follows the part of the ad that displays colorful images and graphics.
- **The ad should direct the reader to seek a doctor's advice about taking the drug.** The drug company should include this statement as a way to ensure that a consumer will not think he or she is qualified to make the prescribing decision.
- **Information sources in ads**. Product claim ads may provide sources of further information, such as a website and toll-free telephone number.

CORRECT REMINDER AD

Reminder ads give the drug's name but not the drug's use. The assumption behind reminder ads is that the audience knows what the drug is for and does not need to be told. A reminder ad does not contain risk information about the drug because the ad does not discuss the condition treated or how well the drug works.

Reminder ads are not appropriate for drugs whose labeling has a "boxed warning" about certain very serious drug risks.

- **The ad does not describe or name the condition the drug treats or make dosage recommendations.** Notice that neither allergies nor any allergy symptoms are mentioned or pictured.
- **Reminder ads must identify the drug's brand name (if it has one) and its generic name.**

CORRECT HELP-SEEKING AD

Help-seeking ads describe a disease or condition but do not recommend or suggest specific drugs. Help-seeking ads may include a drug company's name and may also provide a telephone number to call for more information. The FDA does not regulate lawful help-seeking ads. They are regulated by the Federal Trade Commission (FTC). However, if an apparent help-seeking ad references a particular drug, it is no longer a help-seeking ad, and the FDA regulates it.

- The help-seeking ad should not show an image of a specific drug.
- This help-seeking ad should identify the symptoms of a condition without identifying a possible drug treatment.
- Any help-seeking ad may recommend that readers seek the advice of their health-care provider.
- While this ad may not name a drug, it may identify the company sponsoring the ad and provide a telephone number to call or a website to visit for more information.[6]

---

[6] "Prescription Drug Advertising," U.S. Food and Drug Administration (FDA), July 8, 2019. Available online. URL: www.fda.gov/drugs/information-consumers-and-patients-drugs/prescription-drug-advertising. Accessed February 16, 2024.

Section 37.6 | Imported Drugs Raise Safety Concerns

Under the Federal Food, Drug, and Cosmetic (FD&C) Act, the interstate shipment of any prescription drug that lacks required U.S. Food and Drug Administration (FDA) approval is illegal. Interstate shipment includes importation—bringing drugs from a foreign country into the United States.

Drugs sold in the United States must also have proper labeling that conforms with the FDA's requirements and must be made in accordance with good manufacturing practices. As part of the FDA's high standards, drugs can be manufactured only at plants registered with the agency, whether those facilities are domestic or foreign. If a foreign firm is listed as a manufacturer or supplier of a drug's ingredients on a new drug application, the FDA generally travels to that site to inspect it.

After the FDA approves a drug, manufacturers are still subject to FDA inspections and must continue to comply with good manufacturing practices. "With an unapproved drug, you can't be sure that it has been shipped, handled, and stored under conditions that meet U.S. requirements," Joe McCallion, a Consumer Safety Officer (CSO) in the FDA's Office of Regulatory Affairs (ORA), says.

Along with legal requirements on manufacturing, U.S. pharmacists and wholesalers must be licensed or authorized in the states where they operate and limits on how drugs can be distributed lessen the likelihood that counterfeit or poor-quality drugs will turn up. It is because of such safeguards that the process of getting drugs onto U.S. pharmacy shelves is commonly referred to as a "closed distribution system."

Counterfeit drugs—phony replicas of pharmaceuticals—can surface anywhere. Historically, they have been more common in foreign countries than in the United States. And, while the Internet has given customers the convenience of buying drugs from the privacy of their own homes, it has also opened up windows for crooks to crawl through.

In an investigation that ended in the indictment of seven people and five companies in the spring of 2002, undercover agents in the Manhattan District Attorney's Office in New York bought more than 25,000 counterfeit Viagra pills. They pretended to sell the impotence pills and uncovered four supply streams from China and India.

Some of the little blue pills arrived in the mail stuffed inside a teddy bear and stereo speakers. The exporters used a machine to punch the pills with Pfizer's logo, and intermediaries sold the pills over the Internet to brokers and consumers.

In this case, all the counterfeit pills tested had some of Viagra's active ingredient (sildenafil citrate) with varying potency, according to Barbara Thompson, a spokeswoman for the Manhattan District Attorney's Office. "With fake drugs, you could be getting some of an active ingredient, or you could be getting nothing at all," she says.

That is what happened with a batch of Viagra worth $150,000 that Health Authority Law Enforcement Task Force (HALT), an organization of police officers and other law enforcement personnel with special training in pharmaceuticals, seized from Los Angeles gift shops. "It looked perfect," says Daniel Hancz, a pharmacist with the HALT. "But there was nothing there—just lactose, dye, and other filling agents."

LIMITS ON REIMPORTATION

The FD&C Act also states that prescription drugs made in the United States and exported to a foreign country can only be reimported by the drug's original manufacturer. Even when original manufacturers reimport drugs, the drugs must be real, properly handled, and relabeled for sale in the United States if necessary.

The Medicine Equity and Drug Safety (MEDS) Act, enacted in 2000, would have allowed prescription drugs manufactured in the United States and exported to certain foreign countries to be reimported from those countries for sale to American consumers. Supporters of the bill hoped that lower drug pricing in other countries would be passed along to consumers. But former U.S. Department of Health and Human Services (HHS) Secretary Tommy G. Thompson responded by saying that, while he believed strongly in access to affordable drugs, he could not implement the act because it would sacrifice public safety by opening up the closed distribution system in the United States.

Though the law was enacted in 2000, before the bill can take effect, one provision requires that the HHS secretary determines whether adequate safety could be maintained and whether costs could be reduced significantly. Both Thompson and his predecessor, Donna Shalala, concluded that these conditions could not be guaranteed.

"Once an FDA-approved prescription drug is exported for sale in another country, it is no longer subject to U.S. requirements, and it can no longer be monitored by U.S. regulators," Thompson wrote in a letter to Sen. James Jeffords, Ind-Vt., one of the bill's sponsors. "In addition, it may not have the U.S.-approved labeling. Instead, it may have labeling for the country to which it is exported."

GUIDANCE ON PERSONAL USE

Although importing unapproved prescription drugs is illegal, the FDA's guidance on importing prescription drugs for personal use recognizes that there may be circumstances in which the FDA can exercise discretion to not take action against the illegal importation.

The personal use guidance was first adopted in 1954, and it was modified in 1988 in response to concerns that certain acquired immunodeficiency syndrome (AIDS) treatments were not available in the United States. The guidance allows individuals with serious conditions, such as a rare form of cancer, to get treatments that are legally available in foreign countries but are not approved in the United States.

The policy is not a law or a regulation but serves as guidance for FDA personnel. The importation of certain unapproved prescription medications for personal use may be allowed in some circumstances if all the following factors apply:

- if the intended use is for a serious condition for which effective treatment may not be available domestically
- if the product is not considered to represent an unreasonable risk
- if the individual seeking to import the drug affirms in writing that it is for the patient's own use and provides the name and address of the U.S.-licensed doctor responsible for his or her treatment with the drug or

provides evidence that the drug is for continuation of a treatment begun in a foreign country
- if the product is for personal use and is a three-month supply or less and not for resale, since larger amounts would lend themselves to commercialization
- if there is no known commercialization or promotion to U.S. residents by those involved in distribution of the product

That means if you buy your high blood pressure (HBP) or other medication from a foreign country because it is cheaper—even though a drug with the same name is approved for sale in the United States—generally the drug will be considered unapproved and the FDA's personal use guidance will not apply. The U.S. Drug Enforcement Administration (DEA) has additional requirements for controlled drugs.

THE SAME GOES FOR CANADA

Neena Quirion, Director of the Maine Council on Aging (MCOA) in Augusta, has organized bus trips to Canada for her members and estimates that 25 seniors collectively saved about $19,000 on an overnight trip. "Paying for drugs is a real hardship for so many people," she says. "One lady takes about 15 different medications."

Quirion says that they have obtained prescriptions from a doctor who is licensed to practice medicine in both Maine and Canada and who performs a physical examination on each person before writing prescriptions. "Our feeling is that the quality of the drugs is the same," she says. "Everything's very regulated in Canada."

Greg Thompson, PharmD, a pharmacy professor at the University of Southern California (USC), agrees. "Getting drugs from Canada under the doctor's orders is different than getting drugs from Mexico on your own," he says. "Regulations in Mexico aren't as strict."

But even if you obtain drugs from a place or in a manner that you consider to be safe, according to the FDA, you are almost always obtaining unapproved drugs. "The law applies evenly to all countries outside of FDA's jurisdiction," says Thomas McGinnis,

Buying Prescription Drugs

PharmD, Director of Pharmacy Affairs in the FDA's Office of Policy and Planning (OPP).

So what about the belief often mentioned in the media that drugs sold in Canada are exactly the same as drugs sold in the United States—made in the exact same manufacturing plants? Some may be, and some may not. For example, drugs sold and distributed in Canada by Eli Lilly Canada come from the company's manufacturing facilities throughout the world—the United States, Europe, Asia, and South America.

Manufacturing facilities that make drugs for Canadians have been approved and registered by Health Canada's Health Products and Food Branch (HPFB), the federal agency responsible for regulating drugs sold in Canada. This agency is responsible for approving the product labeling, which must be made available in Canada's two official languages, English and French.

However, the FDA does not have authority to approve drugs sold in Canada. And, if a Canadian company is selling drugs only for export to the United States and not to Canadian citizens, Health Canada may not regulate the drugs or the company at all. Drugs coming to the United States from Canada may be coming from some other country and simply passing through Canada. The drugs could also be counterfeit, contaminated, or subpotent, among other things.

Experts at the FDA say it would be hard for you to know whether drugs sold outside the United States meet FDA standards and have been manufactured in a plant listed on an FDA-approved new drug application. "Even if you did know," McCallion says, "existing law requires you to prove it. The burden is on the importer to prove that the drug meets legal requirements—that includes having an FDA-approved label in English." The fact also remains that a drug made in this country can only be reimported back into this country by the original manufacturer, he adds.

Barbara Wells, Executive Director of the National Association of Pharmacy Regulatory Authorities (NAPRA) in Ontario, Canada, says that the practice of U.S. residents filling prescriptions in Canada is an issue that her organization is concerned about. "Our members do not feel that Canadian pharmacists should be breaking laws of jurisdictions in which their patients reside," she says.

INTERNET CHALLENGES

When it comes to buying prescription drugs online, Canada is dealing with some of the same regulatory challenges that occur in the United States.

The NAPRA has signed an agreement with the National Association of Boards of Pharmacy (NABP) in the United States and has developed a program in Canada modeled after the NABP's Verified Internet Pharmacy Practice Sites (VIPPS), a voluntary certification program.

A VIPPS® seal of approval indicates that an online pharmacy complies with state licensing and inspection requirements, along with other VIPPS criteria dealing with such areas as patient rights to privacy and authentication of orders.

The NABP developed the service in 1999 after consumers complained to state pharmacy boards about rogue sites posing as legitimate pharmacies. Sites can pop up overnight and disappear just as quickly, and there is little the U.S. government can do if you get swindled. The FDA suggests you steer clear of foreign websites. If you buy medicine from a domestic site, remember that the legitimate ones require a valid prescription.

The FDA sends warning letters over the Internet to suspicious sites. About 30 percent of Internet sites that receive the FDA's letters stop their illegal activity. The FDA also sends copies of the letters to the home governments of the websites when the locations can be identified.

"We seek out the cooperation of foreign governments because we have limited reach in a foreign land," says David Horowitz, Director of the Office of Compliance (OC) for the FDA's Center for Drug Evaluation and Research (CDER). "That is one of the major challenges of Internet enforcement."

HOW THE U.S. FOOD AND DRUG ADMINISTRATION WORKS WITH U.S. CUSTOMS AND BORDER PROTECTION

The exact amount of imported drugs that come into the United States is hard to track, and the high volume makes it impossible to examine them all. In one pilot program, the FDA and the U.S.

Buying Prescription Drugs

Customs and Border Protection (CBP) examined 1,908 packages of drug products from 19 countries that came through a mail facility in Carson, California, during a five-week period.

The FDA estimates that a total of 16,500 packages could have been set aside if there were enough resources to handle them. Of the 1,908 packages, 721 were detained, and the addressees were notified that the products appeared to violate the FD&C Act.

The FDA's enforcement efforts focus on drugs for commercial use, fraudulent drugs, and products that pose an unreasonable health risk.

If a bag or package arouses suspicion, customs will set it aside and contact the nearest office of the FDA or the DEA for advice on whether to release or detain the drug product. Even though your bag may not be checked, it is against the law not to properly declare imported medications to customs. Failure to declare products could result in penalties. Possession of certain medications without a prescription from a licensed physician may violate federal, state, and local laws.

Prescription drugs should be stored in their original containers, and you should have a copy of your doctor's prescription or letter of instruction. If a drug is detained, the FDA is required by law to send you a written notice asking whether you can show that the product meets legal requirements. If you cannot, the drug could be destroyed or returned to the sender.

POTENTIAL HEALTH RISKS WITH IMPORTED DRUGS
Quality Assurance Concerns
Medications that have not been approved for sale in the United States may not have been manufactured under quality assurance procedures designed to produce a safe and effective product.

Counterfeit Potential
Some imported medications—even those that bear the name of a United States—approved product—may, in fact, be counterfeit versions that are unsafe or even completely ineffective.

Presence of Untested Substances

Imported medications and their ingredients, although legal in foreign countries, may not have been evaluated for safety and effectiveness in the United States. These products may be addictive or contain other dangerous substances.

Risks of Unsupervised Use

Some medications, whether imported or not, are unsafe when taken without adequate medical supervision. You may need a medical evaluation to ensure that the medication is appropriate for you and your condition. Or you may require medical checkups to make sure that you are taking the drug properly, it is working for you, and you are not having unexpected or life-threatening side effects.

Labeling and Language Issues

The medication's label, including instructions for use and possible side effects, may be in a language you do not understand or may make medical claims and suggest specific uses that have not been adequately evaluated for safety and effectiveness.

Lack of Information

An imported medication may lack information that would permit you to be promptly and correctly treated for a dangerous side effect caused by the drug.[7]

---

[7] "Imported Drugs Raise Safety Concerns," U.S. Food and Drug Administration (FDA), March 1, 2018. Available online. URL: www.fda.gov/drugs/information-consumers-and-patients-drugs/imported-drugs-raise-safety-concerns. Accessed February 16, 2024.

Chapter 38 | Generic Drugs

WHAT ARE GENERIC DRUGS?
A generic drug is a medication created to be the same as an already marketed brand-name drug in dosage form, safety, strength, route of administration, quality, performance characteristics, and intended use. These similarities help demonstrate bioequivalence, which means that a generic medicine works in the same way and provides the same clinical benefit as the brand-name medicine. In other words, you can take a generic medicine as an equal substitute for its brand-name counterpart.

HOW DOES THE U.S. FOOD AND DRUG ADMINISTRATION ENSURE GENERIC MEDICINES WORK THE SAME AS BRAND-NAME MEDICINES?
Any generic medicine must perform the same in the body as the brand-name medicine. It must be the same as a brand-name medicine in dosage, form and route of administration, safety, effectiveness, strength, and labeling (with certain limited exceptions). It must also meet the same high standards of quality and manufacturing as the brand-name product, and it must be of the same quality, taken and used in the same way as well. This standard applies to all generic medicines.

Generic medicines use the same active ingredients as brand-name medicines and work the same way, so they have the same risks and benefits as the brand-name medicines. The U.S. Food and Drug Administration (FDA) Generic Drugs Program conducts a rigorous review to ensure generic medicines meet these standards, in addition to conducting inspections of manufacturing plants and monitoring drug safety after the generic medicine has been approved and brought to the market.

A generic drug may have certain minor differences from the brand-name product, such as different inactive ingredients.

It is important to note that there will always be a slight, but not medically significant, level of expected variability—just as there is for one batch of brand-name medicine compared with the next batch of brand-name product. This variability can and does occur during manufacturing, for both brand-name and generic medicines. When a medicine, generic or brand-name, is mass-produced, very small variations in purity, size, strength, and other parameters are permitted. The FDA limits how much variability is acceptable.

For example, a very large research study comparing generics with brand-name medicines found that there were very small differences (approximately 3.5%) in absorption into the body between generic and brand-name medicines. Some generics were absorbed slightly more, some slightly less. This amount of difference is expected and clinically acceptable, whether for one batch of brand-name medicine tested against another batch of the same brand, or for a generic tested against a brand-name medicine.

WHY DOES A GENERIC DRUG LOOK DIFFERENT FROM THE BRAND DRUG?

Trademark laws in the United States do not allow a generic drug to look exactly like other drugs already on the market. Generic medicines and brand-name medicines share the same active ingredient, but other characteristics, such as colors and flavorings, that do not affect the performance, safety, or effectiveness of the generic medicine may be different.

WHY DO GENERIC MEDICINES OFTEN COST LESS THAN THE BRAND-NAME MEDICINES?

Generic drugs are approved only after a rigorous review by the FDA and after a set period of time that the brand product has been on the market exclusively. This is because new drugs, like other new products, are usually protected by patents that prohibit others from making and selling copies of the same drug.

Generic Drugs

Generic drugs tend to cost less than their brand-name counterparts because generic drug applicants do not have to repeat animal and clinical (human) studies that were required of the brand-name medicines to demonstrate safety and effectiveness. This abbreviated pathway is why the application is called an "abbreviated new drug application" (ANDA).

The reduction in upfront research costs means that although generic medicines have the same therapeutic effect as their branded counterparts, they are typically sold at substantial discounts, an estimated 80–85 percent less, compared with the price of the brand-name medicine. According to the IMS Health Institute, generic drugs saved the U.S. health-care system nearly $2.2 trillion from 2009 to 2019.

When multiple generic companies are approved to market a single product, more competition exists in the marketplace, which typically results in lower prices for patients.

Bringing more drug competition to the market and addressing the high cost of medicines is one of the FDA's top priorities. In 2017, the FDA announced the Drug Competition Action Plan (DCAP) to further encourage robust and timely market competition for generic drugs and help bring greater efficiency and transparency to the generic drug review process, without sacrificing the scientific rigor underlying our generic drug program.

WHAT STANDARDS MUST GENERIC MEDICINES MEET TO RECEIVE THE U.S. FOOD AND DRUG ADMINISTRATION APPROVAL?

Drug companies must submit an ANDA to the FDA for approval to market a generic drug that is the same as (or bioequivalent to) the brand product. The FDA reviews the application to ensure drug companies have demonstrated that the generic medicine can be substituted for the brand-name medicine that it copies.

An ANDA must show the generic medicine is equivalent to the brand in the following ways:
- The active ingredient is the same as that of the brand-name drug/innovator drug.
  - An active ingredient in a medicine is the component that makes it pharmaceutically active—effective against the illness or condition it is treating.

- Generic drug companies must provide scientific evidence that shows that their active ingredient is the same as that of the brand-name medicine they copy, and the FDA must review that evidence.
- The generic medicine is the same strength.
- The medicine is the same type of product (such as a tablet or an injectable).
- The medicine has the same route of administration (such as oral or topical).
- It has the same usage indications.
- The inactive ingredients of the medicine are acceptable.
  - Some differences, which must be shown to have no effect on how the medicine functions, are allowed between the generic and the brand-name product.
  - Generic drug companies must submit evidence that all the ingredients used in their products are acceptable, and the FDA must review that evidence.
- It lasts for at least the same amount of time.
  - Most medicines break down, or deteriorate, over time.
  - Generic drug companies must do months-long "stability tests" to show that their products last for at least the same amount of time as the brand-name product.
- It is manufactured under the same strict standards as the brand-name medicine.
  - It meets the same batch requirements for identity, strength, purity, and quality.
  - The manufacturer is capable of making the medicine correctly and consistently.
    - Generic drug manufacturers must explain how they intend to manufacture the medicine and must provide evidence that each step of the manufacturing process will produce the same result each time. FDA scientists review those procedures, and FDA inspectors go to the generic drug manufacturer's facility to verify that the manufacturer is capable of making the medicine

Generic Drugs

consistently and to check that the information the manufacturer has submitted to the FDA is accurate.
- Often, different companies are involved (such as one company manufacturing the active ingredient and another company manufacturing the finished medicine). Generic drug manufacturers must produce batches of the medicines they want to market and provide information about the manufacturing of those batches for the FDA to review.
- The container in which the medicine will be shipped and sold is appropriate.
- The label is the same as the brand-name medicine's label.
  - The drug information label for the generic medicine should be the same as the brand-name label. One exception is if the brand-name drug is approved for more than one use and that use is protected by patents or exclusivities. A generic medicine can omit the protected use from its labeling and only be approved for a use that is not protected by patents or exclusivities, so long as that removal does not take away information needed for safe use. Labels for generic medicines can also contain certain changes when the drug is manufactured by a different company, such as a different lot number or company name.
  - Relevant patents or exclusivities are addressed.
  - As an incentive to develop new medicines, drug companies are awarded patents and exclusivities that may delay FDA approval of applications for generic medicines. The FDA must comply with the delays in approval that the patents and exclusivities impose.

The ANDA process does not, however, require the drug applicant to repeat costly animal and clinical (human) studies on ingredients or dosage forms already approved for safety and effectiveness. This allows generic medicines to be brought to market more quickly and at lower cost, allowing for increased access to medications by the public.

IS A GENERIC OF YOUR BRAND-NAME MEDICINE AVAILABLE?

In addition to asking your local pharmacist for assistance, there are following ways to find out if there is a generic of your brand-name medicine available:
- Use Drugs@FDA (www.accessdata.fda.gov/scripts/cder/daf), a catalog of FDA-approved drug products, including their drug labeling.
  - First, search by brand name.
  - Second, select the brand name product and note which products are listed under the section labeled "Therapeutic Equivalents for ..."
  - Products that include an ANDA (not NDA) number next to the name are generic products.
- Use the online version of the Orange Book (www.accessdata.fda.gov/scripts/cder/ob/index.cfm).
  - First, search by proprietary or brand name. Note the active ingredient name.
  - Second, search again by the active ingredient name.
  - Scroll right to find the dosage form (e.g., tablet) and strength.
  - Next, scroll right to the TE Code column. If the TE column contains a code beginning with "A," the FDA has approved generic equivalents.
  - Finally, look at the column "Appl No." If the letter "A" appears before the number, that product is an FDA-approved generic for the brand-name drug.
  - For very recent approvals, consult First Generic Drug Approvals (www.fda.gov/drugs/drug-and-biologic-approval-and-ind-activity-reports/first-generic-drug-approvals).

If you are unable to locate a generic of your brand-name medicine, it may be that the brand-name medicine is still within the period of time when it has exclusive rights to the marketplace, which allows drug companies to recoup their costs for the initial research and marketing of the brand-name or innovator drug. It is only after both patent and other periods of exclusivity are resolved that the FDA can approve a generic of the brand-name medicine.

HOW DOES THE U.S. FOOD AND DRUG ADMINISTRATION MONITOR SIDE EFFECTS OR SAFETY ISSUES WITH GENERIC MEDICINES?

The FDA takes several actions to ensure safety and quality before and after a new or generic medicine is approved. When a generic drug application is submitted, the FDA conducts a thorough examination of the data submitted by the applicant and evaluates information obtained by FDA investigators while inspecting the related testing and manufacturing facilities to ensure that every generic drug is safe, effective, of high quality, and substitutable to the brand-name drug.

FDA staff continually monitors all approved drug products, including generics, to make certain the medicines at all levels of the supply chain, from active pharmaceutical ingredients (APIs) to products being sold to consumers, are safe, effective, and of high quality.

The FDA also monitors and investigates reports of negative patient side effects or other reactions. The investigations may lead to changes in how a product (brand name and generic) is used or manufactured, and the FDA will make recommendations to healthcare professionals and the public if the need arises.

MedWatch (www.fda.gov/safety/medwatch-fda-safety-information-and-adverse-event-reporting-program) is the FDA's medical product safety reporting program. Health professionals, patients, and consumers can use MedWatch to voluntarily report a serious adverse event, product quality problem, product use/medication error, or therapeutic inequivalence/failure that is suspected to be associated with the use of an FDA-regulated drug, biologic, medical device, dietary supplement, or cosmetic.[1]

---

[1] "Generic Drugs: Questions & Answers," U.S. Food and Drug Administration (FDA), March 16, 2021. Available online. URL: www.fda.gov/drugs/frequently-asked-questions-popular-topics/generic-drugs-questions-answers. Accessed February 21, 2024.

Chapter 39 | Other Types of Drugs

Chapter Contents
Section 39.1—Biosimilars 385
Section 39.2—Precision Medicine 387

Section 39.1 | Biosimilars

Biosimilars are a type of biologic medication that are safe and effective for treating many illnesses. The U.S. Food and Drug Administration (FDA) has approved biosimilar medications to treat conditions such as chronic skin and bowel diseases, arthritis, kidney conditions, macular degeneration, and some cancers.

BIOLOGICS: MEDICATIONS FROM LIVING ORGANISMS

Biologics include medicines that generally come from living organisms, which can include animal cells and microorganisms, such as yeast and bacteria. That makes biologics different from conventional medications, which are commonly made from chemicals.

Biologics (including insulin) generally come from living organisms, so their nature varies, and their structures are generally more complex. Manufacturing biologics can be a more complicated process than making conventional drugs.

A biosimilar is a biologic that is highly similar to another biologic that is already FDA-approved (known as the "original biologic"). It is both normal and expected for both biosimilars and original biologics to have minor differences between batches of the same medication. This means that biologics cannot be copied exactly, and that is why biosimilars are not identical to their original biologic.

Biosimilars must have no clinically meaningful differences from their original biologic. On top of that, biosimilars must:
- be given the same way (same route of administration)
- have the same strength and dosage form
- have the same potential side effects

This means that biosimilars provide the same treatment benefits and have the same risks as the original biologic.

BIOSIMILARS ARE SAFE AND EFFECTIVE

Biosimilars are as safe and effective as the original biologic. Both are rigorously and thoroughly evaluated by the FDA before approval.

For biosimilars to be approved by the FDA, manufacturers must show that patients taking biosimilars do not have any new or worsening side effects as compared to people taking the original biologics.

As it does with all medication approvals, the FDA carefully reviews the data provided by manufacturers and takes several steps to ensure that all biosimilars meet standards for patient use. The FDA's thorough evaluation makes sure that all biosimilar medications are as safe and effective as their original biologic and meet the FDA's high standards for approval. This means you can expect the same safety and effectiveness from the biosimilar over the course of treatment as you would from the original product.

In addition, the FDA closely regulates the manufacturing of biosimilars. The same quality manufacturing standards that apply to the original biologic also apply to the biosimilar. It must be manufactured in accordance with Current Good Manufacturing Practice (CGMP) requirements, which cover:

- methods
- facilities
- controls for the manufacturing, processing, packaging, or holding of a medication

This helps prevent manufacturing mistakes or unacceptable impurities and ensure consistent product quality.

INTERCHANGEABLE BIOSIMILAR MEDICATIONS

An interchangeable biosimilar is a biosimilar that meets additional requirements outlined by the law that allows for the FDA to approve biosimilar and interchangeable biosimilar medications.

An interchangeable biosimilar product may be substituted for the original product without consulting the prescriber, much like how generic drugs are routinely substituted for brand-name drugs. This is commonly called "pharmacy-level substitution" and is subject to state pharmacy laws.

Both biosimilars and interchangeable biosimilars are as safe and effective as the original biologic they were compared to, and they can both be used in its place. This means that health-care

Other Types of Drugs

professionals can prescribe either a biosimilar or interchangeable biosimilar product instead of the original biologic.

DO BIOSIMILARS SAVE MONEY?
Similar to generic drugs, biosimilars may cost less because manufacturers rely on the FDA's finding that the original biologics are safe and effective. The lower cost is not a reflection of the effectiveness or safety of biosimilars. Because of the lower cost, biosimilars may be covered by more insurance companies and offer patients additional treatment options.

The FDA does not control the cost of drugs, but you can learn more about the price of a specific biosimilar by contacting your pharmacy or insurance company. If you are covered by Medicare or Medicaid, check with the Centers for Medicare & Medicaid Services (CMS) and your plan provider.

Biologics are among the fastest growing, and most expensive, segments of the prescription medication market. The FDA approval of additional biosimilar and interchangeable biosimilar medications may help stimulate competition, which would give patients more treatment options and potentially less expensive alternatives.[1]

Section 39.2 | Precision Medicine

WHAT IS PRECISION MEDICINE?
According to the Precision Medicine Initiative (PMI), precision medicine is "an emerging approach for disease treatment and prevention that takes into account individual variability in genes, environment, and lifestyle for each person." This approach will allow doctors and researchers to predict more accurately which treatment and prevention strategies for a particular disease will work in which

---

[1] "Biosimilar and Interchangeable Biologics: More Treatment Choices," U.S. Food and Drug Administration (FDA), August 17, 2023. Available online. URL: www.fda.gov/consumers/consumer-updates/biosimilar-and-interchangeable-biologics-more-treatment-choices. Accessed February 21, 2024.

groups of people. It is in contrast to a one-size-fits-all approach, in which disease treatment and prevention strategies are developed for the average person, with less consideration for the differences between individuals.

Although the term precision medicine is relatively new, the concept has been a part of health care for many years. For example, a person who needs a blood transfusion is not given blood from a randomly selected donor; instead, the donor's blood type is matched to the recipient to reduce the risk of complications. Although examples can be found in several areas of medicine, the role of precision medicine in day-to-day health care is relatively limited. Researchers hope that this approach will expand to many areas of health and health care in coming years.

WHAT IS THE DIFFERENCE BETWEEN PRECISION MEDICINE AND PERSONALIZED MEDICINE?

There is a lot of overlap between the terms "precision medicine" and "personalized medicine." According to the National Research Council (NRC), "personalized medicine" is an older term with a meaning similar to "precision medicine." However, there was concern that the word "personalized" could be misinterpreted to imply that treatments and preventions are being developed uniquely for each individual; in precision medicine, the focus is on identifying which approaches will be effective for which patients based on genetic, environmental, and lifestyle factors. The Council therefore preferred the term "precision medicine" to "personalized medicine." However, some people still use the two terms interchangeably.

WHAT ABOUT PHARMACOGENOMICS?

Pharmacogenomics is a part of precision medicine. Pharmacogenomics is the study of how genes affect a person's response to particular drugs. This relatively new field combines pharmacology (the science of drugs) and genomics (the study of genes and their functions) to develop effective, safe medications and doses that are tailored to variations in a person's genes.

Other Types of Drugs

WHAT IS THE PRECISION MEDICINE INITIATIVE?

The PMI is a long-term research endeavor, involving the National Institutes of Health (NIH) and multiple other research centers, which aims to understand how a person's genetics, environment, and lifestyle can help determine the best approach to prevent or treat disease.

The PMI has both short- and long-term goals. The short-term goals involve expanding precision medicine in the area of cancer research. Researchers at the National Cancer Institute (NCI) hope to use an increased knowledge of the genetics and biology of cancer to find new, more effective treatments for various forms of this disease. The long-term goals of the PMI focus on bringing precision medicine to all areas of health and health care on a large scale. The NIH has launched a study, known as the "All of Us Research Program," which involves a group (cohort) of at least 1 million volunteers from around the United States. Participants are providing genetic data, biological samples, and other information about their health. To encourage open data sharing, participants can access their health information, as well as research that uses their data, during the study. Researchers can use these data to study a large range of diseases, with the goals of better predicting disease risk, understanding how diseases occur, and finding improved diagnosis and treatment strategies.

WHAT ARE SOME POTENTIAL BENEFITS OF PRECISION MEDICINE AND THE PRECISION MEDICINE INITIATIVE?

Precision medicine holds promise for improving many aspects of health and health care. Some of these benefits will be apparent soon, as the All of Us Research Program continues and new tools and approaches for managing data are developed. Other benefits will result from long-term research in precision medicine and may not be realized for years.

Potential benefits of the PMI include the following:
- new approaches for protecting research participants, particularly patients' privacy and the confidentiality of their data

- design of new tools for building, analyzing, and sharing large sets of medical data
- improvement of the U.S. Food and Drug Administration (FDA) oversight of tests, drugs, and other technologies to support innovation while ensuring that these products are safe and effective
- new partnerships of scientists in a wide range of specialties, as well as people from the patient advocacy community, universities, pharmaceutical companies, and others
- opportunity for a million people to contribute to the advancement of scientific research

Potential long-term benefits of research in precision medicine:
- wider ability of doctors to use patients' genetic and other molecular information as part of routine medical care
- improved ability to predict which treatments will work best for specific patients
- better understanding of the underlying mechanisms by which various diseases occur
- improved approaches to preventing, diagnosing, and treating a wide range of diseases
- better integration of electronic health records (EHRs) in patient care, which will allow doctors and researchers to access medical data more easily

WHAT ARE SOME OF THE CHALLENGES RELATED TO PRECISION MEDICINE AND THE PRECISION MEDICINE INITIATIVE?

Precision medicine is a growing field. Many of the technologies that are needed to meet the goals of the PMI have only recently been developed. For example, researchers needed to standardize the collection of clinic and hospital data from more than 1 million volunteers around the country. They also needed databases to store large amounts of patient data efficiently.

The PMI also raises ethical, social, and legal issues. It is critical to protect participants' privacy and the confidentiality of their

Other Types of Drugs

personal and health information. Participants need to understand the risks and benefits of participating in research, which means researchers must have a rigorous process of informed consent.

Cost is also an issue with precision medicine. The PMI itself will cost many millions of dollars in federal funding, and the ongoing initiative will require Congress to approve funding over multiple years. Technologies such as sequencing large amounts of deoxyribonucleic acid (DNA) are expensive to carry out (although the cost of sequencing is decreasing). Additionally, drugs that are developed to treat conditions based on molecular or genetic variations are likely to be expensive. Reimbursement from third-party payers (such as private insurance companies) for these targeted drugs is also likely to become an issue.

If precision medicine approaches are to become part of routine health care, doctors and other health-care providers will need to know more about molecular genetics and biochemistry. They will increasingly need to interpret the results of genetic tests, understand how that information is relevant to treatment or prevention approaches, and convey this knowledge to patients.[2]

---

[2] MedlinePlus, "What Is Precision Medicine?" National Institutes of Health (NIH), May 17, 2022. Available online. URL: https://medlineplus.gov/genetics/understanding/precisionmedicine/definition. Accessed February 21, 2024.

Chapter 40 | Taking Medicine

Chapter Contents
Section 40.1—Tips for Taking Medications 395
Section 40.2—Know When Antibiotics Work 396
Section 40.3—Kids Are Not Just Small Adults: Advice on
 Giving Medicine to Your Child 399

Section 40.1 | Tips for Taking Medications

Sticking to your medication routine (or medication adherence) means taking your medications as prescribed—the right dose, at the right time, and in the right way and frequency. Not taking your medicine as prescribed by a doctor or instructed by a pharmacist could lead to your disease getting worse, hospitalization, and even death.

Many patients do not follow health-care provider instructions on how to take medications for various reasons, such as not understanding the directions, forgetfulness, multiple medications with different regimens, unpleasant side effects, or the medication does not seem to be working. Cost can also be a factor causing medication nonadherence—patients cannot afford to fill their prescriptions or decide to take less than the prescribed dose to make the prescription last longer. "However, to help you get the best results from your medications taking your medicine as instructed is very important," says Kimberly DeFronzo, RPh, MS, MBA, a Consumer Safety Officer (CSO) in the Center for Drug Evaluation and Research (CDER) of the U.S. Food and Drug Administration (FDA).

TIPS TO HELP YOU TAKE YOUR MEDICINE

Taking your medicine as prescribed or medication adherence is important for controlling chronic conditions, treating temporary conditions, and overall long-term health and well-being. A personal connection with your health-care provider or pharmacist is an important part of medication adherence. "Because your pharmacist is an expert in medications, they can help suggest how best to take your medications," says DeFronzo. However, you play the most important part by taking all of your medications as directed.

Here are tips that may help:
- Take your medication at the same time every day.
- Tie taking your medications with a daily routine such as brushing your teeth or getting ready for bed. Before choosing mealtime for your routine, check if

your medication should be taken on a full or empty stomach.
- Keep a "medicine calendar" with your pill bottles and note each time you take a dose.
- Use a pill container. Some types have sections for multiple doses at different times, such as morning, lunch, evening, and night.
- When using a pill container, refill it at the same time each week. For example, every Sunday morning after breakfast.
- Purchase timer caps for your pill bottles and set them to go off when your next dose is due. Some pillboxes also have timer functions.
- When traveling, be certain to bring enough of your medication, plus a few days extra, in case your return is delayed.
- If you are flying, keep your medications in your carry-on bag to avoid lost luggage. Temperatures inside the cargo hold could damage your medication.[1]

Section 40.2 | Know When Antibiotics Work

Antibiotic resistance is one of the most urgent threats to the public's health. Antibiotic resistance happens when germs, such as bacteria and fungi, develop the ability to defeat the drugs designed to kill them. That means the germs are not killed and continue to grow. More than 2.8 million antibiotic-resistant infections occur in the United States each year, and more than 35,000 people die as a result.

Antibiotics can save lives, but any time antibiotics are used, they can cause side effects and contribute to the development of antibiotic resistance. Each year, at least 28 percent of antibiotics

---

[1] "Why You Need to Take Your Medications as Prescribed or Instructed," U.S. Food and Drug Administration (FDA), February 16, 2016. Available online. URL: www.fda.gov/drugs/special-features/why-you-need-take-your-medications-prescribed-or-instructed. Accessed February 20, 2024.

are prescribed unnecessarily in U.S. doctors' offices and emergency rooms (ERs), which makes improving antibiotic prescribing and use a national priority.

Helping health-care professionals improve the way they prescribe antibiotics, and improving the way we take antibiotics, helps keep us healthy now, helps fight antibiotic resistance, and ensures that these lifesaving drugs will be available for future generations.

WHEN ANTIBIOTICS ARE NEEDED

Antibiotics are only needed for treating certain infections caused by bacteria, but even some bacterial infections get better without antibiotics. We rely on antibiotics to treat serious, life-threatening conditions such as pneumonia and sepsis, the body's extreme response to an infection. Effective antibiotics are also needed for people who are at high risk for developing infections. Some of those at high risk for infections include patients undergoing surgery, patients with end-stage renal disease (ESRD), or patients receiving cancer therapy (chemotherapy).

WHEN ANTIBIOTICS ARE NOT NEEDED

Antibiotics do not work on viruses, such as those that cause colds, flu, or coronavirus disease (COVID-19).

Antibiotics are also not needed for many sinus infections and some ear infections.

When antibiotics are not needed, they would not help you, and the side effects could still cause harm. Common side effects of antibiotics can include:
- rash
- dizziness
- nausea
- diarrhea
- yeast infections

More serious side effects can include:
- *Clostridioides difficile* (also called "*difficile*" or "*C. diff*") infection, which causes severe diarrhea that can lead to severe colon damage and death

- severe and life-threatening allergic reactions, such as wheezing, hives, shortness of breath, and anaphylaxis, which also includes feeling like your throat is closing or choking, or your voice is changing

Antibiotic use can also lead to the development of antibiotic resistance.

WHAT YOU CAN DO TO FEEL BETTER
- Ask your health-care professional about the best way to feel better while your body fights off the virus.
- If you need antibiotics, take them exactly as prescribed. Talk with your health-care professional if you have any questions about your antibiotics.
- Talk with your health-care professional if you develop any side effects, especially severe diarrhea, since that could be a *C. diff* infection, which needs to be treated immediately.
- Do your best to stay healthy and keep others healthy:
  - Clean hands by washing with soap and water for at least 20 seconds or use a hand sanitizer that contains at least 60 percent alcohol.
  - Cover your mouth and nose with a tissue when you cough or sneeze.
  - Stay home when sick.
  - Get recommended vaccines, such as the flu vaccine.[2]

---

[2] "Be Antibiotics Aware: Smart Use, Best Care," Centers for Disease Control and Prevention (CDC), November 12, 2021. Available online. URL: www.cdc.gov/patientsafety/features/be-antibiotics-aware.html. Accessed February 20, 2024.

Section 40.3 | Kids Are Not Just Small Adults: Advice on Giving Medicine to Your Child

Use care when giving any medicine to an infant or a child. Even over-the-counter (OTC) medicines that you buy are serious medicines. The following is advice for giving OTC medicine to your child, from the U.S. Food and Drug Administration (FDA) and the makers of OTC medicines:

- **Always read and follow the Drug Facts label on your OTC medicine.** This is important for choosing and safely using all OTC medicines. Read the label every time, before you give the medicine. Be sure you clearly understand how much medicine to give and when the medicine can be taken again.
- **Know the "active ingredient" in your child's medicine.** This is what makes the medicine work and is always listed at the top of the Drug Facts label. Sometimes an active ingredient can treat more than one medical condition. For that reason, the same active ingredient can be found in many different medicines that are used to treat different symptoms. For example, a medicine for a cold and a medicine for a headache could each contain the same active ingredient. Therefore, if you are treating a cold and a headache with two medicines and both have the same active ingredient, you could be giving two times the normal dose. If you are confused about your child's medicines, check with a doctor, nurse, or pharmacist.
- **Give the right medicine, in the right amount, to your child.** Not all medicines are right for an infant or a child. Medicines with the same brand name can be sold in many different strengths, such as infant, child, and adult formulas. The amount and directions are also different for children of different ages or weights. Always use the right medicine and follow the directions exactly. Never use more medicine than directed, even if your child seems sicker than the last time.

- **Talk to your doctor, pharmacist, or nurse to find out what mixes well and what does not.** Medicines, vitamins, supplements, foods, and beverages do not always mix well with each other. Your health-care professional can help.
- **Use the dosing tool that comes with the medicine, such as a dropper or a dosing cup.** A different dosing tool, or a kitchen spoon, could hold the wrong amount of medicine.
- **Know the difference between a tablespoon (tbsp.) and a teaspoon (tsp.).** Do not confuse them! A tbsp. holds three times as much medicine as a tsp. On measuring tools, a tsp. is equal to "5 cc" or "5 mL."
- **Know your child's weight.** Directions on some OTC medicines are based on weight. Never guess the amount of medicine to give to your child or try to figure it out from the adult dose instructions. If a dose is not listed for your child's age or weight, call your doctor or other members of your health-care team.
- **Prevent a poison emergency by always using a child-resistant cap.** Relock the cap after each use. Be especially careful with any products that contain iron; they are the leading cause of poisoning deaths in young children.
- **Store all medicines in a safe place.** Medicines are tasty, colorful, and many can be chewed. Kids may think that these products are candy. To prevent an overdose or poisoning emergency, store all medicines and vitamins in a safe place out of your child's (and even your pet's) sight and reach. If your child takes too much, call the Poison Center Hotline at 800-222-1222 (open 24 hours every day, 7 days a week) or call 911.
- **Check the medicine three times.** First, check the outside packaging for such things as cuts, slices, or tears. Second, once you are at home, check the label on the inside package to be sure you have the right medicine. Make sure the lid and seal are not

Taking Medicine

broken. Third, check the color, shape, size, and smell of medicine. If you notice anything different or unusual, talk to a pharmacist or another health-care professional.[3]

---

[3] "Kids Aren't Just Small Adults—Medicines, Children, and the Care Every Child Deserves," U.S. Food and Drug Administration (FDA), December 20, 2017. Available online. URL: www.fda.gov/drugs/information-consumers-and-patients-drugs/kids-arent-just-small-adults-medicines-children-and-care-every-child-deserves. Accessed February 20, 2024.

Chapter 41 | Adverse Drug Reactions

Drugs approved by the U.S. Food and Drug Administration (FDA) for sale in the United States must be safe and effective—which means that the benefits of the drug must be greater than the known risks. However, both prescription and over-the-counter (OTC) drugs have side effects. Side effects, also known as "adverse reactions," are unwanted undesirable effects that are possibly related to a drug. Side effects can vary from minor problems such as a runny nose to life-threatening events such as a heart attack or liver damage.

Several things can affect who does and does not have a side effect when taking a drug—age; use of other drugs, vitamins, or dietary supplements; or other underlying diseases or conditions (e.g., diseases that weaken the immune system or affect the function of the kidneys or liver).

Common side effects include upset stomach, dry mouth, and drowsiness. A side effect is considered serious if the result is death, life-threatening, hospitalization, disability or permanent damage, or exposure prior to conception or during pregnancy that caused birth defect.

Side effects can happen when you:
- start taking a new drug or dietary supplement (e.g., vitamins)
- stop taking a drug that you have been on for a while
- increase or decrease the dose (amount) of a drug that you take

REDUCING YOUR RISK

There are several ways to learn about side effects for your prescription drugs and to reduce your risk of experiencing a side effect.

- **Ask your health-care professional about any possible side effects and what, if any, steps should be taken to reduce the risk when you are prescribed a drug.** For example, your health-care professional may recommend taking the drug with food to lower the chance of getting nausea or to not take the drug with other drugs.
- **Ask your health-care professional for information about the drug when you receive your prescription (FDA-approved labeling for patients includes Medication Guides and Patient Information).** These documents will include possible common and serious side effects.
- **Read the pharmacy label and any stickers that may be attached to the prescription bottle or box.** The label and stickers may have information on how to take the drug and possible side effects.

Prescription drug information on side effects is available on the FDA's Drugs@FDA (www.accessdata.fda.gov/scripts/cder/daf/index.cfm) database and the FDA's FDALabel (https://nctr-crs.fda.gov/fdalabel/ui/search) database. For OTC drugs, read the Drug Facts label.

WHEN A SIDE EFFECT OCCURS

Should you experience a side effect, you may be able to lessen or eliminate the effects. Work with your health-care professional to see if adjusting the dosage or switching to a different medication will ease or eliminate the side effect. Other options, such as a lifestyle or dietary change, may be suggested by your health-care professional.

REPORTING SIDE EFFECTS

When side effects do occur, you are encouraged to report them to the FDA's MedWatch (www.accessdata.fda.gov/scripts/medwatch/

Adverse Drug Reactions

index.cfm?action=reporting.home), a program for reporting serious problems with human medical products, including drugs.

MedWatch has a consumer reporting form, FDA 3500B. Written in plain language and designed to be consumer friendly, the form starts off with a page of some commonly asked questions and answers to help guide you in submitting the form and then asks simple questions about the problem. In addition to formal reports, MedWatch has a toll-free line (800-332-1088) to answer questions.

Be an active member of your health-care team. By taking time to learn about the possible side effects of a drug and working with your health-care provider and pharmacist, you will be better prepared to reduce your chance of experiencing a side effect or coping with any side effect that you may experience.

WHERE CAN YOU FIND DETAILED SIDE EFFECT INFORMATION FOR A DRUG?

The FDA's FDALabel database is used to perform customizable searches of thousands of drug labeling, including searching for side effects for a drug. Please use these instructions to find side effect information about a particular drug:
- Go to the FDA's FDALabel website: https://nctr-crs.fda.gov/fdalabel/ui/search.
- If you are looking for a prescription drug for humans, click on "Human Rx":
  - Go to the "Product Name(s)" search box and enter the entire or part of the drug name.
  - Consider looking for the trade name of the drug you are looking for and then click on "Structured Product Labeling (SPL) Document" in that row.
  - Go to the "6 Adverse Reactions" to find the side effects for the drug.
- If you are looking for an OTC drug for humans, click on "Human OTC":
  - Go to the "Product Name(s)" search box and enter the entire or part of the drug name.

- Consider looking for the trade name of the drug you are looking for and then click on "SPL Document" in that row.
- Go to the "Warnings" to find the side effects for the drug.[1]

---

[1] "Finding and Learning about Side Effects (Adverse Reactions)," U.S. Food and Drug Administration (FDA), August 8, 2022. Available online. URL: www.fda.gov/drugs/information-consumers-and-patients-drugs/finding-and-learning-about-side-effects-adverse-reactions. Accessed February 22, 2024.

Chapter 42 | Drug Interactions: What You Should Know

There are more opportunities today than ever before to learn about your health and to take better care of yourself. It is also more important than ever to know about the medicines you take. If you take several different medicines, see more than one doctor, or have certain health conditions, you and your doctors need to be aware of all the medicines you take. Doing so will help you avoid potential problems such as drug interactions.

Drug interactions may make your drug less effective, cause unexpected side effects, or increase the action of a particular drug. Some drug interactions can even be harmful to you. Reading the label every time you use a nonprescription or prescription drug and taking the time to learn about drug interactions may be critical to your health. You can reduce the risk of potentially harmful drug interactions and side effects with a little bit of knowledge and common sense. Drug interactions fall into three broad categories:

- **Drug-drug interactions**. This occurs when two or more drugs react with each other. This drug-drug interaction may cause you to experience an unexpected side effect. For example, mixing a drug you take to help you sleep (a sedative) and a drug you take for allergies (an antihistamine) can slow your reactions and make driving a car or operating machinery dangerous.
- **Drug-food/beverage interactions**. This results from drugs reacting with foods or beverages. For example,

mixing alcohol with some drugs may cause you to feel tired or slow your reactions.
- **Drug-condition interactions.** This may occur when an existing medical condition makes certain drugs potentially harmful. For example, if you have high blood pressure (HBP), you could experience an unwanted reaction if you take a nasal decongestant.

DRUG INTERACTIONS AND OVER-THE-COUNTER MEDICINES

Over-the-counter (OTC) drug labels contain information about ingredients, uses, warnings, and directions that is important to read and understand. The label also includes important information about possible drug interactions. Further, drug labels may change as new information becomes known. That is why it is especially important to read the label every time you use a drug.
- The "Active Ingredients" and "Purpose" sections list provides:
  - the name and amount of each active ingredient
  - the purpose of each active ingredient
- The "Uses" section of the label:
  - tells you what the drug is used for
  - helps you find the best drug for your specific symptoms
- The "Warnings" section of the label provides important drug interaction and precaution information such as:
  - when to talk to a doctor or pharmacist before use
  - the medical conditions that may make the drug less effective or not safe
  - under what circumstances the drug should not be used
  - when to stop taking the drug
- The "Directions" section of the label tells you:
  - the length of time and the amount of the product that you may safely use
  - any special instructions on how to use the product

Drug Interactions: What You Should Know

- The "Other Information" section of the label tells you:
  - required information about certain ingredients, such as sodium content, for people with dietary restrictions or allergies
- The "Inactive Ingredients" section of the label tells you:
  - the name of each inactive ingredient (such as colorings, binders, etc.)
- The "Questions?" or "Questions or Comments?" section of the label (if included):
  - provides telephone numbers of a source to answer questions about the product

LEARNING MORE ABOUT DRUG INTERACTIONS

Talk to your doctor or pharmacist about the drugs you take. When your doctor prescribes a new drug, discuss all OTC and prescription drugs, dietary supplements, vitamins, botanicals, minerals, and herbals you take, as well as the foods you eat. Ask your pharmacist for the package insert for each prescription drug you take. The package insert provides more information about potential drug interactions.

Before taking a drug, ask your doctor or pharmacist the following questions:
- Can I take it with other drugs?
- Should I avoid certain foods, beverages, or other products?
- What are possible drug interaction signs I should know about?
- How will the drug work in my body?
- Is there more information available about the drug or my condition (on the Internet or in health and medical literature)?

Know how to take drugs safely and responsibly. Remember, the drug label will tell you:
- what the drug is used for
- how to take the drug
- how to reduce the risk of drug interactions and unwanted side effects

If you still have questions after reading the drug product label, ask your doctor or pharmacist for more information.

Remember that different OTC drugs may contain the same active ingredient. If you are taking more than one OTC drug, pay attention to the active ingredients used in the products to avoid taking too much of a particular ingredient. Under certain circumstances—such as if you are pregnant or breastfeeding—you should talk to your doctor before you take any medicine. Also, make sure you know what ingredients are contained in the medicines you take. Doing so will help you avoid possible allergic reactions.[1]

---

[1] "Drug Interactions: What You Should Know," U.S. Food and Drug Administration (FDA), September 25, 2013. Available online. URL: www.fda.gov/drugs/resources-drugs/drug-interactions-what-you-should-know. Accessed February 22, 2024.

Chapter 43 | Preventing Medication Errors

A medication error is defined as "any preventable event that may cause or lead to inappropriate medication use or patient harm while the medication is in the control of the health-care professional, patient, or consumer," according to the National Coordinating Council for Medication Error Reporting and Prevention (NCC MERP).

Medication errors can occur throughout the medication-use system, such as when prescribing a drug, upon entering information into a computer system, when the drug is being prepared or dispensed, or when the drug is given to or taken by a patient.

The U.S. Food and Drug Administration (FDA) receives more than 100,000 U.S. reports each year associated with a suspected medication error. The FDA reviews the reports and classifies them to determine the cause and type of error. The reports come from drug manufacturers, health-care professionals, and consumers through MedWatch, the agency's safety information and adverse event reporting program. Serious harmful results of a medication error may include:
- death
- life-threatening situation
- hospitalization
- disability
- birth defect

LOOKING FOR WAYS TO REDUCE MEDICATION ERRORS

The FDA looks for ways to prevent medication errors. Before drugs are approved for marketing, the FDA reviews the drug name,

labeling, packaging, and product design to identify and revise information that may contribute to medication errors. For example, the FDA reviews:
- proposed proprietary (brand) names to minimize confusion among drug names (With the help of simulated prescriptions and computerized models, the FDA determines the acceptability of proposed proprietary names to minimize medication errors associated with product name confusion.)
- container labels to help health-care providers and consumers select the right drug product (If a drug is made in multiple strengths—e.g., 5 mg, 10 mg, and 25 mg—the labels of those three containers should be easy to differentiate. The label design may use different colors or identify the strength in large bold numbers and letters.)
- prescribing and patient information to ensure the directions for prescribing, preparing, and use are clear and easy to read

After drugs are approved for marketing in the United States, the FDA monitors and evaluates medication error reports. The FDA may require a manufacturer to revise the labels, labeling, packaging, product design, or proprietary name to prevent medication errors. The FDA may also issue communications alerting the public about a medication error safety issue, by way of drug safety communications, drug safety alerts, medication guides, and drug safety podcasts.

The FDA collaborates with external stakeholders, regulators, patient safety organizations (PSOs) such as the Institute for Safe Medication Practices (ISMP), standard-setting organizations such as the U.S. Pharmacopeia (USP), and researchers to understand the causes of medication errors and the effectiveness of interventions to prevent them and to address broader safety issues that may contribute to medication errors.

GETTING THE RIGHT DRUG TO THE RIGHT PATIENT

The FDA also put into place rules requiring barcodes on certain drug and biological product labels. Barcodes allow health-care professionals to use barcode scanning equipment to verify that the right drug—in the right dose and right route of administration—is being given to the right patient at the right time. This system is intended to help reduce the number of medication errors that occur in hospitals and other health-care settings.

The FDA has published several guidances to help manufacturers design their drug labels, labeling, packaging, and select drug names in a way to minimize or eliminate hazards that can contribute to medication errors. For example, in 2016, the FDA issued a final guidance titled, *Safety Considerations for Product Design to Minimize Medication Errors,* to avoid errors and encourage safe use of drugs. The guidance recommendations include the following:

- **Tablets and other oral dosage forms should have distinct and legible imprint codes**. So health-care providers and consumers can verify the drug product and strength.
- **Oral syringes and other dosing devices copackaged with a liquid oral dosage form should be appropriate for the doses to be measured**. Dosing errors have been reported when an oral syringe is labeled in milligrams, but the dose is prescribed in milliliters.
- **The package design should protect the consumer against incorrect use**. Medications applied to the skin (topical) should not be packaged in containers that look similar to the containers usually associated with eye, ear, nasal, or oral products. Similar looking containers have resulted in people putting a topical product in the eye, ear, nose, and mouth.

OVER-THE-COUNTER AND PRESCRIPTION DRUG LABELING

According to a Harris Interactive Market Research Poll conducted for the National Council on Patient Information and Education (NCPIE) and released in January 2002, consumers tend to overlook important label information on over-the-counter (OTC) drugs. In response to that report, the FDA now requires a standardized Drug Facts label on more than 100,000 OTC drug products. Modeled after the Nutrition Facts label on foods, the Drug Facts label helps consumers compare and select OTC medicines and follow the instructions. The label clearly lists active ingredients, inactive ingredients, uses, warnings, dosage, directions, and other information, such as how to store the medicine.

In 2006, the FDA revised its rules for the content and format of prescribing information for prescription drug and biological products. The revised look helps health-care professionals find the information they need more easily and quickly. The FDA also makes updated prescribing information available on the web at Drugs@FDA (www.accessdata.fda.gov/scripts/cder/daf/index.cfm).

CONSUMERS PLAY AN IMPORTANT ROLE

Consumers can also play an important role in reducing medication errors. Here are some drug safety tips:

- **Know the various risks and causes for medication errors.**
- **Find out what drug you are taking and what it is for.** Rather than simply letting the doctor write you a prescription and send you on your way, be sure to ask the name of the drug and the purpose of the drug.
- **Find out how to take the drug and make sure you understand the directions.** Ask if the medicine needs to be kept in the refrigerator.
- **Check the container's label every time you take a drug.** This is especially important if you are taking several drugs because it will lower your risk of accidentally taking the wrong medicine.
- **Keep drugs stored in their original containers.** Many pills look alike so keeping them in their original containers will help know the name of the drug and how to take them. If you are having trouble keeping multiple medications straight, ask your doctor or pharmacist about helpful aids.
- **Keep an updated list of all medications taken for health reasons, including OTC drugs, supplements, medicinal herbs, and other substances.** Give a copy of this list to your health-care provider.

Preventing Medication Errors

- **Be aware of the risk of drug-drug or drug-food interactions.**
- **If in doubt or you have questions about your medication, ask your pharmacist or other health-care provider.**
- **Report suspected medication errors to MedWatch (www.accessdata.fda.gov/scripts/medwatch/index.cfm?action=reporting.home).**[1]

---

[1] "Working to Reduce Medication Errors," U.S. Food and Drug Administration (FDA), August 23, 2019. Available online. URL: www.fda.gov/drugs/information-consumers-and-patients-drugs/working-reduce-medication-errors. Accessed February 29, 2024.

Chapter 44 | Unapproved, Counterfeit, and Misused Drugs

Chapter Contents
Section 44.1—Unapproved Drugs and Counterfeit Drugs....... 419
Section 44.2—Misuse of Prescription Pain Relievers 424

Section 44.1 | Unapproved Drugs and Counterfeit Drugs

UNAPPROVED DRUGS
Unapproved prescription drugs pose significant risks to patients because they have not been reviewed by the U.S. Food and Drug Administration (FDA) for safety, effectiveness, or quality. Without FDA review, there is no way to know if these drugs are safe and effective for their intended use, whether they are manufactured in a way that ensures consistent drug quality, or whether their label is complete and accurate. Unapproved drugs have resulted in patient harm, and the agency works to protect patients from the risks posed by these drugs.

Preserving Patient Access to Medically Necessary Drugs
The agency balances its goal to eliminate unapproved prescription drugs from the market with patient access to medically necessary drugs. The FDA carefully considers the possible effects on patient access, including whether any action would likely lead to a disruption in the drug supply, before initiating an action against an unapproved drug.

The U.S. Food and Drug Administration Approval Is Required by Law
Federal law requires all new drugs in the United States be shown to be safe and effective for their intended use prior to marketing. However, some drugs are available in the United States even though they have never received the required FDA approval. Many healthcare professionals and patients are unaware that some of the drugs prescribed are not FDA approved.

The FDA permits some unapproved prescription drugs to be marketed if:
- the drug is subject to an open Drug Efficacy Study Implementation (DESI) program proceeding

- health-care professionals rely on the drug to treat serious medical conditions when there is no FDA-approved drug to treat the condition
- there is insufficient supply of an FDA-approved drug

The law allows some unapproved prescription drugs to be lawfully marketed if they meet the criteria of generally recognized as safe and effective (GRASE) or grandfathered. However, the agency is not aware of any human prescription drug that is lawfully marketed as grandfathered.

Risk-Based Approach

The agency has a two-prong approach to help assure patient safety. First, the agency encourages manufacturers of unapproved drugs to obtain approval to be legally marketed in the United States. Second, the FDA has worked to remove unapproved drugs from the market. Many potentially unsafe drugs have been removed from the market since 2006, including several drugs with significant safety concerns. The agency uses a risk-based approach, giving enforcement priority to drugs that pose the highest risk to public health, without imposing undue burden on patients or unnecessarily disrupting the availability of drugs on the market.

Search Marketed Drugs Listed with the U.S. Food and Drug Administration, Including Unapproved Drugs

Drugs marketed in the United States, with or without FDA approval, can be identified in the following databases:
- **National Drug Code (NDC) Directory (www.fda.gov/drugs/drug-approvals-and-databases/national-drug-code-directory).** This publishes data derived from information submitted to the agency as part of drug listing requirements, including information on unapproved drugs. NDC numbers are provided for all listed drugs, regardless of approval status. Information in the directory does not indicate that the FDA has verified the information provided.

Unapproved, Counterfeit, and Misused Drugs

- **Drugs@FDA (www.accessdata.fda.gov/scripts/cder/daf)**. This lists information on FDA-approved drugs since 1998, including patient information, labels, and approval letters.
- **Orange Book (www.fda.gov/drugs/drug-approvals-and-databases/approved-drug-products-therapeutic-equivalence-evaluations-orange-book)**. This identifies FDA-approved drugs.

Unapproved Drugs and Drug Prices

There are many factors that contribute to drug pricing. When there is a sole source of an FDA-approved drug, market dynamics may enable the company that sought approval to set a higher price than when the drug faces competition. Patients and health-care professionals can, however, have confidence that the FDA-approved version has been shown to be safe and effective for its intended use and that it is manufactured according to federal quality standards.

While the FDA does not have the authority to regulate drug prices, it is keenly aware of price fluctuations that can occur on the heels of its regulatory actions and takes steps within its authority to minimize the duration, if not the extent, of those price hikes. Although following the FDA approval process may result in cost increases for a drug over the short term, the risks to the individual patient are substantially reduced, and the benefits are assured for the long term.[1]

COUNTERFEIT MEDICINE

Counterfeit (fake or falsified) medicines may be harmful to your health because while being passed off as authentic, they may contain the wrong ingredients; contain too much, too little, or no active ingredient at all; or contain other harmful ingredients.

The U.S. drug supply is among the safest in the world. The United States has federal and state laws that create a "closed" drug

---

[1] "Unapproved Drugs," U.S. Food and Drug Administration (FDA), June 2, 2021. Available online. URL: www.fda.gov/drugs/enforcement-activities-fda/unapproved-drugs. Accessed February 29, 2024.

distribution system to help ensure the U.S. drug supply is safe. The FDA remains vigilant in protecting the U.S. drug supply from counterfeit drugs. However, there has been an increase in overdose deaths that are related to fentanyl-laced counterfeit drugs. The FDA takes reports of suspect counterfeits seriously and works closely with other federal agencies and the private sector to help protect the nation's drug supply.

Possible Signs of Counterfeit Drugs

Health-care providers and consumers need to be aware of how they could be exposed to counterfeit medicines. Watch out for possible signs of a counterfeit drug:
- Does the drug or packaging look different from what you normally receive?
- Have you experienced a new or unusual side effect after using the drug?
- Did you buy the drug from an online pharmacy?

Consumers, health-care providers, and supply chain stakeholders should only buy from state-licensed pharmacies to ensure they are getting safe, effective, and high-quality drugs that have been approved by the FDA.

Company Reports of Counterfeit Drugs

Companies report counterfeit drugs to the FDA, and the agency provides this information to consumers:
- Novo Nordisk warns consumers about counterfeit Ozempic (semaglutide) injection 1 mg in the United States.
- Novo Nordisk warns of counterfeit Ozempic (semaglutide injection) pen found in the United States.
- Bausch + Lomb alerts about the counterfeit versions of Muro 128 (sodium chloride hypertonicity ophthalmic ointment, 5%) and Muro 128 (sodium chloride

hypertonicity ophthalmic solution, 5%) found in the United States.
- Janssen alerts that counterfeit Symtuza is being distributed in the United States.

Report Suspected Unsafe Products to the U.S. Food and Drug Administration
- Report sales of medicine by unsafe online pharmacies to the FDA (www.fda.gov/safety/report-problem-fda/reporting-unlawful-sales-medical-products-internet).
- Report adverse effects caused by any medicine to the FDA's MedWatch program (www.fda.gov/safety/medwatch-fda-safety-information-and-adverse-event-reporting-program).
- Report suspected criminal counterfeit activity to the FDA's Office of Criminal Investigations (OCI; www.accessdata.fda.gov/scripts/email/oc/oci/contact.cfm).

Global Perspective
Many counterfeit drugs are made abroad and arrive in the United States through the mail or are smuggled into the country. The FDA works with U.S. Customs and Border Protection (CBP) and focuses on areas that present the most substantial threat to our drug supply.

Drug safety and quality do not begin or end at the U.S. border. The U.S. government works with foreign regulatory counterparts, when possible, to disrupt or close illegal operations involving the production and distribution of counterfeit drugs.

The U.S. Food and Drug Administration Actions to Protect against Counterfeit Drugs
- Works with industry and stakeholders to create a tighter, closed prescription drug distribution system to prevent harmful drugs from entering the supply chain, detect

harmful drugs if they do enter the supply chain, and enable rapid response when such drugs are found.
- Electronically screens all FDA-regulated drugs imported into the United States to ensure imported drugs must meet the FDA's rigorous standards for quality, safety, and effectiveness as drugs made in the United States.
- The FDA's OCI conducts criminal investigations of illegal activities involving FDA-regulated products, arresting those responsible and bringing them before U.S. Department of Justice (DOJ) for prosecution. This includes activities such as cybercrime and distributing counterfeit, unapproved, and misbranded drugs.[2]

Section 44.2 | Misuse of Prescription Pain Relievers

Prescription pain relievers, when used correctly and under a doctor's supervision, are safe and effective. But abuse them, or mix them with illegal drugs or alcohol, and you could wind up in the morgue. Even using prescription pain relievers with other prescription drugs (such as antidepressants) or over-the-counter (OTC) medications (such as cough syrups and antihistamines) can lead to life-threatening respiratory failure.

DRUGS TO WATCH OUT FOR

The most dangerous prescription pain relievers are those containing drugs known as "opioids," such as morphine and codeine. Some common drugs containing these substances include Darvon, Demerol, Dilaudid, OxyContin, Tylenol with Codeine, and Vicodin. Some slang names for these drugs include: ac/dc, coties,

---

[2] "Counterfeit Medicine," U.S. Food and Drug Administration (FDA), December 22, 2023. Available online. URL: www.fda.gov/drugs/buying-using-medicine-safely/counterfeit-medicine. Accessed February 29, 2024.

demmies, dillies, hillbilly heroin, o.c, oxy, oxycotton, percs, and vics to name a few. Whatever you call them, remember one thing—they can be killers.

SYMPTOMS OF OVERDOSE

If you or any of your friends have taken prescription pain relievers, here are the danger signs to watch for:
- slow breathing (Less than 10 breaths a minute is a sign of serious trouble.)
- small, pinpoint pupils
- confusion
- being tired, nodding off, or passing out
- dizziness
- weakness
- apathy (They do not care about anything.)
- cold and clammy skin
- nausea
- vomiting
- seizures

A lot of these symptoms can make people think someone who has overdosed on prescription pain relievers is drunk. And you may be tempted to let them sleep it off or tell their parents or other adults they had too much to drink. Do not do this. Be honest about what drugs the person has ingested. Without proper treatment, people who overdose on prescription pain relievers could go to sleep and never wake up.

WHAT YOU CAN DO IF A FRIEND IS OVERDOSING

Make an anonymous call to 911 or your friend's parents if you are too scared to identify yourself. Try to get your friend to respond to you by calling out his or her name. Make your friend wake up and talk to you. Shake him or her if you have to. Otherwise, your friend could suffer brain damage, fall into a coma, or die.

ADDICTION CAN BE A LIVING DEATH

If you abuse prescription pain relievers and are lucky enough to cheat death, you are still in big trouble. Prescription pain relievers can be addictive. The longer you take them, the more your body needs them. Try to stop and you could experience withdrawal symptoms.

Addiction to prescription pain relievers is similar to that of being hooked on heroin, and the withdrawal is not much different: bone and muscle pain, diarrhea, vomiting, cold flashes, and insomnia.

If you or someone you know is abusing or is addicted, get professional help. You can also ask for help from parents, doctors, relatives, teachers, or school guidance counselors. Substance abuse ruins lives. Do not let it happen to your friends—or to you.[3]

---

[3] "Misuse of Prescription Pain Relievers: The Buzz Takes Your Breath Away… Permanently," U.S. Food and Drug Administration (FDA), January 10, 2018. Available online. URL: www.fda.gov/drugs/resources-drugs/misuse-prescription-pain-relievers-buzz-takes-your-breath-away-permanently. Accessed February 29, 2024.

Part 6 | Managing Chronic Disease

Chapter 45 | Self-Management of Chronic Illness

Chapter Contents
Section 45.1—Take Charge of Your Health 431
Section 45.2—Adopt a Healthy Eating Plan 433
Section 45.3—Stress and Your Health 438
Section 45.4—Exercise Can Improve Some
　　　　　　　Chronic Disease Conditions 442
Section 45.5—Tips for Dealing with Pain 448
Section 45.6—The Health Benefits of Having Pets 450

Section 45.1 | Take Charge of Your Health

Health care is a team effort, and you are the most important member of the team. Your team also includes doctors, nurses, pharmacists, and insurance providers.

To take charge of your health care:
- keep track of important health information
- know your family's health history
- see a doctor regularly for checkups
- be prepared for medical appointments
- ask your doctor, nurse, or pharmacist questions
- follow up after your appointment

KEEP TRACK OF IMPORTANT HEALTH INFORMATION

Keeping all your health information in one place will make it easier to manage your health care. Take this information with you to every medical appointment.

To start your own personal health record, write down:
- the name and phone number of a friend or relative to call if there is an emergency
- phone numbers and addresses of all the places where you get medical care, including your pharmacy
- your blood type
- dates and results of checkups and screening tests
- all the vaccines (shots) you have had and the dates that you got them
- medicines you take, how much you take, and why you take them
- any health conditions you have, including allergies
- any health conditions that run in your family

If you are not sure about some of this information, check with your doctor's office.

GET REGULAR CHECKUPS

Getting regular checkups with your doctor or nurse can help you stay healthy. Regular checkups can help find problems early when they may be easier to treat. If you do not have a doctor or nurse, check out the tips available at https://health.gov/myhealthfinder/doctor-visits/regular-checkups/choosing-doctor-quick-tips for choosing a doctor you can trust.

COST AND INSURANCE

Under the Affordable Care Act (ACA), insurance plans must cover many preventive services, such as screenings and vaccines. Plans must also cover well-child visits through the age of 21 and well-woman visits. Depending on your insurance plan, you may be able to get preventive services at no cost to you.

Medicare also covers certain health services at no cost. If you do not have insurance, you may still be able to get free or low-cost health services.

MAKE THE MOST OF DOCTOR VISITS

Take your list of questions and personal health record with you to the appointment. You may also want to ask a family member or friend to go with you to help take notes.

Be sure to talk about any changes since your last visit, such as:
- new medicines you are taking, including over-the-counter (OTC) medicines
- herbs, home remedies, and vitamins you are taking
- recent illnesses or surgeries
- important changes in your life, such as losing your job or a death in the family
- health concerns or issues

FOLLOW UP AFTER YOUR APPOINTMENT

It can take time and hard work to make the healthy changes you talked about with your doctor or nurse. Remember to:
- call if you have any questions or if you experience side effects from a medicine

Self-Management of Chronic Illness

- schedule follow-up appointments for tests or lab work if you need to
- contact the doctor to get test results if you need to[1]

Section 45.2 | Adopt a Healthy Eating Plan

Good nutrition is essential in keeping current and future generations of Americans healthy across the lifespan. Fewer than 1 in 10 children and adults eat the recommended daily amount of vegetables. Only 4 in 10 children and fewer than 1 in 7 adults eat enough fruit.

Breastfeeding helps protect against childhood illnesses, including ear and respiratory infections, asthma, and sudden infant death syndrome (SIDS). People with healthy eating patterns live longer and are at lower risk for serious health problems, such as heart disease, type 2 diabetes, and obesity. For people with chronic diseases, healthy eating can help manage these conditions and prevent complications.[2]

Healthy eating emphasizes fruits, vegetables, whole grains, dairy, and protein. Dairy recommendations include low-fat or fat-free milk, lactose-free milk, and fortified soy beverages. Other plant-based beverages do not have the same nutritional properties as animal's milk and soy beverages. Protein recommendations include seafood, lean meats and poultry, eggs, legumes (beans, peas, and lentils), soy products, nuts, and seeds.

Most people in the United States need to adjust their eating patterns to increase their intake of dietary fiber, calcium, vitamin D, and potassium, according to the *Dietary Guidelines for Americans, 2020–2025* (DGA). At the same time, we need to consume less

---

[1] Office of Disease Prevention and Health Promotion (ODPHP), "Take Charge of Your Health Care," U.S. Department of Health and Human Services (HHS), December 22, 2022. Available online. URL: https://health.gov/myhealthfinder/doctor-visits/talking-doctor/take-charge-your-health-care. Accessed March 6, 2024.

[2] "Nutrition—Why It Matters," Centers for Disease Control and Prevention (CDC), January 25, 2021. Available online. URL: www.cdc.gov/nutrition/about-nutrition/why-it-matters.html. Accessed March 6, 2024.

added sugar, saturated fat, and sodium. Here are some ways to get started.

EAT MORE FIBER

Fiber helps maintain digestive health and helps us feel fuller longer. Fiber also helps control blood sugar and lowers cholesterol levels. Fresh fruits and vegetables, whole grains, legumes, nuts, and seeds are good sources of fiber.

To bump up fiber, try the following:
- Slice up raw vegetables to use as quick snacks. Storing celery and carrots in water in the refrigerator will keep them crisp longer.
- Start your day off with a whole grain cereal such as oatmeal or food made with bulgur or teff. For even more fiber, top your cereal with berries, pumpkin seeds, or almonds.
- Add half a cup of beans or lentils to your salad to add fiber, texture, and flavor.
- Enjoy whole fruit—maybe a pear, apple, melon slice, or passion fruit—with a meal or as dessert.

INCREASE CALCIUM AND VITAMIN D

Calcium and vitamin D work together to promote optimal bone health. Our bodies can make vitamin D from sunshine, but some individuals may have difficulty producing enough vitamin D and too much sun exposure can increase the risk of skin cancer. While very few foods naturally contain vitamin D, several foods and beverages are fortified with this essential nutrient. To increase calcium and vitamin D intake, try the following:
- **Drink a fortified dairy beverage with your meals.**
- **When you pack your lunch, include a packet of salmon or can of sardines once a week.** Salmon and sardines with bones have more calcium than salmon and sardines without bones.
- **Include spinach, collard greens, bok choy, mushrooms, and taro root in your vegetable dishes.**

- **Look for foods that are fortified with calcium and vitamin D.** Soy beverages, soy yogurt, orange juice, and some whole-grain cereals may have these added nutrients.

ADD MORE POTASSIUM

Potassium helps the kidneys, heart, muscles, and nerves function properly. Not getting enough potassium can increase blood pressure, deplete calcium in bones, and increase the risk of kidney stones.

People with chronic kidney disease (CKD) and people taking certain medications may have too much potassium in their blood. But most people in the United States need more potassium in their eating patterns.

To add more potassium, try the following:
- Try new recipes that use beet greens, lima beans, or Swiss chard.
- Put some variety in your beverages with one cup of 100 percent prune juice or 100 percent pomegranate juice.
- Have a banana as a snack.
- Enjoy 100 percent orange juice or a recommended dairy product with your meals.

LIMIT ADDED SUGARS

Too much added sugar in your diet can contribute to weight gain, obesity, type 2 diabetes, and heart disease. Some foods such as fruit and milk contain natural sugars. Added sugars are sugars and syrups that are added to foods and drinks when they are processed or prepared. Added sugars have many different names, such as cane juice, corn syrup, dextrose, and fructose. Table sugar, maple syrup, and honey are also considered added sugars. Sugary drinks are a common source of added sugars.

To limit added sugars, try the following:
- Drink water instead of sugary drinks. Add berries or slices of lime, lemon, or cucumber for more flavor.
- Add fruit to your cereal or yogurt for sweetness.

- Do not stock up on sugary drinks and snacks. Instead, drink water and keep fruit and vegetable slices handy for snacks.
- At coffee shops, skip the flavored syrups and whipped cream. Ask for low-fat or fat-free milk or an unsweetened, fortified soy beverage. Or get back to basics with black coffee.
- Read Nutrition Facts labels (www.cdc.gov/nutrition/strategies-guidelines/nutrition-facts-label.html) and choose foods with no or lower amounts of added sugars.

REPLACE SATURATED FATS

Replacing saturated fat with healthier unsaturated fats can help protect your heart. Common sources of saturated fat are fatty meats such as beef ribs and sausage, whole milk, full-fat cheese, butter, and cream cheese.

We need some dietary fat to give us energy, help us develop healthy cells, and help us absorb some vitamins and minerals. But unsaturated fat is better for us than saturated fat.

To replace saturated fats with unsaturated fats, try the following:
- Replace whole milk in a smoothie with low-fat yogurt and an avocado.
- Sprinkle nuts or seeds on salads instead of cheese.
- Use beans or seafood instead of meat as a source of protein.
- Cook with canola, corn, olive, peanut, safflower, soybean, or sunflower oil instead of butter or margarine.
- Replace full-fat milk and cheese with low-fat or fat-free versions.

CUT BACK ON SODIUM

Eating too much sodium can raise your risk of high blood pressure (HBP), heart attack, and stroke. More than 70 percent of the sodium Americans consume comes from packaged and prepared foods. While sodium has many forms, 90 percent of the sodium we consume is from salt.

Self-Management of Chronic Illness

To cut back on sodium, try the following:
- Instead of using salt, add flavor to your meals with a squeeze of lemon juice, a dash of no-salt spice blends, or fresh herbs.
- Eat high-sodium processed and prepackaged food less frequently. Many common foods, including breads, pizza, and deli meats, have high amounts of sodium.
- At the grocery store, read the Nutrition Facts label to find low-sodium products.
- Buy unprocessed food, such as fresh or frozen vegetables, to prepare at home without salt.

AIM FOR A VARIETY OF COLORS

A good practice is to aim for a variety of colors on your plate. Fruits and vegetables such as dark, leafy greens; oranges; and tomatoes—even fresh herbs—are loaded with vitamins, fiber, and minerals.

To make your plate more colorful, try the following:
- Sprinkle fresh herbs over a salad or whole wheat pasta.
- Make a red sauce with fresh tomatoes (or canned tomatoes with low sodium or no salt added), fresh herbs, and spices.
- Add diced veggies—such as peppers, broccoli, or onions—to stews and omelets to give them a boost of color and nutrients.
- Top low-fat, unsweetened yogurt with your favorite fruit.[3]

---

[3] National Center for Chronic Disease Prevention and Health Promotion (NCCDPHP), "Healthy Eating Tips," Centers for Disease Control and Prevention (CDC), July 11, 2022. Available online. URL: www.cdc.gov/nccdphp/dnpao/features/healthy-eating-tips/index.html. Accessed March 6, 2024.

Section 45.3 | **Stress and Your Health**

Not all stress is bad. But long-term stress can lead to health problems. Preventing and managing long-term stress can lower your risk for other conditions—such as heart disease, obesity, high blood pressure (HBP), and depression.

CAUSES OF STRESS

Stress is how the body reacts to a challenge or demand. Change is often a cause of stress. Even positive changes, such as having a baby or getting a job promotion, can be stressful. Stress can be short term or long term.

Common causes of short-term stress:
- needing to do a lot in a short amount of time
- having a lot of small problems in the same day, such as getting stuck in a traffic jam or running late
- getting ready for a work or school presentation
- having an argument

Common causes of long-term stress:
- having problems at work or at home
- having money problems
- having a long-term illness
- taking care of someone with an illness
- dealing with the death of a loved one

SIGNS OF STRESS

When you are under stress, you may feel:
- worried
- angry
- irritable
- depressed
- unable to focus

Self-Management of Chronic Illness

HEALTH EFFECTS OF STRESS
Stress also affects your body. Physical signs of stress include:
- headaches
- trouble sleeping or sleeping too much
- upset stomach
- weight gain or loss
- tense muscles

Stress can also lead to a weakened immune system (the system in the body that fights infections), which could make you more likely to get sick. Stress is different for everyone.

PREVENTION OF STRESS
You can prevent or reduce stress by:
- planning ahead
- deciding which tasks to do first
- preparing for stressful events

MANAGEMENT OF STRESS
Some stress is hard to avoid. You can find ways to manage stress by:
- noticing when you feel stressed
- taking time to relax
- getting active and eating healthy
- finding solutions to problems you are having
- talking to friends and family

BENEFITS OF MANAGING STRESS
Over time, long-term stress can lead to health problems. Managing stress can help you:
- sleep better
- control your weight
- have less muscle tension
- be in a better mood
- get along better with family and friends

TIPS FOR PREVENTING AND MANAGING STRESS

You cannot always avoid stress, but you can take steps to deal with stress in a positive way. Following are tips for preventing and managing stress.

Plan and Prepare

Being prepared and feeling in control of your situation might help lower your stress.
- **Plan your time.** Think ahead about how you are going to use your time. Write a to-do list and figure out what is most important—then do that thing first. Be realistic about how long each task will take.
- **Prepare yourself.** Prepare ahead for stressful events such as a hard conversation with a loved one. You can:
  - picture what the room will look like and what you will say
  - think about different ways the conversation could go and how you could respond
  - have a plan for ending the conversation early if you need time to think

Relax

The following techniques can help relax your mind and body:
- **Deep breathing and meditation.** This can help relax your muscles and clear your mind.
- **Stretching or taking a hot shower.** Stress causes tension in your muscles. Try stretching or taking a hot shower to help you relax.

Get Active

Regular physical activity can help prevent and manage stress. It can also help relax your muscles and improve your mood. So get active with the following activities:
- **Aerobic activities.** Aim for 150 minutes a week of moderate-intensity aerobic activities—such as going for a bike ride or taking a walk.

Self-Management of Chronic Illness

- **Strengthening activities.** Do strengthening activities—such as push-ups or lifting weights—at least two days a week.

Remember, any amount of physical activity is better than none.

Food and Alcohol
Give your body plenty of energy by eating healthy—including vegetables, fruits, grains, and proteins. Avoid using alcohol or other drugs to manage stress. If you choose to drink, drink only in moderation. This means:
- one drink or less in a day for women
- two drinks or less in a day for men

Get Support
Stress is a normal part of life. But, if your stress does not go away or keeps getting worse, you may need help. Over time, stress can lead to serious problems such as depression or anxiety.
- If you are feeling stressed, tell your friends and family. They may be able to help.
- If you are feeling down or hopeless, talk with your doctor about depression.
- If you are feeling anxious, find out how to get help for anxiety (www.nimh.nih.gov/health/topics/anxiety-disorders).
- If you have lived through a traumatic event (such as a major accident, crime, or natural disaster), find out about treatment for posttraumatic stress disorder (PTSD; www.nimh.nih.gov/health/topics/post-traumatic-stress-disorder-ptsd).

A mental health professional (such as a psychologist or social worker) can help treat these conditions with talk therapy (also called "psychotherapy") or medicine.[4]

---

[4] Office of Disease Prevention and Health Promotion (ODPHP), "Manage Stress," U.S. Department of Health and Human Services (HHS), July 20, 2022. Available online. URL: https://health.gov/myhealthfinder/health-conditions/heart-health/manage-stress. Accessed March 6, 2024.

Section 45.4 | Exercise Can Improve Some Chronic Disease Conditions

Regular physical activity helps improve your overall health, fitness, and quality of life (QOL). It also helps reduce your risk of chronic conditions, such as obesity, type 2 diabetes, heart disease, many types of cancer, depression and anxiety, and dementia.

Everyone can benefit from physical activity—no matter your age, sex, race or ethnicity, health condition, shape, or size.

WHAT ARE THE TYPES OF PHYSICAL ACTIVITY?

There are two types of physical activity:
- **Cardio or aerobic activity.** This activity involves moderate or vigorous intensity exercises that get you breathing harder and your heart beating faster (e.g., brisk walking, biking, dancing, and yard work).
- **Muscle-strengthening activity.** This activity works best when you work all your body's major muscle groups, including your legs, hips, back, chest, abs, shoulders, and arms (e.g., heavy gardening or carrying heavy loads, including groceries).

HOW MUCH PHYSICAL ACTIVITY DO YOU NEED?

Fitting regular physical activity into your schedule may seem hard at first, but you can reach your goals through different types and amounts of physical activity each week.

Adults

Adults should do at least 150 minutes of moderate-intensity aerobic activity every week, plus muscle-strengthening activities at least two days a week. Adults aged 65 and older also need balance-improving activities. Adults try walking 30 minutes a day, five days a week. Older adults practice standing on one foot or walking heel to toe.

Self-Management of Chronic Illness

Kids
Kids between the ages of 6 and 17 should be physically active and do at least 60 minutes (one hour) or more physical activity each day.

Preschool-Aged Children
Children between the ages of three and five should be physically active throughout the day with plenty of opportunities for active play.

TIPS TO GET AND STAY ACTIVE
- Talk to your doctor if you have a chronic condition such as type 2 diabetes or heart disease.
- Get the support of your friends and family and invite them to get active with you.
- Start slowly and add time, frequency, or intensity every week.
- Schedule physical activity for times in the day or week when you are most energetic.
- Plan ahead. Make physical activity part of your daily or weekly schedule.
- Walk instead of drive to nearby destinations or park the car farther away and fit in a walk to your destination.
- Support improvements in your neighborhood that make it easier to walk or bike to where you want to go.[5]

BENEFITS OF PHYSICAL ACTIVITY
Regular physical activity is one of the most important things you can do for your health. Being physically active can improve your brain health, help manage weight, reduce the risk of disease, strengthen bones and muscles, and improve your ability to do everyday activities.

---

[5] National Center for Chronic Disease Prevention and Health Promotion (NCCDPHP), "Physical Activity Helps Prevent Chronic Diseases," Centers for Disease Control and Prevention (CDC), May 8, 2023. Available online. URL: www.cdc.gov/chronicdisease/resources/infographic/physical-activity.htm. Accessed March 6, 2024.

Adults who sit less and do any amount of moderate-to-vigorous physical activity gain some health benefits. Only a few lifestyle choices have as large an effect on your health as physical activity.

Everyone can experience the health benefits of physical activity—age, abilities, ethnicity, shape, or size do not matter.

Immediate Benefits

Some benefits of physical activity on brain health happen right after a session of moderate-to-vigorous physical activity. Benefits include improved thinking or cognition for children aged 6–13 and reduced short-term feelings of anxiety for adults. Regular physical activity can help keep your thinking, learning, and judgment skills sharp as you age. It can also reduce your risk of depression and anxiety and help you sleep better.

Weight Management

Both eating patterns and physical activity routines play a critical role in weight management. You gain weight when you consume more calories through eating and drinking than the amount of calories you burn, including those burned during physical activity.

- **Maintain your weight.** Work your way up to 150 minutes a week of moderate physical activity, which could include dancing or yard work. You could achieve the goal of 150 minutes a week with 30 minutes a day, five days a week. People vary greatly in how much physical activity they need for weight management. You may need to be more active than others to reach or maintain a healthy weight.
- **Lose weight and keep it off**. You will need a high amount of physical activity unless you also adjust your eating patterns and reduce the amount of calories you are eating and drinking. Getting to and staying at a healthy weight requires both regular physical activity and healthy eating.

Self-Management of Chronic Illness

Reduce Your Health Risk
CARDIOVASCULAR DISEASE
Heart disease and stroke are two leading causes of death in the United States. Getting at least 150 minutes a week of moderate physical activity can put you at a lower risk for these diseases. You can reduce your risk even further with more physical activity. Regular physical activity can also lower your blood pressure and improve your cholesterol levels.

TYPE 2 DIABETES AND METABOLIC SYNDROME
Regular physical activity can reduce your risk of developing type 2 diabetes and metabolic syndrome. Metabolic syndrome is some combination of too much fat around the waist, high blood pressure (HBP), low high-density lipoproteins (HDLs) cholesterol, high triglycerides, or high blood sugar. People start to see benefits at levels from physical activity even without meeting the recommendations for 150 minutes a week of moderate physical activity. Additional amounts of physical activity seem to lower risk even more.

INFECTIOUS DISEASES
Physical activity may help reduce the risk of serious outcomes from infectious diseases, including coronavirus disease 2019 (COVID-19), the flu, and pneumonia.
- **People who do little or no physical activity are more likely to get very sick from COVID-19 than those who are physically active.** A systemic review by the Centers for Disease Control and Prevention (CDC) found that physical activity is associated with a decrease in COVID-19 hospitalizations and deaths, while inactivity increases that risk.
- **People who are more active may be less likely to die from flu or pneumonia.** A CDC study found that adults who meet the aerobic and muscle-strengthening physical activity guidelines are about half as likely to die from flu and pneumonia as adults who meet neither guideline.

SOME CANCERS
Being physically active lowers your risk for developing several common cancers. Adults who participate in greater amounts of physical activity have reduced risks of developing cancers of the:
- bladder
- breast
- colon (proximal and distal)
- endometrium
- esophagus (adenocarcinoma)
- kidney
- lung
- stomach (cardia and noncardia adenocarcinoma)

If you are a cancer survivor, getting regular physical activity not only helps give you a better QOL but also improves your physical fitness.

Strengthen Your Bones and Muscles
As you age, it is important to protect your bones, joints, and muscles—they support your body and help you move. Keeping bones, joints, and muscles healthy can help ensure that you are able to do your daily activities and be physically active.

Muscle-strengthening activities such as lifting weights can help you increase or maintain your muscle mass and strength. This is important for older adults who experience reduced muscle mass and muscle strength with aging. Slowly increasing the amount of weight and number of repetitions you do as part of muscle-strengthening activities will give you even more benefits, no matter your age.

Improve Your Ability to do Daily Activities and Prevent Falls
Everyday activities include climbing stairs, grocery shopping, or playing with your grandchildren. Being unable to do everyday activities is called a "functional limitation." Physically active middle-aged or older adults have a lower risk of functional limitations than people who are inactive.

Self-Management of Chronic Illness

For older adults, doing a variety of physical activities improves physical function and decreases the risk of falls or injury from a fall. Include physical activities such as aerobic, muscle-strengthening, and balance training. Multicomponent physical activity can be done at home or in a community setting as part of a structured program.

Hip fracture is a serious health condition that can result from a fall. Breaking a hip has life-changing negative effects, especially if you are an older adult. Physically active people have a lower risk of hip fracture than inactive people.

Increase Your Chances of Living Longer

An estimated 110,000 deaths per year could be prevented if U.S. adults aged 40 and older increased their moderate-to-vigorous physical activity by a small amount. Even 10 minutes more a day would make a difference.

Taking more steps a day also helps lower the risk of premature death from all causes. For adults under the age of 60, the risk of premature death leveled off at about 8,000–10,000 steps per day. For adults aged 60 and older, the risk of premature death leveled off at about 6,000–8,000 steps per day.

Manage Chronic Health Conditions and Disabilities

Regular physical activity can help people manage existing chronic conditions and disabilities. For example, regular physical activity can:

- reduce pain and improve function, mood, and QOL for adults with arthritis
- help control blood sugar levels and lower risk of heart disease and nerve damage for people with type 2 diabetes
- help support daily living activities and independence for people with disabilities[6]

---

[6] "Benefits of Physical Activity," Centers for Disease Control and Prevention (CDC), August 1, 2023. Available online. URL: www.cdc.gov/physicalactivity/basics/pa-health/index.htm. Accessed March 6, 2024.

Section 45.5 | Tips for Dealing with Pain

Most people experience some kind of pain during their lives. Pain serves an important purpose: It warns the body when it is in danger. However, ongoing pain causes distress and affects the quality of life (QOL). Pain is the number one reason people see a doctor.

NONDRUG PAIN MANAGEMENT

There are many nondrug treatments that can help with pain. It is important to check with your health-care provider before trying any of the following treatments:

- **Acupuncture**. It involves stimulating acupuncture points. These are specific points on your body. There are different acupuncture methods. The most common one involves inserting thin needles through the skin. Others include using pressure, electrical stimulation, and heat. Acupuncture is based on the belief that qi (vital energy) flows through the body along paths, called "meridians." Practitioners believe that stimulating the acupuncture points can rebalance the qi. Research suggests that acupuncture can help manage certain pain conditions.
- **Biofeedback techniques**. These techniques use electronic devices to measure body functions such as breathing and heart rate. This teaches you to be more aware of your body functions, so you can learn to control them. For example, a biofeedback device may show you measurements of your muscle tension. By watching how these measurements change, you can become more aware of when your muscles are tense and learn to relax them. Biofeedback may help control pain, including chronic headaches and back pain.
- **Electrical stimulation**. This involves using a device to send a gentle electric current to your nerves or muscles. This can help treat pain by interrupting or blocking the pain signals. Types include:
    - transcutaneous electrical nerve stimulation (TENS)

Self-Management of Chronic Illness

- implanted electric nerve stimulation
- deep brain or spinal cord stimulation
- **Massage therapy.** It is a treatment in which the soft tissues of the body are kneaded, rubbed, tapped, and stroked. Among other benefits, it may help people relax and relieve stress and pain.
- **Meditation.** It is a mind-body practice in which you focus your attention on something, such as an object, word, phrase, or breathing. This helps you minimize distracting or stressful thoughts or feelings.
- **Physical therapy.** This uses techniques such as heat, cold, exercise, massage, and manipulation. It can help control pain, as well as condition muscles and restore strength.
- **Psychotherapy (talk therapy).** This uses methods such as discussion, listening, and counseling to treat mental and behavioral disorders. It can also help people who have pain, especially chronic pain, by:
  - teaching them coping skills to be able to better deal with the stress that pain can cause
  - addressing negative thoughts and emotions that can make pain worse
  - providing them with support
- **Relaxation therapy.** It can help reduce muscle tension and stress, lower blood pressure, and control pain. It may involve tensing and relaxing muscles throughout the body. It may be used with guided imagery (focusing the mind on positive images) and meditation.
- **Surgery.** It can sometimes be necessary to treat severe pain with surgery, especially when it is caused by back problems or serious musculoskeletal injuries. There are always risks to getting surgery, and it does not always work to treat pain. So it is important to go through all the risks and benefits with your health-care provider.[7]

---

[7] MedlinePlus, "Non-Drug Pain Management," National Institutes of Health (NIH), August 28, 2018. Available online. URL: https://medlineplus.gov/nondrugpainmanagement.html. Accessed March 6, 2024.

Section 45.6 | The Health Benefits of Having Pets

Nothing compares to the joy of coming home to a loyal companion. The unconditional love of a pet can do more than keep you company. Pets may also decrease stress, improve heart health, and even help children with their emotional and social skills. Research on human-animal interactions is still relatively new. Some studies have shown positive health effects, but the results have been mixed. Interacting with animals has been shown to decrease levels of cortisol (a stress-related hormone) and lower blood pressure. Other studies have found that animals can reduce loneliness, increase feelings of social support, and boost your mood.

ANIMALS HELPING PEOPLE

Animals can serve as a source of comfort and support. Therapy dogs are especially good at this. They are sometimes brought into hospitals or nursing homes to help reduce patients' stress and anxiety.

"Dogs are very present. If someone is struggling with something, they know how to sit there and be loving," says Dr. Ann Berger, a physician and researcher at the National Institutes of Health (NIH) Clinical Center (CC) in Bethesda, Maryland. "Their attention is focused on the person all the time." Dr. Berger works with people who have cancer and terminal illnesses. She teaches them about mindfulness to help decrease stress and manage pain.

"The foundations of mindfulness include attention, intention, compassion, and awareness," Dr. Berger says. "All of those things are things that animals bring to the table. People kind of have to learn it. Animals do this innately."

Researchers are studying the safety of bringing animals into hospital settings because animals may expose people to more germs. Scientists will be testing the children's hands to see if there are dangerous levels of germs transferred from the dog after the visit.

Self-Management of Chronic Illness

Dogs may also aid in the classroom. A study found that dogs can help children with attention deficit hyperactivity disorder (ADHD) focus their attention. Researchers enrolled two groups of children diagnosed with ADHD into 12-week group therapy sessions. The first group of kids read to a therapy dog once a week for 30 minutes. The second group read to puppets that resembled dogs.

Kids who read to the real animals showed better social skills and more sharing, cooperation, and volunteering. They also had fewer behavioral problems.

Another study found that children with autism spectrum disorder (ASD) were calmer while playing with guinea pigs in the classroom. When the children spent 10 minutes in a supervised group playtime with guinea pigs, their anxiety levels dropped. The children also had better social interactions and were more engaged with their peers. The researchers suggest that the animals offered unconditional acceptance, making them a calm comfort to the children.

Animals may help you in other unexpected ways. A study showed that caring for fish helped teens with diabetes better manage their disease. Researchers had a group of teens with type 1 diabetes care for a pet fish twice a day by feeding and checking water levels. The caretaking routine also included changing the tank water each week. This was paired with the children reviewing their blood glucose (blood sugar) logs with their parents.

Researchers tracked how consistently these teens checked their blood glucose. Compared with teens who were not given a fish to care for, fish-keeping teens were more disciplined about checking their own blood glucose levels, which is essential for maintaining their health.

While pets may bring a wide range of health benefits, an animal may not work for everyone. Studies suggest that early exposure to pets may help protect young children from developing allergies and asthma. But for people who are allergic to certain animals, having pets in the home can do more harm than good.

HELPING EACH OTHER

Pets also bring new responsibilities. Knowing how to care for and feed an animal is part of owning a pet. Remember that animals can feel stressed and fatigued, too. It is important for kids to be able to recognize signs of stress in their pets and know when not to approach them. Animal bites can cause serious harm.[8]

---

[8] *NIH News in Health*, "The Power of Pets," National Institutes of Health (NIH), February 2018. Available online. URL: https://newsinhealth.nih.gov/2018/02/power-pets. Accessed March 6, 2024.

Chapter 46 | Caring for Children

Chapter Contents
Section 46.1—Children's Health 455
Section 46.2—Developmental and Behavioral
Screening Tests 456
Section 46.3—Vaccines for Children 460
Section 46.4—Caring for a Seriously Ill Child 473

Section 46.1 | Children's Health

When we talk about a child's growth, we often think first about height and weight. These are two important parts of your child's physical health. Each time you visit your doctor, your child's growth since your last visit will be measured. You can access the growth charts your doctor uses on the following website: www.cdc.gov/growthcharts.

Your child's health is the foundation of all growth and development. Of course, your child's health includes more than physical growth. Some other important parts of your child's health include their cognitive (learning and thinking) development, social and emotional growth, and mental health. All aspects of health and development work together to form your child's overall well-being.

As a parent or caregiver, you are the most important person to support and promote your child's health and wellness, so it is important to find quality health-care services and professionals. Expect professionals to answer your questions, listen to your input, and be available. You know your child best, and you are his or her primary advocate.

Some of the most important parts of children's health and wellness are as follows:
- Brain development (learning and thinking)
  - supporting your child's brain development
- Physical health
  - making sure that you have a medical home
  - ensuring that your child receives well-child physical exams
  - using healthy habits to prevent illness
  - managing illness
- Nutrition
  - making informed decisions about breastfeeding and formula feeding
  - offering nutritious meals that meet your child's needs and give him or her energy to learn
- Social, emotional, and mental health:
  - helping your child understand and lean to share his or her feelings

- helping your child learn to have positive relationships
- encouraging your child to explore and learn
- learning strategies for parenting in tough times and coping with depression or other difficult feelings
- building resilience in yourself and your child
- Oral health
  - encouraging oral and dental health, so children are better able to eat, speak, and focus on learning
- Active living
  - providing age-appropriate amounts of physical activity in your child's daily routines to support physical health and positive behaviors
- Safety and injury prevention
  - creating and maintaining safe environments
  - educating your child on ways to avoid injuries
  - identifying and reporting suspected child abuse and neglect[1]

Section 46.2 | Developmental and Behavioral Screening Tests

WHAT ARE DEVELOPMENTAL AND BEHAVIORAL SCREENING TESTS?

Developmental and behavioral screening tests look at how a child is developing. The screenings are made up of checklists and questionnaires for parents. They include questions about their child's language, movement, thinking, behavior, and emotions.

Many of the questions are based on developmental milestones. Developmental milestones are skills and behaviors that show up in babies and children at certain ages as they grow. They include smiling for the first time, rolling over, and walking. The screening compares your child's milestones to those of other children of the

---

[1] ChildCare.gov, "Supporting Children's Physical Health," Administration for Children and Families (ACF), January 19, 2018. Available online. URL: https://childcare.gov/consumer-education/your-childs-health. Accessed March 27, 2024.

same age. If the screening shows your child is developing at a slower rate, it may be a sign of a developmental disability. Developmental disabilities are conditions that cause problems in physical and/or mental functions, including the following:

- **Intellectual disabilities (IDs)**. IDs cause below-average mental abilities. People with IDs often have problems with learning and daily living skills.
- **Autism spectrum disorder (ASD)**. ASD is a disorder that affects behavior, communication, and social skills.
- **Cerebral palsy (CP)**. CP is a condition that affects movement, coordination, and balance.
- **Deafness or other hearing problems**. Hearing disorders make it hard, but not impossible, to hear. They can often be helped. Deafness can keep you from hearing sound at all.

Developmental and behavioral screening tests do not diagnose these conditions. But a screening can show if your child is not developing on schedule. When developmental disabilities are found and treated early, they can make a big difference in a child's life. Early treatment, known as "early intervention," helps children learn important skills, make the most of their strengths, and improve their quality of life (QOL).

WHAT ARE DEVELOPMENTAL AND BEHAVIORAL SCREENING TESTS USED FOR?

Developmental and behavioral screening tests are used to see if a child is meeting his or her developmental milestones. Some examples of milestones for infants and toddlers are as follows:

- **Birth to four months**. Includes smiling, cooing, and bringing hands to mouth.
- **Six months**. Includes playing with others, looking at themselves in the mirror, sitting without support, and rolling over.
- **Nine months**. Includes making sounds such as "mama" and "dada," understanding the word "no," crawling, and pulling to a stand.

- **One year.** Includes playing peekaboo, following simple directions, and walking while holding onto furniture.
- **One and a half years.** Includes speaking and understanding several words, eating with a spoon, walking, and walking up and down stairs.
- **Two to three years.** Includes recognizing labels and colors, naming pictures of common objects, getting dressed and undressed, and walking and running easily.

Developmental milestones are general guidelines. Children grow at different rates. There is a range in what is considered normal development. But looking at milestones can help identify potential problems early.

WHY DOES YOUR CHILD NEED A DEVELOPMENTAL AND BEHAVIORAL SCREENING TEST?

The American Academy of Pediatrics (AAP) recommends developmental and behavioral screenings for all children during regular well-child checkups at the following ages:
- 9 months
- 18 months
- 30 months

The AAP also recommends that all children should be screened for ASD during regular checkups at 18 and 24 months.

Also, talk to your provider about screening if you think there is a problem with your child's development. As a parent, you will probably be the first to notice any problems with the way your child interacts, learns, speaks, or moves.

WHAT HAPPENS DURING A DEVELOPMENT AND BEHAVIORAL SCREENING TEST?

Screenings may be done by your child's provider and/or by you with guidance from your child's provider.

There are many different types of developmental and behavioral screening tests. Each test asks questions about a child's development.

Caring for Children

You may be asked about your child's social interactions, language skills, and/or gross and fine motor skills. Motor skills are the ability to move muscles. Gross motor skills involve moving large muscles for movements such as walking and jumping. Fine motor skills are the ability to move small muscles with precision, such as picking up a toy or using a fork.

The following are the common tests:
- **Ages and stages questionnaire.** This test is designed for children between the ages of one month and five and a half years. It contains a series of questions with answer choices of "yes," "sometimes," and "not yet."
- **Parents' evaluation of developmental status (PEDS).** The PEDS test is designed for children from birth to the age of eight. It is a brief test that can be completed in about five minutes.
- **Child development inventories (CDIs).** CDIs are three different tests. They are geared to age groups from infancy to preschool. Each contains 60 yes or no questions.
- **Modified checklist for autism in toddlers (M-CHAT).** The M-CHAT test is for toddlers between the ages of 16 and 30 months. It includes a series of yes or no questions.

ARE THERE ANY SPECIAL PREPARATIONS NEEDED FOR THIS SCREENING?
There are no special preparations needed for this screening.

ARE THERE ANY RISKS TO THE SCREENING?
There is no risk in taking a questionnaire.

WHAT DO THE RESULTS MEAN?
If the results show that your child is not developing at the same rate as other children of the same age, it does not necessarily mean there is a problem. But your child may be referred to a specialist for further testing and treatment. If you have questions about the results, talk to your child's provider.

IS THERE ANYTHING ELSE YOU NEED TO KNOW ABOUT DEVELOPMENTAL AND BEHAVIORAL SCREENING TESTS?

If screening tests show a problem with your child's development, your child's provider may recommend at-home developmental monitoring. Developmental monitoring is a way to look at how your child grows and changes over time. Parents and other caregivers use brief checklists to track the child's development.[2]

Section 46.3 | Vaccines for Children

Vaccines work by preparing the body's immune system for future exposure to disease-causing viruses or bacteria. Vaccines contain antigens, which are weakened bacteria or viruses or parts of bacteria or viruses, which mimic the disease-causing agents. As a result of vaccination, the body's immune system thinks the antigens from the vaccine are foreign and should not be in the body, but the antigens do not cause disease in the person receiving the vaccine. After receiving the vaccine, if the virus or bacterium that causes the real disease then enters the body in the future, the immune system is prepared and responds quickly and forcefully to attack the disease-causing agent to prevent the person from getting sick with the disease. Vaccines are commonly administered through injection (a shot), but some are available in oral forms or as nasal sprays.

There are various types of vaccines that are routinely given to children:

- **Attenuated (weakened) live viruses.** These vaccines contain a live virus that has been weakened during the manufacturing process so that they do not cause the actual disease in the person being vaccinated. However, because they contain a small amount of the weakened live virus, people with weakened immune

---

[2] MedlinePlus, "Developmental and Behavioral Screening Tests," National Institutes of Health (NIH), July 26, 2021. Available online. URL: https://medlineplus.gov/lab-tests/developmental-and-behavioral-screening-tests. Accessed March 27, 2024.

systems should talk to their health-care provider before receiving them. Examples include vaccines that prevent chickenpox, rotavirus, and measles, mumps, and rubella (MMR).
- **Inactivated (killed) viruses**. These vaccines contain a virus that has been killed so as not to cause disease, but the body still recognizes it and stimulates the production of antibodies against the virus. They can be given to individuals with weakened immune systems. Examples include vaccines to prevent polio and hepatitis A.
- **Subunits**. In some cases, the entire virus or bacterium is not required for an immune response to prevent disease; just the important parts, a portion or a "subunit" of the disease-causing bacteria or virus, are needed to provide protection. The vaccine to prevent influenza (the flu) that is given as a shot is an example of a subunit vaccine because it is made with parts of the influenza virus.
- **Toxoids**. Some bacteria cause illness in people by secreting a poison (a toxin). Scientists discovered that detoxified toxins do not cause illness. Examples of vaccines that contain toxoids include those to prevent tetanus and diphtheria disease.
- **Recombinant**. These vaccines are made by genetic engineering, the process and method of manipulating the genetic material of an organism. An example of this type of vaccine is those that prevent certain diseases, such as cervical cancer, that are caused by human papillomavirus (HPV). In this case, the genes that code for a specific protein from each of the virus types of HPV included in the vaccine are expressed in yeast to create large quantities of the protein. The protein that is produced is purified and then used to make the vaccine. Because the vaccine only contains a protein and not the entire virus, the vaccine cannot cause the HPV infection. It is the body's immune response to the recombinant protein(s) that then protects against diseases caused by the naturally occurring virus.

- **Polysaccharides.** To protect against certain disease-causing bacteria, the main antigens in a vaccine are sugar-like substances called "polysaccharides." These are purified from the bacteria to make polysaccharide vaccines. However, vaccines composed solely of purified polysaccharides are only effective in older children and adults. Pneumovax 23, a vaccine for the prevention of pneumococcal disease caused by 23 different strains, is an example of a polysaccharide vaccine.
- **Conjugates.** Vaccines made only with polysaccharides do not work very well in young children because their immune system has not fully developed. To make vaccines that protect young children against diseases caused by certain bacteria, the polysaccharides are connected to a protein so that the immune system can recognize and respond to the polysaccharide. The protein acts as a "carrier" for the part of the vaccine that will make protective antibodies in the body. Examples of conjugate vaccines include those to prevent invasive disease caused by *Haemophilus influenzae* type b (Hib).

ROUTINELY ADMINISTERED VACCINES FOR CHILDREN

Some of the most commonly administered vaccines are briefly discussed as follows.

Diphtheria and Tetanus Toxoids and Acellular Pertussis Vaccine Adsorbed

Brand names: Daptacel® and Infanrix®
- **What it is for.** This vaccine prevents the bacterial diseases diphtheria, tetanus (lockjaw), and pertussis (whooping cough). This combination vaccine is given as a series in infants and children aged six weeks through six years, prior to their seventh birthday. The bacteria that cause diphtheria can infect the throat,

causing a thick covering that can lead to problems with breathing, paralysis, or heart failure. Tetanus can cause painful tightening (spasms) of the muscles, seizures, paralysis, and death. Pertussis, also known as "whooping cough," has the initial symptoms of runny nose, sneezing, and a mild cough, which may seem like a typical cold. Usually, the cough slowly becomes more severe. Eventually, the patient may experience bouts of rapid coughing followed by the "whooping" sound that gives the disease its common name as they try to inhale. While the coughing fit is occurring, the patient may vomit or turn blue from lack of air. Patients gradually recover over weeks to months.
- **Common side effects.** It causes fever, drowsiness, fussiness or irritability, and redness, soreness, or swelling at the injection site.
- **Tell your health-care provider beforehand.** Inform your health-care provider if the child is moderately or severely ill, has had swelling of the brain within seven days after a previous dose of vaccine, has a neurologic disorder such as epilepsy, or has had a severe allergic reaction to a previous shot.

Tetanus Toxoid, Reduced Diphtheria Toxoid, and Acellular Pertussis Vaccine Adsorbed

Brand names: Adacel® and Boostrix®
- **What it is for.** This is a booster shot for children aged 10 or 11 to prevent the bacterial infections diphtheria, tetanus (lockjaw), and pertussis (whooping cough). In addition, Boostrix is approved for all individuals aged 10 and older (including the elderly). Adacel is approved for use in people aged 10–64.
- **Common side effects.** It causes pain, redness, and swelling at the injection site; headache; and tiredness.
- **Tell your health-care provider beforehand.** Inform your health-care provider if the child is moderately or severely ill, has had swelling of the brain within seven

days after a previous dose of the pertussis vaccine, or has any allergic reaction to any vaccine that protects against diphtheria, tetanus, or pertussis diseases.

Haemophilus B Conjugate Vaccine
Brand names: ActHIB®, Hiberix®, and PedvaxHIB®
- **What it is for.** This vaccine prevents Hib invasive disease. Before the availability of Hib vaccines, Hib disease was the leading cause of bacterial meningitis among children under the age of five in the United States. Meningitis is an infection of the tissue covering the brain and spinal cord, which can lead to lasting brain damage and deafness. Hib disease can also cause pneumonia, severe swelling in the throat, infections of the blood, joints, bones, and tissue covering of the heart, as well as death. Both ActHIB® and PedvaxHIB® are approved for infants and children beginning at two months. ActHIB® can be given through five years of age, and PedvaxHIB® can be given through 71 months of age. Hiberix is approved for children aged six weeks through four years (prior to their fifth birthday).
- **Common side effects.** It causes fussiness, sleepiness, soreness, and swelling and redness at the injection site.
- **Tell your health-care provider beforehand.** Inform your health-care provider if the child is moderately or severely ill or has ever had an allergic reaction to a previous dose of the Hib vaccine.

Hepatitis A Vaccine
Brand names: Havrix® and Vaqta®
- **What it is for.** This vaccine prevents disease caused by the hepatitis A virus. People infected with hepatitis A may not have any symptoms, and if they do have symptoms, they may feel like they have a mild "flu-like" illness, or they may have jaundice (yellow skin or eyes),

Caring for Children

tiredness, stomachache, nausea, and diarrhea. Young children may not have any symptoms, so when a child's caregiver becomes sick, that is when it is recognized that the child is infected. Hepatitis A is most often spread by an object contaminated with the feces of a person with hepatitis A, such as when a parent or caregiver does not properly wash his or her hands after changing diapers or cleaning up the stool of an infected person. Both vaccines are approved for use in children aged one and older.
- **Common side effects**. It causes soreness and redness at the injection site and loss of appetite.
- **Tell your health-care provider beforehand**. Inform your health-care provider if the child is moderately to severely ill or has ever had an allergic reaction to a previous dose of the vaccine.

Hepatitis B Vaccine
Brand names: Engerix-B® and Recombivax HB®
- **What it is for**. This vaccine prevents infection caused by the hepatitis B virus. Hepatitis B is spread when body fluid infected with hepatitis B enters the body of a person who is not infected. Hepatitis B can lead to chronic hepatitis (liver inflammation), liver cancer, and death. The vaccines are approved for individuals of all ages, including newborns. It is particularly important for those at an increased risk of exposure to the hepatitis B virus, such as a baby born to a mom who is infected with the virus, to be vaccinated.
- **Common side effects**. It causes soreness, redness, and swelling at the injection site; irritability; fever; diarrhea; fatigue or weakness; loss of appetite; and headache.
- **Tell your health-care provider beforehand**. Inform your health-care provider if the child is moderately or severely ill or has ever had a life-threatening allergic reaction to yeast or to a previous dose of the vaccine.

Human Papillomavirus Vaccine
Brand name: Gardasil 9®
- **What it is for.** This vaccine is for use in females and males aged 9–45. It prevents cervical, vulvar, vaginal, and anal cancers caused by any of the following HPV types: 16, 18, 31, 33, 45, 52, and 58. Overall, it has the potential to prevent approximately 90 percent of cervical, vulvar, vaginal, and anal cancers. It is also approved for the prevention of genital warts caused by types 6 and 11 in both males and females.
- **Common side effects.** It causes headache, fever, nausea, dizziness, fainting, and pain, swelling, redness, itchiness, or bruising at the injection site.
- **Tell your health-care provider beforehand.** Inform your health-care provider if the individual has had an allergic reaction to yeast or to a previous dose of the vaccine.

Influenza Vaccine (Administered with a Needle)
Brand names: Afluria Quadrivalent®, Fluarix Quadrivalent®, Flucelvax Quadrivalent®, FluLaval Quadrivalent®, and Fluzone Quadrivalent®
- **What it is for.** Different vaccines are approved for different age groups to prevent influenza disease, caused by the strains of the influenza virus that are included in the vaccine. Influenza, commonly called "flu," is a contagious respiratory virus that can cause mild-to-severe illness. The elderly, young children, and people with certain health conditions (such as asthma, diabetes, or heart disease) are at high risk for serious influenza-related complications. Complications may include pneumonia, ear infections, sinus infections, dehydration, and worsening of certain medical conditions, such as congestive heart failure, asthma, or diabetes. The strains of the influenza virus that cause disease in people frequently change, so yearly vaccination is needed to provide protection against the influenza viruses likely to cause illness each winter.

- **Common side effects.** It causes pain, redness, and swelling at the injection site; low-grade fever; muscle aches; headache; fatigue; and a general feeling of being unwell.
- **Tell your health-care provider beforehand.** Inform your health-care provider if the child is moderately or severely ill, has a weakened immune system, has asthma or recurrent wheezing, or has a history of Guillain-Barré syndrome (GBS), a neurological disorder that causes severe muscle weakness. Also, tell your health-care provider about any allergies, including severe allergies to eggs and any allergic reaction to a previous dose of any influenza vaccine. In addition, because of the association of Reye syndrome with aspirin and wild-type influenza infection, the health-care provider should be made aware if the child is currently receiving aspirin or aspirin-containing therapy.

Influenza Vaccine, Intranasal (Nasal Spray)
Brand name: FluMist Quadrivalent®
- **What it is for.** This vaccine protects against four different strains of the influenza virus included in the vaccine for children and adults aged 2–49.
- **Common side effects.** It causes a runny or stuffy nose and cough.
- **Tell your health-care provider beforehand.** Inform your health-care provider if the child is moderately or severely ill, has a weakened immune system, has asthma or recurrent wheezing, or has a history of GBS, a neurological disorder that causes severe muscle weakness. Also, tell your health-care provider about any allergies, including severe allergies to eggs and any allergic reaction to a previous dose of any influenza vaccine. In addition, because of the association of Reye syndrome with aspirin and wild-type influenza infection, the health-care provider should be made

aware if the child is currently receiving aspirin or aspirin-containing therapy.

Measles, Mumps, and Rubella Vaccine
Brand name: M-M-R II®
- **What it is for**. This vaccine prevents MMR in children aged one and older. Measles is a respiratory disease that causes a skin rash all over the body and fever, cough, and runny nose. Measles can be severe, causing ear infections, pneumonia, seizures, and swelling of the brain. Mumps causes fever, headache, loss of appetite, and the well-known sign of swollen cheeks and jaw which is from the swelling of the salivary glands. Rare complications include deafness, meningitis (infection of the lining that surrounds the brain and spinal cord), and painful swelling of the testicles or ovaries. Rubella, also called "German measles," causes fever, a rash, and—mainly in women—arthritis. Rubella infection during pregnancy can lead to birth defects.
- **Common side effects**. It causes fever, mild rash, fainting, headache, dizziness, irritability, and burning/stinging, redness, swelling, and tenderness at the injection site.
- **Tell your health-care provider beforehand**. Inform your health-care provider if the child is ill and has a fever; has ever had an allergic reaction to gelatin, the antibiotic neomycin, or a previous dose of the vaccine; or has immune system problems, cancer, or problems with the blood or lymph system.

Meningococcal Vaccine
There are two different types of meningococcal vaccines. One type protects against four groups of meningococcal bacteria called groups "A," "C," "W-135," and "Y." The U.S. Food and Drug Administration (FDA) has approved two vaccines of this type. The other type protects against a meningococcal bacterium called

Caring for Children

"group B." The FDA has also approved two meningococcal group B vaccines, but they are only recommended for routine use in certain high-risk groups.

Brand names: Bexsero®, Menactra®, Menveo®, and Trumenba®

- **What it is for.** This vaccine prevents certain types of meningococcal disease, a life-threatening illness caused by the bacterium *Neisseria meningitidis* that infects the bloodstream and the lining that surrounds the brain and spinal cord (meningitis). *N. meningitidis* is a leading cause of meningitis in young children. Even with appropriate antibiotics and intensive care, between 10 and 15 percent of people who develop meningococcal disease die from the infection. Another 10–20 percent suffer from complications, such as brain damage or loss of limb or hearing. Bexsero and Trumenba are approved for use in those aged 10–25 to prevent invasive meningococcal disease caused by *N. meningitidis* serogroup B. Menactra® and Menveo® prevent meningococcal disease caused by *N. meningitidis* serogroups A, C, Y, and W-135. Menactra® is approved for use in those aged 9 months through 55 years. Menveo® is approved for use in those aged 2 months through 55 years.
- **Common side effects.** It causes tenderness, pain, redness, and swelling at the injection site; irritability; headache; fever; tiredness; chills; diarrhea; and loss of appetite for a short while.
- **Tell your health-care provider beforehand.** Inform your health-care provider if the child is moderately or severely ill, has had a severe allergic reaction to a previous dose of the meningococcal vaccine, or has a known sensitivity to vaccine components.

Pneumococcal 13-Valent Conjugate Vaccine
Brand name: Prevnar 13®

- **What it is for.** This vaccine prevents invasive disease caused by 13 different types of the bacterium *Streptococcus pneumoniae* in infants, children, and adolescents aged

6 weeks through 17 years. In infants and children aged six weeks through five years, it is also approved for the prevention of otitis media (ear infection) caused by seven different types of the bacterium. *S. pneumoniae* can cause infections of the blood, middle ear, and the covering of the brain and spinal cord, as well as pneumonia. Prevnar 13 is also approved for adults aged 18 and older.
- **Common side effects.** This causes pain, redness, and swelling at the injection site; irritability; decreased appetite; and fever.
- **Tell your health-care provider beforehand.** Inform your health-care provider if the child is moderately or severely ill and has ever had an allergic reaction to a previous dose or component of the vaccine, including diphtheria toxoid (i.e., diphtheria, tetanus, and pertussis (DTaP) vaccine).

Poliovirus Vaccine
Brand name: Ipol®
- **What it is for.** This vaccine prevents polio in infants as young as six weeks of age. Polio is a disease that can cause paralysis or death.
- **Common side effects.** It causes redness, hardening, and pain at the injection site; fever; irritability; sleepiness; fussiness; and crying.
- **Tell your health-care provider beforehand.** Inform your health-care provider if the child is moderately or severely ill, including illness with a fever, and has ever had a severe allergic reaction to a previous dose of the polio vaccine, any component of the vaccine, or an allergic reaction to the antibiotics neomycin, streptomycin, or polymyxin B.

Rotavirus Vaccine
Brand names: Rotarix® and RotaTeq®
- **What it is for.** This vaccine prevents gastroenteritis caused by rotavirus infection in infants as young as

six weeks of age. Rotavirus disease is the leading cause of severe diarrhea and dehydration in infants worldwide. In the United States, the disease occurs more often during the winter. Before rotavirus vaccines were available, most children in the United States were infected with the rotavirus before the age of two. In addition, the rotavirus resulted in about 55,000–70,000 hospitalizations and 20–60 infant deaths in the United States each year.
- **Common side effects.** It causes fussiness or irritability, cough or runny nose, fever, and loss of appetite.
- **Tell your health-care provider beforehand.** Inform your health-care provider if the child has an illness with a fever; has a weakened immune system because of a disease; has a blood disorder; has any type of cancer; has gastrointestinal problems; has had stomach surgery or ever had intussusception, which is a form of blockage of the intestines; is allergic to any of the ingredients of the vaccine; has ever had an allergic reaction to a previous dose of the vaccine; or has regular close contact with a member of a family or household who has a weak immune system.

Varicella Virus Vaccine
Brand name: Varivax®
- **What it is for.** This vaccine prevents varicella (chickenpox) in children aged one and older. Chickenpox usually causes a blister-like itchy rash, tiredness, headache, and fever. It can be serious, particularly in babies, adolescents, adults, and people with weak immune systems, causing less common but more serious complications, such as skin infection, scarring, pneumonia, brain swelling, Reye syndrome (which affects the liver and brain), and death.
- **Common side effects.** It causes soreness, pain, redness, or swelling at the injection site; fever; irritability; and chickenpox-like rash on the body or at the site of the shot.

- **Tell your health-care provider beforehand.** Inform your health-care provider if the child is moderately or severely ill, including a fever; has a weak immune system; has received a blood or plasma transfusion or immune globulin within the last five months; takes any medicines; and has allergies, including any life-threatening allergic reaction to gelatin, the antibiotic neomycin, or a previous dose of chickenpox or any other vaccine.[3]

COVID-19 Vaccine

There are two types of coronavirus disease 2019 (COVID-19) vaccines licensed or authorized in the United States. None of the COVID-19 vaccines are preferred over another when more than one licensed or authorized, recommended, and age-appropriate vaccine is available.

MRNA COVID-19 VACCINES

Pfizer-BioNTech and Moderna COVID-19 vaccines are messenger ribonucleic acid (mRNA) vaccines. mRNA vaccines use mRNA created in a laboratory to teach our cells how to make a protein—or even just a piece of a protein—that triggers an immune response inside our bodies. The mRNA from the vaccines is broken down within a few days after vaccination and discarded from the body.

As of September 12, 2023, the 2023–2024 updated Pfizer-BioNTech and Moderna COVID-19 vaccines were recommended by the CDC for use in the United States:
- **Pfizer-BioNTech COVID-19 Vaccine (2023–2024 Formula).** This vaccine is authorized for children aged 6 months to 11 years; COMIRNATY is the licensed Pfizer-BioNTech product for people aged 12 and older.
- **Moderna COVID-19 Vaccine (2023–2024 Formula).** This vaccine is authorized for children aged 6 months to 11 years; SPIKEVAX is the licensed Moderna product for people aged 12 and older.

---

[3] "Vaccines for Children—A Guide for Parents and Caregivers," U.S. Food and Drug Administration (FDA), August 15, 2019. Available online. URL: www.fda.gov/vaccines-blood-biologics/consumers-biologics/vaccines-children-guide-parents-and-caregivers. Accessed March 27, 2024.

PROTEIN SUBUNIT COVID-19 VACCINES

Novavax COVID-19 vaccine is a protein subunit vaccine. Protein subunit vaccines contain pieces (proteins) of the virus that causes COVID-19. The virus pieces are the spike protein. The Novavax COVID-19 vaccine contains another ingredient called an "adjuvant." It helps the immune system respond to that spike protein. After learning how to respond to the spike protein, the immune system will be able to respond quickly to the actual virus spike protein and protect you against COVID-19.

As of October 3, 2023, the 2023–2024 updated Novavax COVID-19 Vaccine, Adjuvanted was recommended by the CDC for use in the United States for people aged 12 and older.[4]

Section 46.4 | Caring for a Seriously Ill Child

When a child is seriously ill, each person in the family is affected differently. That is why it is important that you, your child, and your family get the support and care you need during this difficult time. A special type of care called "palliative care" can help. Palliative care is a key part of care for children living with a serious illness. It is also an important source of support for their families.

WHAT IS PALLIATIVE CARE?

Palliative care can ease the symptoms, discomfort, and stress of serious illness for your child and family. Palliative care can help with your child's illness and give support to your family. It can:
- ease your child's pain and other symptoms of illness
- provide emotional and social support that respects your family's cultural values

---

[4] "Overview of COVID-19 Vaccines," Centers for Disease Control and Prevention (CDC), January 12, 2024. Available online. URL: www.cdc.gov/coronavirus/2019-ncov/vaccines/different-vaccines/overview-COVID-19-vaccines.html. Accessed March 27, 2024.

- help your child's health-care providers work together and communicate with one another to support your goals
- start open discussions with you, your child, and your health-care team about options for care

Palliative care provides comfort for your child. Palliative care can help children and teenagers living with many serious illnesses, including genetic disorders, cancer, neurologic disorders, heart and lung conditions, and others. Palliative care is important for children at any age or stage of serious illness. It can begin as soon as you learn about your child's illness. Palliative care can help prevent symptoms and give relief from much more than physical pain. It can also enhance your child's quality of life (QOL).

Palliative care gives you and your family an added layer of support. Serious illness in a child affects everyone in the family, including parents and siblings of all ages. Palliative care gives extra support for your whole family. It can ease the stress on all of your children, your spouse, and you during a hard time.

Palliative care surrounds your family with a team of experts who work together to support all of you. It is a partnership between your child, your family, and the health-care team. This team listens to your preferences and helps you think through the care options for your family. They will work with you and your child to make a care plan for your family. They can also help when your child moves from one care setting (e.g., the hospital) to another (e.g., outpatient care or care at home).

DOES ACCEPTING PALLIATIVE CARE MEAN YOUR FAMILY IS GIVING UP ON OTHER TREATMENTS?

The purpose of palliative care is to ease your child's pain and other symptoms and provide emotional and other support to your entire family. Palliative care can help children, from newborns to young adults, and their families—at any stage of a serious illness. Palliative care works alongside other treatments your child may be receiving. In fact, your child can start getting palliative care as soon as you learn about your child's illness.

Caring for Children

HOW DOES PALLIATIVE CARE BENEFIT YOUR CHILD?
Palliative care helps your child live a more comfortable life. Palliative care can provide direct support for your child by providing relief from distressing symptoms, such as:
- pain
- shortness of breath
- fatigue
- depression
- anxiety
- nausea
- loss of appetite
- problems with sleep

Palliative care can help your child deal with side effects from medicines and treatments. Perhaps most importantly, palliative care can help enhance your child's QOL. For example, helping cope with concerns about school and friends might be very valuable to your child.

Palliative care may also include direct support for families such as assistance with:
- including siblings in conversations
- providing respite care for parents to be able to spend time with their other children
- locating community resources for services such as counseling and support groups

Palliative care is effective. Scientists have studied how palliative care can help children living with serious illnesses. Studies show that patients who get palliative care say that it helps with:
- pain and other distressing symptoms, such as nausea or shortness of breath
- communication between health-care providers and family members
- emotional support

Other studies show that palliative care:
- helps patients get the kinds of care they want
- meets the emotional, developmental, and spiritual needs of patients

HOW DO YOU KNOW IF YOUR CHILD OR FAMILY NEEDS PALLIATIVE CARE?

Children living with a serious illness often experience physical and emotional distress related to their disease. Emotional distress is also common among their parents, siblings, and other family members. If your child has a genetic disorder, cancer, neurological disorder, heart or lung condition, or another serious illness, palliative care may help reduce pain and enhance QOL.

Ask your child's health-care provider about palliative care if your child or any member of your family (including you):

- suffers from pain or other symptoms due to serious illness
- experiences physical pain or emotional distress that is not under control
- needs help understanding your child's health condition
- needs support coordinating your child's care

WHEN CAN YOU START PALLIATIVE CARE FOR YOUR CHILD?

Palliative care can start as soon as your child needs it. It is never too early to start palliative care. In fact, palliative care can take place at the same time as other treatments for your child's illness. It does not depend on the course or stage of your child's illness.

If you feel your child, your family, or you could benefit from palliative care, ask your child's health-care provider about getting a referral for palliative care services. There is no reason to wait. The sooner you and your child seek palliative care services, the sooner a palliative care team can help your family manage the pain and other symptoms and emotions that may come with a serious illness.

HOW DOES YOUR PALLIATIVE CARE TEAM WORK?

The palliative care team works with you, your child, and your care team. Together with your child's health-care providers, palliative care professionals will work with you and your child to make a care plan that is right for your child, your family, and you. The team will help you and your child include pain and other symptom management into every part of your child's care.

Caring for Children

Palliative care experts spend as much time with you and your family as it takes to help you fully understand your child's condition, care options, and other needs. They also make sure your child experiences a smooth transition between the hospital and other services, such as getting care at home.

Your team will listen to your preferences and work with you and your child to plan care for all of your child's symptoms throughout the illness. This will include care for your child's current needs and flexibility for future changes.

Your child's palliative care team is unique. Every palliative care team is different. Your child's palliative care team may include:
- doctors
- nurses
- social workers
- pharmacists
- chaplains
- counselors
- child life specialists
- nutritionists
- art and music therapists

IF YOUR CHILD IS PUT IN PALLIATIVE CARE, CAN YOUR CHILD STILL SEE THE SAME PRIMARY HEALTH-CARE PROVIDER?

Your child does not have to change to a new primary health-care provider when starting palliative care. The palliative care team and your child's health-care provider work together to help you and your child decide the best care plan for your child.

WHAT IF YOUR CHILD'S HEALTH-CARE PROVIDER IS UNSURE ABOUT REFERRING PALLIATIVE CARE SERVICES?

Some parents are afraid they might offend their child's current health-care providers by asking about palliative care, but this is unlikely. Most health-care providers appreciate the extra time and information the palliative care team provides to their patients. Occasionally, a clinician may not refer a patient for palliative care services. If this happens, ask for an explanation. Let your child's health-care provider know why you think palliative care could help your family.

WHO PAYS FOR PALLIATIVE CARE?

Many insurance plans cover palliative care. If you have questions or concerns about costs, you can ask your health-care team to put you in touch with a social worker, care manager, or financial advisor at your hospital or clinic to look at payment options.

WHERE CAN YOUR CHILD GET PALLIATIVE CARE?

Your palliative care team will help you know what services are available in your community. Your child and family may receive palliative care in a hospital, during clinic visits, or at home. You and your child will likely first meet with your palliative care team in the hospital or at a clinic. After the first visit, some visits may still occur in the clinic or hospital. But many palliative care programs offer services at home and in the community. Home services can occur through telephone calls or home visits.

If palliative care starts in the hospital, your care team can help your child make a successful move to your home or other health-care setting.

Home may feel most comfortable and safe to you and your child. Depending on your child's condition and treatment, the palliative care team may be able to help you find a nursing agency or community care agency to support palliative care for your child at home.

HOW CAN YOUR CHILD'S PAIN BE MANAGED?

The palliative care team can bring your child comfort in many ways. Treating pain often involves medication, but there are also other methods to address a child's discomfort. Your child may feel better with changes such as low lighting, comfortable room temperatures, pleasant smells, guided relaxation, and deep breathing techniques. Your child may welcome additional activities such as video chats, social media, soothing music, and massage and art therapy that may help decrease pain and anxiety.

Caring for Children

If your child has an illness that causes pain that is not relieved by drugs such as acetaminophen (Tylenol®) or ibuprofen (Motrin® or Advil®), your child's palliative care team may recommend trying stronger medicines. There is no reason to wait before beginning these medications. Should your child's pain increase, the dose may be safely increased over time to provide relief.

Pain relief can be offered in a hospital, at home, or in other health-care settings. Your palliative care team will partner with you and your child to learn what is causing discomfort and how best to handle it.[5]

---

[5] "Palliative Care for Children," National Institute of Nursing Research (NINR), July 2015. Available online. URL: www.ninr.nih.gov/sites/default/files/docs/NINR_508cBrochure_2015-7-7.pdf. Accessed March 27, 2024.

Chapter 47 | **Preventing Infection at Home and Work**

Germs are a part of everyday life and are found in the air, soil, and water and in and on our bodies. Some germs are helpful; others are harmful. Many germs live in and on our bodies without causing harm, and some even help us stay healthy. Only a small portion of germs are known to cause infection.

HOW DOES INFECTION OCCUR?
An infection occurs when germs enter the body, increase in number, and cause a reaction in the body.

The following three things are necessary for an infection to occur:
- **Source**. Places where infectious agents (germs) live (e.g., sinks, surfaces, and human skin).
- **Susceptible person**. A way for germs to enter the body.
- **Transmission**. A way germs are moved to the susceptible person.

Source
A source is an infectious agent or germ and refers to a virus, bacteria, or other microbe.

In health-care settings, germs are found in many places. People are one source of germs, including:
- patients
- health-care workers
- visitors and household members

People can be sick with symptoms of an infection or colonized with germs (not have symptoms of an infection but able to pass the germs to others).

Germs are also found in the health-care environment. Examples of environmental sources of germs include:
- dry surfaces in patient care areas (e.g., bed rails, medical equipment, countertops, and tables)
- wet surfaces, moist environments, and biofilms (e.g., cooling towers, faucets and sinks, and equipment such as ventilators)
- indwelling medical devices (e.g., catheters and intravenous (IV) lines)
- dust or decaying debris (e.g., construction dust or wet materials from water leaks)

Susceptible Person

A susceptible person is someone who is not vaccinated or otherwise immune or a person with a weakened immune system who has a way for the germs to enter the body. For an infection to occur, germs must enter a susceptible person's body and invade tissues, multiply, and cause a reaction.

Devices such as IV catheters and surgical incisions can provide an entryway, whereas a healthy immune system helps fight infection.

When patients are sick and receive medical treatment in health-care facilities, the following factors can increase their susceptibility to infection:
- Patients in health care who have underlying medical conditions such as diabetes, cancer, and organ transplantation are at increased risk for infection because often these illnesses decrease the immune system's ability to fight infection.

Preventing Infection at Home and Work

- Certain medications used to treat medical conditions, such as antibiotics, steroids, and certain cancer-fighting medications, increase the risk of some types of infections.
- Lifesaving medical treatments and procedures used in health care, such as urinary catheters, tubes, and surgery, increase the risk of infection by providing additional ways that germs can enter the body.

Recognizing the factors that increase patients' susceptibility to infection allows providers to recognize risks and perform basic infection prevention measures to prevent infection from occurring.

Transmission

Transmission refers to the way germs are moved to the susceptible person.

Germs do not move themselves. Germs depend on people, the environment, and/or medical equipment to move in health-care settings.

There are a few general ways that germs travel in health-care settings—through contact (i.e., touching), sprays and splashes, inhalation, and sharps injuries (i.e., when someone is accidentally stuck with a used needle or sharp instrument).

- **Contact**. This moves germs by touch (e.g., methicillin-resistant *Staphylococcus aureus* (MRSA) or vancomycin-resistant enterococcus (VRE)). For example, health-care provider hands become contaminated by touching germs present on medical equipment or high-touch surfaces and then carry the germs on their hands and spread to a susceptible person when proper hand hygiene is not performed before touching the susceptible person.
- **Sprays and splashes**. These occur when an infected person coughs or sneezes, creating droplets that carry germs short distances (within approximately 6 feet). These germs can land on a susceptible person's eyes,

nose, or mouth and can cause infection (e.g., pertussis or meningitis).
- Close-range inhalation occurs when a droplet containing germs is small enough to breathe in but not durable over distance.
- **Inhalation.** This occurs when germs are aerosolized in tiny particles that survive on air currents over great distances and time and reach a susceptible person. Airborne transmission can occur when infected patients cough, talk, or sneeze germs into the air (e.g., tuberculosis (TB) or measles) or when germs are aerosolized by medical equipment or by dust from a construction zone (e.g., nontuberculous mycobacteria or *Aspergillus*).
- **Sharps injuries.** These can lead to infections (e.g., human immunodeficiency virus (HIV), hepatitis B virus (HBV), and hepatitis C virus (HCV)) when blood-borne pathogens enter a person through a skin puncture by a used needle or sharp instrument.[1]

HANDWASHING TO STAY HEALTHY

Handwashing is one of the best ways to protect yourself and your family from getting sick. Learn when and how you should wash your hands to stay healthy.

How Germs Spread

Washing hands can keep you healthy and prevent the spread of respiratory and diarrheal infections. Germs can spread from person to person or from surface to person when you:
- touch your eyes, nose, and mouth with unwashed hands
- prepare or eat food and drinks with unwashed hands
- touch surfaces or objects that have germs on them

---

[1] "How Infections Spread," Centers for Disease Control and Prevention (CDC), January 7, 2016. Available online. URL: www.cdc.gov/infectioncontrol/spread/index.html. Accessed February 16, 2024.

Preventing Infection at Home and Work

- blow your nose, cough, or sneeze into your hands and then touch other people's hands or common objects

Key Times to Wash Hands

You can help yourself and your loved ones stay healthy by washing your hands often, especially during the following key times when you are likely to get and spread germs:
- before, during, and after preparing food
- before and after eating food
- before and after caring for someone at home who is sick with vomiting or diarrhea
- before and after treating a cut or wound
- after using the toilet
- after changing diapers or cleaning up a child who has used the toilet
- after blowing your nose, coughing, or sneezing
- after touching an animal, animal feed, or animal waste
- after handling pet food or pet treats
- after touching garbage

If soap and water are not readily available, use a hand sanitizer with at least 60 percent alcohol to clean your hands.

Follow Five Steps to Wash Your Hands the Right Way

Washing your hands is easy, and it is one of the most effective ways to prevent the spread of germs. Clean hands can help stop germs from spreading from one person to another and in communities—including homes, workplaces, schools, and childcare facilities.

Follow the five steps listed here every time:
- Wet your hands with clean, running water (warm or cold); turn off the tap; and apply soap.
- Lather your hands by rubbing them together with the soap. Lather the backs of your hands, between your fingers, and under your nails.
- Scrub your hands for at least 20 seconds.
- Rinse your hands well under clean, running water.
- Dry your hands using a clean towel or an air dryer.

Use Hand Sanitizer When You Cannot Use Soap and Water

Washing hands with soap and water is the best way to get rid of germs in most situations. If soap and water are not readily available, you can use an alcohol-based hand sanitizer that contains at least 60 percent alcohol. You can tell if the sanitizer contains at least 60 percent alcohol by looking at the product label.

Sanitizers can quickly reduce the number of germs on hands in many situations. However, hand sanitizers:
- do not get rid of all types of germs
- may not be as effective when hands are visibly dirty or greasy
- might not remove harmful chemicals such as pesticides from hands

Swallowing alcohol-based hand sanitizer can cause alcohol poisoning if more than a couple of mouthfuls are swallowed. Keep it out of reach of young children and supervise their use.

How to Use Hand Sanitizer
- Apply the gel product to the palm of one hand (read the label to learn the correct amount).
- Cover all surfaces of hands.
- Rub your hands and fingers together until they are dry. This should take around 20 seconds.[2]

---

[2] "When and How to Wash Your Hands," Centers for Disease Control and Prevention (CDC), November 15, 2022. Available online. URL: www.cdc.gov/handwashing/when-how-handwashing.html. Accessed February 16, 2024.

Chapter 48 | Chronic Illness and Depression

CHRONIC ILLNESS AND MENTAL HEALTH
Chronic illnesses such as cancer, heart disease, or diabetes may make you more likely to have or develop a mental health condition.

It is common to feel sad or discouraged after having a heart attack, receiving a cancer diagnosis, or when trying to manage a chronic condition such as pain. You may be facing new limits on what you can do and may feel stressed or concerned about treatment outcomes and the future. It may be hard to adapt to a new reality and to cope with the changes and ongoing treatment that come with the diagnosis. Favorite activities, such as hiking or gardening, may be harder to do.

Temporary feelings of sadness are expected, but if these and other symptoms last longer than a couple of weeks, you may have depression. Depression affects your ability to carry on with daily life and to enjoy family, friends, work, and leisure. The health effects of depression go beyond mood: Depression is a serious medical illness with many symptoms, including physical ones. Some symptoms of depression include:
- persistent sad, anxious, or empty mood
- feeling hopeless or pessimistic
- feeling irritable, easily frustrated, or restless
- feeling guilty, worthless, or helpless
- loss of interest or pleasure in hobbies and activities
- decreased energy, fatigue, or feeling slowed down
- difficulty concentrating, remembering, or making decisions

- difficulty sleeping, early morning awakening, or oversleeping
- changes in appetite or weight
- aches or pains, headaches, cramps, or digestive problems without a clear physical cause that do not ease even with treatment
- suicide attempts or thoughts of death or suicide

People with Other Chronic Medical Conditions Are at Higher Risk of Depression

The same factors that increase the risk of depression in otherwise healthy people also raise the risk in people with other medical illnesses, particularly if those illnesses are chronic (long-lasting or persistent). These risk factors include a personal or family history of depression or family members who have died by suicide.

However, some risk factors for depression are directly related to having another illness. For example, conditions such as Parkinson disease (PD) and stroke cause changes in the brain. In some cases, these changes may have a direct role in depression. Illness-related anxiety and stress can also trigger symptoms of depression.

Depression is common among people who have chronic illnesses such as:
- Alzheimer disease (AD)
- autoimmune diseases, including systemic lupus erythematosus (SLE), rheumatoid arthritis (RA), and psoriasis
- cancer
- coronary heart disease
- diabetes
- epilepsy
- human immunodeficiency virus/acquired immunodeficiency syndrome (HIV/AIDS)
- hypothyroidism
- multiple sclerosis (MS)
- Parkinson disease (PD)
- stroke

Chronic Illness and Depression

Some people may experience symptoms of depression after being diagnosed with a medical illness. Those symptoms may decrease as they adjust to or treat the other condition. Certain medications used to treat the illness can also trigger depression.

Research suggests that people who have depression and another medical illness tend to have more severe symptoms of both illnesses. They may have more difficulty adapting to their medical condition, and they may have higher medical costs than those who do not have both depression and a medical illness. Symptoms of depression may continue even as a person's physical health improves.

A collaborative care approach that includes both mental and physical health care can improve overall health. Research has shown that treating depression and chronic illness together can help people better manage both their depression and their chronic disease.

CHILDREN AND ADOLESCENTS WITH CHRONIC ILLNESSES

Children and adolescents with chronic illnesses often face more challenges than their healthy peers in navigating adolescence. Chronic illnesses can affect physical, cognitive, social, and emotional development, and they can take a toll on parents and siblings. These limitations put children and adolescents at higher risk than their healthy peers of developing a mental illness.

Children and adolescents with chronic illnesses experience many forms of stress. Parents and health-care providers should be on the lookout for signs of depression, anxiety, and adjustment disorders (a group of conditions that can occur when someone has difficulty coping with a stressful life event) in young people and their families.

People with Depression Are at Higher Risk for Other Medical Conditions

It may come as no surprise that adults with a medical illness are more likely to experience depression. The reverse is also true: People of all ages with depression are at higher risk of developing certain physical illnesses.

People with depression have an increased risk of cardiovascular disease (CVD), diabetes, stroke, pain, and AD, for example. Research also suggests that people with depression may be at higher risk for osteoporosis. The reasons are not yet clear. One factor with some of these illnesses is that many people with depression may have less access to good medical care. They may have a more challenging time caring for their health—for example, seeking care, taking prescribed medication, eating well, and exercising.

Scientists are also exploring whether physiological changes seen in depression may play a role in increasing the risk of physical illness. In people with depression, scientists have found changes in the way several different systems in the body function that could have an effect on physical health, including:
- increased inflammation
- changes in the control of heart rate and blood circulation
- abnormalities in stress hormones
- metabolic changes such as those seen in people at risk for diabetes

There is some evidence that these changes, seen in depression, may raise the risk of other medical illnesses. It is also clear that depression has a negative effect on mental health and everyday life.

Depression Is Treatable Even When Another Illness Is Present

Depression is a common complication of chronic illness, but it does not have to be a normal part of having a chronic illness. Effective treatment for depression is available and can help even if you have another medical illness or condition.

If you or a loved one think you have depression, it is important to tell your health-care provider and explore treatment options. You should also inform your health-care provider about all your present treatments or medications for your chronic illness or depression (including prescribed medications and dietary supplements). Sharing information can help avoid problems with multiple medicines interfering with each other. It also helps your

Chronic Illness and Depression

health-care provider stay informed about your overall health and treatment issues.

Recovery from depression takes time, but treatment can improve your quality of life (QOL) even if you have a medical illness.

Treating depression with medication, psychotherapy (also called "talk therapy"), or a combination of the two may also help improve the physical symptoms of a chronic illness or reduce the risk of future problems. Likewise, treating the chronic illness and getting symptoms under control can help improve symptoms of depression.

Depression affects each individual differently. There is no "one-size-fits-all" for treatment. It may take some trial and error to find the treatment that works best.[1]

---

[1] "Chronic Illness and Mental Health: Recognizing and Treating Depression," National Institute of Mental Health (NIMH), 2021. Available online. URL: www.nimh.nih.gov/health/publications/chronic-illness-mental-health. Accessed March 7, 2024.

Chapter 49 | Technologies in Disease Management

Chapter Contents
Section 49.1—Rehabilitative and Assistive Technology............ 495
Section 49.2—Artificial Pancreas... 499
Section 49.3—Artificial Intelligence 504
Section 49.4—Biosensors and Biomaterials............................... 507

Section 49.1 | Rehabilitative and Assistive Technology

Rehabilitative and assistive technologies are tools, equipment, or products that can help people with disabilities function successfully at school, home, work, and in the community.

Assistive technology can be as simple as a magnifying glass or as complex as a digital communication system. An assistive device can be as large as a power wheelchair lift for a van or as small as a handheld hook that assists with buttoning a shirt.

Tools to help people recover or improve their functioning after injury or illness are sometimes called "rehabilitative technology." But the term is often used interchangeably with the term "assistive technology."

Rehabilitative engineers use scientific principles to study how people with disabilities function in society. They study barriers to optimal function and design solutions so that people with disabilities can interact successfully in their environments.

The *Eunice Kennedy Shriver* National Institute of Child Health and Human Development (NICHD) supports research on developing and evaluating technologies, devices, instruments, and other aids to help people with disabilities achieve their full potential.

WHAT ARE SOME TYPES OF ASSISTIVE DEVICES, AND HOW ARE THEY USED?

Some examples of assistive technologies are as follows:
- mobility aids, such as wheelchairs, scooters, walkers, canes, crutches, prosthetic devices, and orthotic devices
- hearing aids to help people hear or hear more clearly
- cognitive aids, including computer or electrical assistive devices, to help people with memory, attention, or other challenges in their thinking skills
- computer software and hardware, such as voice recognition programs, screen readers, and screen enlargement applications, to help people with mobility and sensory impairments use computers and mobile devices

- tools, such as automatic page-turners, bookholders, and adapted pencil grips, to help learners with disabilities participate in educational activities
- closed captioning to allow people with hearing problems to watch movies, television programs, and other digital media
- physical modifications in the built environment, including ramps, grab bars, and wider doorways, to enable access to buildings, businesses, and workplaces
- lightweight, high-performance mobility devices that enable persons with disabilities to play sports and be physically active
- adaptive switches and utensils to allow those with limited motor skills to eat, play games, and accomplish other activities
- devices and features of devices to help perform tasks, such as cooking, dressing, and grooming (e.g., specialized handles and grips, devices that extend reach, and lights on telephones and doorbells)

WHAT ARE SOME TYPES OF REHABILITATIVE TECHNOLOGIES?

Rehabilitative technologies and techniques help people recover or improve function after injury or illness. Examples include the following:
- **Robotics**. Specialized robots help people regain and improve function in their arms or legs after a stroke.
- **Virtual reality**. People who are recovering from injury can restrain themselves to perform motions within a virtual environment.
- **Musculoskeletal modeling and simulations**. These computer simulations of the human body can pinpoint underlying mechanical problems in a person with a movement-related disability. This technique can help improve assistive aids or physical therapies.
- **Transcranial magnetic stimulation (TMS)**. TMS sends magnetic impulses through the skull to stimulate

the brain. This system can help people who have had a stroke recover movement and brain function.
- **Transcranial direct current stimulation (tDCS).** In tDCS, a mild electrical current travels through the skull and stimulates the brain. This can help recover movement in patients recovering from stroke or other conditions.
- **Motion analysis.** This captures video of human motion with specialized computer software that analyzes the motion in detail. The technique gives health-care providers a detailed picture of a person's specific movement challenges to guide proper therapy.

HOW DOES REHABILITATIVE TECHNOLOGY BENEFIT PEOPLE WITH DISABILITIES?

Rehabilitative technology can help restore or improve function in people who have developed a disability due to disease, injury, or aging. Appropriate assistive technology often helps people with disabilities compensate, at least in part, for a limitation.

For example, assistive technology enables students with disabilities to compensate for certain impairments. This specialized technology promotes independence and decreases the need for other support.

Rehabilitative and assistive technology can enable individuals to:
- care for themselves and their families
- work
- learn in typical school environments and other educational institutions
- access information through computers and reading
- enjoy music, sports, travel, and the arts
- participate fully in community life

Assistive technology also benefits employers, teachers, family members, and everyone who interacts with people who use the technology.

Assistive technologies become more commonplace, and people without disabilities are benefiting from them. For example, people for whom English is a second language are taking advantage of screen readers. Older individuals are using screen enlargers and magnifiers.

The person with a disability, along with his or her caregivers and a team of professionals and consultants, usually decides which type of rehabilitative or assistive technology would be most helpful. The team is trained to match particular technologies to specific needs to help the person function better or more independently. The team may include family doctors, regular and special education teachers, speech-language pathologists, rehabilitation engineers, occupational therapists, and other specialists, including representatives from companies that manufacture assistive technology.

WHAT CONDITIONS MAY BENEFIT FROM ASSISTIVE DEVICES?

Some disabilities are quite visible, while others are "hidden." Most disabilities can be grouped into the following categories:

- **Cognitive disability**. Intellectual and learning disabilities/disorders, distractability, reading disorders, and inability to remember or focus on large amounts of information.
- **Hearing disability**. Hearing loss or impaired hearing.
- **Physical disability**. Paralysis, difficulties with walking or other movement, inability to use a computer mouse, slow response time, and difficulty controlling movement.
- **Visual disability**. Blindness, low vision, and color blindness.
- **Mental conditions**. Posttraumatic stress disorder (PTSD), anxiety disorders, mood disorders, eating disorders, and psychosis.

Hidden disabilities are those that might not be immediately apparent when you look at someone. They can include visual impairments, movement problems, hearing impairments, and mental health conditions.

Technologies in Disease Management

Some medical conditions may also contribute to disabilities or may be categorized as hidden disabilities under the Americans with Disabilities Act (ADA). For example, epilepsy, diabetes, sickle cell conditions, human immunodeficiency virus (HIV)/acquired immunodeficiency syndrome (AIDS), cystic fibrosis (CF), cancer, and heart, liver, or kidney problems may lead to problems with mobility or daily function and may be viewed as disabilities under the law. The conditions may be short term or long term, stable or progressive, constant or unpredictable, and changing, treatable, or untreatable. Many people with hidden disabilities can benefit from assistive technologies for certain activities or during certain stages of their diseases or conditions.

People who have spinal cord injuries (SCIs), traumatic brain injury (TBI), cerebral palsy (CP), muscular dystrophy (MD), spina bifida, osteogenesis imperfecta (OI), multiple sclerosis (MS), demyelinating diseases, myelopathy, progressive muscular atrophy (PMA), amputations, or paralysis often benefit from complex rehabilitative technology. The assistive devices are individually configured to help each person with his or her own unique disability.[1]

Section 49.2 | Artificial Pancreas

An artificial pancreas is a system made of three parts that work together to mimic how a healthy pancreas controls blood glucose, also called "blood sugar," in the body. An artificial pancreas is mainly used to help people with type 1 diabetes.

In type 1 diabetes, the pancreas does not produce insulin. People with type 1 diabetes control their blood glucose level by checking it and taking insulin, either by injection or through an insulin infusion pump, several times a day. An artificial pancreas automatically monitors your blood glucose level, calculates the amount of insulin you need at different points during the day, and delivers it.

---

[1] "Rehabilitative and Assistive Technology," *Eunice Kennedy Shriver* National Institute of Child Health and Human Development (NICHD), October 24, 2018. Available online. URL: www.nichd.nih.gov/health/topics/rehabtech. Accessed April 3, 2024.

Most artificial pancreas systems require you to count and enter the amount of carbohydrates you consume at mealtime. These are called "hybrid artificial pancreas systems" because some of the insulin is given automatically and some is given based on the information you enter. These systems help control blood glucose levels throughout the day and night, making it easier for people with type 1 diabetes to keep their blood glucose levels in range. Keeping blood glucose levels within range will prevent other health problems from developing and may improve daily life for people with type 1 diabetes.

HOW DO ARTIFICIAL PANCREAS SYSTEMS WORK?
The following three devices make up an artificial pancreas system:
- **Continuous glucose monitor (CGM).** A CGM tracks blood glucose levels every few minutes using a tiny sensor that is inserted under the skin. The sensor wirelessly sends the information to a program stored on a smartphone or on an insulin infusion pump.
- **Control algorithm.** This computer program calculates how much insulin is needed and signals the insulin infusion pump when insulin needs to be delivered.
- **Insulin infusion pump.** This pump will deliver small doses of insulin throughout the day when blood glucose levels are not in your target range. There are different types of insulin pumps:
  - One type of pump is worn outside the body on a belt or in a pocket or pouch. Insulin flows from the pump through a plastic tube that connects to a smaller tube, called a "catheter," which has a needle that is inserted under the skin and stays in place for several days.
  - Another type of pump attaches directly to the skin with an adhesive pad and gives insulin through a catheter inserted under the skin. This kind of pump is replaced every few days.

ARE THERE OTHER NAMES FOR THE ARTIFICIAL PANCREAS?
Other names for the artificial pancreas include:
- automated insulin delivery system
- closed-loop system
- bionic pancreas

WHAT ARE THE DIFFERENT TYPES OF ARTIFICIAL PANCREAS SYSTEMS?
There are several types of artificial pancreas systems.

Threshold Suspend and Predictive Suspend Systems
The threshold suspend and predictive suspend systems can temporarily stop or "suspend" delivering insulin if your blood glucose level gets low.

The threshold suspend system stops delivering insulin when your blood glucose level drops to a preset level. The predictive suspend system calculates your blood glucose level and will stop delivering insulin before your blood glucose level gets too low. Neither system automatically increases insulin doses.

Stopping insulin delivery at the right moment can help a person with type 1 diabetes avoid low blood sugar, or hypoglycemia, a condition when a person's blood glucose level is lower than their target range. These systems may help people with type 1 diabetes who develop hypoglycemia overnight, particularly children.

Insulin-Only Systems
Insulin-only systems keep your blood glucose level within your target range by automatically increasing or decreasing the amount of insulin delivered to your body based on your CGM values. Insulin-only systems can increase insulin doses if your blood glucose level is higher than your target range.

One type of insulin-only system is the hybrid system. The hybrid insulin-only system automatically adjusts insulin doses in response to your CGM values. But you must still count carbohydrate levels and calculate insulin doses for all meals and snacks.

Dual-Hormone Systems

Researchers are currently developing and testing systems that use two hormones—insulin to lower glucose levels and glucagon to raise blood glucose levels. Using two hormones to control blood glucose is similar to the way the pancreas works in people who do not have diabetes. These systems may be able to tightly control glucose levels without causing hypoglycemia. Researchers are also testing how well other combinations, such as rapid-acting insulin and pramlintide, can control blood glucose levels.

WHO CAN USE AN ARTIFICIAL PANCREAS?

You need a prescription from your doctor to get an artificial pancreas. Together, you and your doctor will consider which system can best control your blood glucose levels and fit your lifestyle. Other factors to consider are:

- age (Some models are approved for children as young as two years old, while others are approved for people aged six and older.)
- whether you can place the devices in the correct position without help, check that they are working properly, and adjust them or enter carbohydrate data as needed
- whether you prefer an insulin pump with tubing or one that attaches directly to your skin
- whether you have access to a wireless fidelity (Wi-Fi) network so that information can flow between the parts of the system

Parents or guardians of children with type 1 diabetes should talk about appropriate artificial pancreas systems with the child's doctor.

Researchers continue to develop new and different types of artificial pancreas systems that will meet the needs of people with type 1 diabetes and other types of diabetes.

How much an artificial pancreas will cost you depends on your health insurance provider. Private insurance plans or government plans may not cover all artificial pancreas systems available for people with type 1 diabetes.

WHAT ARE THE BENEFITS OF AN ARTIFICIAL PANCREAS?

An artificial pancreas may help people with type 1 diabetes reach their target blood glucose levels and improve their quality of life (QOL).

With an artificial pancreas system, your glucose levels will be monitored continuously. The computer program improves blood glucose control by automatically adjusting the amount of insulin it delivers to keep your blood glucose levels in range. The system helps you avoid hypoglycemia and hyperglycemia.

Doctors can monitor insulin doses remotely and recommend dosage adjustments for people who need closer supervision. Also, parents or guardians can monitor blood glucose levels from their own smartphones throughout the day and night.

WHAT ARE THE LIMITS OF AN ARTIFICIAL PANCREAS?

Artificial pancreas systems are not completely "hands off." You have to regularly maintain the devices to be sure they are working properly and enter meal sizes into the system every time you eat. You will also need to do the following:

- Check the CGM and infusion pump catheter to be sure they are in place and change them when needed.
- Check the CGM for accuracy and replace the CGM sensor from time to time.
- Count the number of mealtime carbohydrates and enter them into the system.
- Adjust the computer program settings to make sure you get the right amount of insulin to keep your blood glucose level in your target range.
- Reboot or reconnect the CGM, infusion pump, and computer program if there are problems.
- Manage high or low blood glucose levels if the system is not able to keep your blood glucose within range.

The adhesive patches used with these systems may cause skin redness or irritation. Some medicines you take might also interfere with the glucose monitor.[2]

Section 49.3 | Artificial Intelligence

WHAT IS ARTIFICIAL INTELLIGENCE AND MACHINE LEARNING?

Artificial intelligence (AI) is a machine-based system that can, for a given set of human-defined objectives, make predictions, recommendations, or decisions influencing real or virtual environments. AI systems use machine- and human-based inputs to perceive real and virtual environments, abstract such perceptions into models through analysis in an automated manner, and use model inference to formulate options for information or action.

Machine learning (ML) is a set of techniques that can be used to train AI algorithms to improve performance at a task based on data.

Some real-world examples of AI and ML technologies are as follows:
- **Imaging system.** This system uses algorithms to give diagnostic information for skin cancer in patients.
- **Smart sensor device.** This device estimates the probability of a heart attack.[3]

WHAT ARE THE TYPES OF ARTIFICIAL INTELLIGENCE, AND HOW DO THEY DIFFER?
- **Artificial intelligence.** A feature where machines learn to perform tasks rather than simply carrying out computations that are input by human users. Early

---

[2] "Artificial Pancreas," National Institute of Diabetes and Digestive and Kidney Diseases (NIDDK), October 2021. Available online. URL: www.niddk.nih.gov/health-information/diabetes/overview/managing-diabetes/artificial-pancreas. Accessed April 3, 2024.

[3] "Artificial Intelligence and Machine Learning in Software as a Medical Device," U.S. Food and Drug Administration (FDA), March 15, 2024. Available online. URL: www.fda.gov/medical-devices/software-medical-device-samd/artificial-intelligence-and-machine-learning-software-medical-device. Accessed April 3, 2024.

Technologies in Disease Management

applications of AI included machines that could play games such as checkers and chess and programs that could reproduce language.
- **Machine learning.** An approach to AI in which a computer algorithm (a set of rules and procedures) is developed to analyze and make predictions from data that are fed into the system. ML-based technologies are routinely used every day, such as personalized news feeds and traffic prediction maps.
- **Neural networks.** An ML approach modeled after the brain in which algorithms process signals via interconnected nodes called "artificial neurons." By mimicking biological nervous systems, artificial neural networks have been used successfully to recognize and predict patterns of neural signals involved in brain function.
- **Deep learning.** A form of ML that uses many layers of computation to form what is described as a deep neural network, capable of learning from large amounts of complex, unstructured data. Deep neural networks are responsible for voice-controlled virtual assistants as well as self-driving vehicles, which learn to recognize traffic signs.[4]

WHAT IS THE ROLE OF ARTIFICIAL INTELLIGENCE IN MEDICINE AND PUBLIC HEALTH?

Though still in its infancy as a field, AI is poised to transform the practice of medicine and the delivery of health care. Powered by breakthroughs in ML algorithms, enhanced computing power, and increasing data volume and storage capacity, AI has made noteworthy advances over the past decade across many medical subspecialties. Experts predict AI-based medical devices and algorithms

---

[4] "Artificial Intelligence (AI)," National Institute of Biomedical Imaging and Bioengineering (NIBIB), January 9, 2020. Available online. URL: www.nibib.nih.gov/science-education/science-topics/artificial-intelligence-ai. Accessed April 3, 2024.

will play a major role in the delivery of preventive, diagnostic, and therapeutic interventions.[5]

HOW IS ARTIFICIAL INTELLIGENCE BEING USED TO IMPROVE MEDICAL CARE AND BIOMEDICAL RESEARCH?

- **Radiology.** The ability of AI to interpret imaging results may aid in detecting a minute change in an image that a clinician might accidentally miss.
- **Imaging.** One example is the use of AI to evaluate how an individual will look after facial and cleft palate surgery.
- **Telehealth.** Wearable devices allow for constant monitoring of a patient and the detection of physiological changes that may provide early warning signs of an event such as an asthma attack.
- **Clinical care.** A large focus of AI in the health-care sector is in clinical decision support systems, which use health observations and case knowledge to assist with treatment decisions.[6]

WHAT ARE THE STUDIES IN TESTING ARTIFICIAL INTELLIGENCE FOR HEALTH?

The National Institutes of Health (NIH) funds studies to test AI in many areas of health, including:
- predicting who is at high risk for breast cancer
- connecting people with quality medical information via chatbots
- modeling disease spread across countries
- identifying new drug candidates
- diagnosing Alzheimer disease (AD) before symptoms develop
- predicting changes in blood sugar levels before they occur in people with diabetes

---

[5] "Artificial Intelligence in Medicine and Public Health: Prospects and Challenges Beyond the Pandemic," Centers for Disease Control and Prevention (CDC), March 1, 2022. Available online. URL: https://blogs.cdc.gov/genomics/2022/03/01/artificial-intelligence-2. Accessed April 3, 2024.
[6] See foonote [4].

Technologies in Disease Management

- creating "smart clothing" that can reduce back pain by warning the wearer about unsafe movements
- improving colonoscopies, so colon cancers can be detected and treated at earlier stages[7]

Section 49.4 | Biosensors and Biomaterials

BIOSENSORS

Sensors are tools that detect and respond to some type of input from the physical environment. There is a broad range of sensors used in everyday life, which are classified based on the quantities and qualities they detect. Examples include electric current, magnetic or radio sensors, humidity sensors, fluid velocity or flow sensors, pressure sensors, thermal or temperature sensors, optical sensors, position sensors, environmental sensors, and chemical sensors.

In medicine and biomedical research, there are many types of sensors that are used to detect specific biological, chemical, or physical processes that then transmit or report these data to individual users or health-care professionals:

- **Thermometers.** These sensors translate the expansion of a fluid or bending of a metal strip in response to heat into a value that corresponds to body temperature.
- **Wearable technologies.** These sensors such as smartwatches carry sensors that can track, analyze, and transmit data about heart rate and sleep patterns. Researchers are using wearables to monitor the health of individuals and even predict and potentially intervene to prevent acute health events such as stroke or heart attack.

---

[7] *NIH News in Health*, "Artificial Intelligence and Your Health," National Institutes of Health (NIH), January 2024. Available online. URL: https://newsinhealth.nih.gov/2024/01/artificial-intelligence-your-health. Accessed April 3, 2024.

- **Pulse oximeters.** These sensors measure changes in the body's absorption of special types of light to measure heart rate and the amount of oxygen in the blood. These sensors are frequently used in hospitals and clinics and can also be purchased for at-home use.

While many advanced sensors are not practical for routine medical care, they allow researchers to study and learn about the basic foundations of disease, potentially facilitating the development of new technologies.[8]

BIOMATERIALS

Biomaterials play an integral role in medicine today—restoring function and facilitating healing for people after injury or disease. Biomaterials may be natural or synthetic and are used in medical applications to support, enhance, or replace damaged tissue or a biological function. The first historical use of biomaterials dates to antiquity when ancient Egyptians used sutures made from animal sinew. The modern field of biomaterials combines medicine, biology, physics, and chemistry and more recent influences from tissue engineering and materials science. The field has grown significantly in the past decade due to discoveries in tissue engineering, regenerative medicine, and more.

Metals, ceramics, plastic, glass, and even living cells and tissues can all be used in creating a biomaterial. They can be reengineered into molded or machined parts, coatings, fibers, films, foams, and fabrics for use in biomedical products and devices. These may include heart valves, hip joint replacements, dental implants, or contact lenses. They are often biodegradable, and some are bioabsorbable, meaning they are eliminated gradually from the body after fulfilling a function.

Doctors, researchers, and bioengineers use biomaterials for the following broad range of applications:
- medical implants, including heart valves, stents, and grafts; artificial joints, ligaments, and tendons; hearing

---

[8] "Sensors," National Institute of Biomedical Imaging and Bioengineering (NIBIB), April 2022. Available online. URL: www.nibib.nih.gov/sites/default/files/2022-05/Fact-Sheet-Sensors.pdf. Accessed April 3, 2024.

Technologies in Disease Management

- loss implants; dental implants; and devices that stimulate nerves
- methods to promote the healing of human tissues, including sutures, clips, and staples for wound closure, and dissolvable dressings
- regenerated human tissues, using a combination of biomaterial support or scaffolds, cells, and bioactive molecules (Examples include a bone-regenerating hydrogel and a lab-grown human bladder.)
- molecular probes and nanoparticles that break through biological barriers and aid in cancer imaging and therapy at the molecular level
- drug-delivery systems that carry and/or apply drugs to a disease target (Examples include drug-coated vascular stents and implantable chemotherapy wafers for cancer patients.)[9]

---

[9] "Biomaterials," National Institute of Biomedical Imaging and Bioengineering (NIBIB), April 2022. Available online. URL: www.nibib.nih.gov/sites/default/files/2022-05/Fact-Sheet-Biomaterials.pdf. Accessed April 3, 2024.

Chapter 50 | Preventive Care Services

Getting preventive care reduces the risk for diseases, disabilities, and death—yet millions of people in the United States do not get recommended preventive health-care services. Children need regular well-child and dental visits to track their development and find health problems early when they are usually easier to treat. But, for a variety of reasons, many people do not get the preventive care they need. Barriers include cost, not having a primary care provider, living too far from providers, and lack of awareness about recommended preventive services.

Teaching people about the importance of preventive care is key to making sure more people get recommended services. Law and policy changes can also help more people access these critical services.[1]

TIPS TO STAY UP-TO-DATE ON YOUR PREVENTIVE CARE

By making healthy choices, you can reduce your chances of getting a chronic disease and improve your quality of life (QOL). Avoiding chronic conditions, such as heart disease, type 2 diabetes, and obesity, can also lower your risk of severe illness from some infectious diseases, such as the flu and coronavirus disease 2019 (COVID-19).

But healthy behaviors are only part of the picture. Getting routine preventive care can help you stay well and catch problems early, helping you live a longer, healthier life.

---

[1] Office of Disease Prevention and Health Promotion (ODPHP), "Preventive Care," U.S. Department of Health and Human Services (HHS), August 19, 2020. Available online. URL: https://health.gov/healthypeople/objectives-and-data/browse-objectives/preventive-care. Accessed March 8, 2024.

Get Regular Medical and Dental Checkups

Regular checkups are separate from any other doctor's visit for sickness or injury. In addition to physical exams, these visits focus on preventive care, such as:

- screening tests, which are medical tests to check for diseases early when they may be easier to treat
- services, such as vaccines (shots), that improve your health by preventing diseases and other health problems
- dental cleanings
- education and counseling to help you make informed health decisions

Know Your Family Health History

Family health history is a record of the diseases and health conditions in your family. You and your family members share genes. You may also have behaviors in common, such as what you do for physical activity and what you like to eat. You may live in the same area and come into contact with similar harmful things in the environment. Family history includes all of these factors, any of which can affect your health.

If you have a family history of a chronic disease, such as cancer, heart disease, diabetes, or osteoporosis, you are more likely to get that disease yourself.

You cannot change your genes, but you can change unhealthy behaviors that can cause chronic diseases—such as smoking, poor nutrition, physical inactivity, or excessive drinking. If you have a family health history of disease, you may have the most to gain from these lifestyle changes and from preventive care practices, such as regular checkups, vaccinations, and screening tests.

Screen for Cancer Regularly

Cancer screening means checking your body for cancer before you have symptoms. Getting screening tests regularly may find breast, cervical, and colorectal (colon) cancers early when treatment is

Preventive Care Services

likely to work best. Lung cancer screening is recommended for some people who are at high risk.

Get Vaccinated

Vaccination is one of the safest and most convenient ways to protect your health. Vaccines offer protection in different ways, but they all help your body remember how to fight a specific infection in the future. It typically takes a few weeks after vaccination for the body to build up that protection.[2]

---

[2] National Center for Chronic Disease Prevention and Health Promotion (NCCDPHP), "Are You Up to Date on Your Preventive Care?" Centers for Disease Control and Prevention (CDC), April 19, 2023. Available online. URL: www.cdc.gov/chronicdisease/about/preventive-care/index.html. Accessed March 8, 2024.

Chapter 51 | **Palliative and Hospice Care**

Many Americans die in facilities, such as hospitals or nursing homes, receiving care that is not consistent with their wishes. It is important for older adults to plan ahead and let their caregivers, doctors, or family members know their end-of-life preferences in advance. For example, if an older person wants to die at home, receiving end-of-life care for pain and other symptoms, and makes this known to health-care providers and family, it is less likely he or she will die in a hospital receiving unwanted treatments.

If the person is no longer able to make health-care decisions for themselves, a caregiver or family member may have to make those decisions. Caregivers have several factors to consider when choosing end-of-life care, including the older person's desire to pursue life-extending treatments, how long he or she has left to live, and the preferred setting for care.

PALLIATIVE CARE

Palliative care is specialized medical care for people living with a serious illness, such as cancer or heart failure. Patients in palliative care may receive medical care for their symptoms, or palliative care, along with treatment intended to cure their serious illness. Palliative care is meant to enhance a person's current care by focusing on quality of life (QOL) for them and their family.

Who Can Benefit from Palliative Care?

Palliative care is a resource for anyone living with a serious illness, such as heart failure, chronic obstructive pulmonary disease

(COPD), cancer, dementia, Parkinson disease (PD), and many others. Palliative care can be helpful at any stage of illness and is best provided soon after a person is diagnosed.

In addition to improving QOL and helping with symptoms, palliative care can help patients understand their choices for medical treatment. The organized services available through palliative care may be helpful to any older person having a lot of general discomfort and disability very late in life.

Who Makes Up the Palliative Care Team?

A palliative care team is made up of multiple different professionals who work with the patient, family, and the patient's other doctors to provide medical, social, emotional, and practical support. The team comprises palliative care specialist doctors and nurses and includes others, such as social workers, nutritionists, and chaplains. A person's team may vary based on their needs and level of care. To begin palliative care, a person's health-care provider may refer him or her to a palliative care specialist. If he or she does not suggest it, the person can ask a health-care provider for a referral.

Where Is Palliative Care Provided?

Palliative care can be provided in hospitals, nursing homes, outpatient palliative care clinics or certain other specialized clinics, or at home. Medicare, Medicaid, and insurance policies may cover palliative care. Veterans may be eligible for palliative care through the U.S. Department of Veterans Affairs (VA). Private health insurance might pay for some services. Health insurance providers can answer questions about what they will cover.

In palliative care, a person does not have to give up treatment that might cure a serious illness. Palliative care can be provided along with curative treatment and may begin at the time of diagnosis. Over time, if the doctor or the palliative care team believes ongoing treatment is no longer helping, there are two possibilities. Palliative care could transition to hospice care if the doctor believes the person is likely to die within six months. Or the palliative care team could continue to help with increasing emphasis on comfort care.

Palliative and Hospice Care

HOSPICE CARE

Increasingly, people are choosing hospice care at the end-of-life. Hospice care focuses on the care, comfort, and QOL of a person with a serious illness who is approaching the end-of-life.

At some point, it may not be possible to cure a serious illness, or a patient may choose not to undergo certain treatments. Hospice is designed for this situation. The patient beginning hospice care understands that his or her illness is not responding to medical attempts to cure it or to slow the disease's progress.

Like palliative care, hospice provides comprehensive comfort care as well as support for the family, but in hospice, attempts to cure the person's illness are stopped. Hospice is provided for a person with a terminal illness whose doctor believes he or she has six months or less to live if the illness runs its natural course.

It is important for a patient to discuss hospice care options with their doctor. Sometimes people do not begin hospice care soon enough to take full advantage of the help it offers. Perhaps they wait too long to begin hospice, and they are too close to death. Or some people are not eligible for hospice care soon enough to receive its full benefits. Starting hospice early may be able to provide months of meaningful care and quality time with loved ones.

Where Is Hospice Care Provided, and Who Provides It?

Hospice is an approach to care, so it is not tied to a specific place. It can be offered in two types of settings: at home or in a facility such as a nursing home, a hospital, or even a separate hospice center.

Hospice care brings together a team of people with special skills—among them are nurses, doctors, social workers, spiritual advisors, and trained volunteers. Everyone works together with the person who is dying, along with the caregiver and/or the family, to provide the medical, emotional, and spiritual support needed.

A member of the hospice team visits regularly, and someone is usually always available by phone—24 hours a day, seven days a week. Hospice may be covered by Medicare and other insurance companies.

It is important to remember that stopping treatment aimed at curing an illness does not mean discontinuing all treatment. A good example is an older person with cancer. If the doctor determines that the cancer is not responding to chemotherapy and the patient chooses to enter hospice care, then the chemotherapy will be stopped. Other medical care may continue as long as it is helpful. For example, if the person has high blood pressure (HBP), he or she will still get medicine for that.

Although hospice provides a lot of support, the day-to-day care of a person dying at home is provided by family and friends. The hospice team coaches family members on how to care for the dying person and even provides respite care when caregivers need a break. Respite care can be for as short as a few hours or for as long as several weeks.

What Are the Benefits of Hospice Care?

Families of people who received care through a hospice program are more satisfied with end-of-life care than those who did not have hospice services. Also, hospice recipients are more likely to have their pain controlled and less likely to undergo tests or be given medicines they do not need compared with people who do not use hospice care.

What Does the Hospice Six-Month Requirement Mean?

In the United States, people enrolled in Medicare can receive hospice care if their health-care provider thinks they have less than six months to live should the disease take its usual course. Doctors have a hard time predicting how long an older, sick person will live. Health often declines slowly, and some people might need a lot of help with daily living for more than six months before they die.

The person should talk with his or her doctor if he or she thinks a hospice program might be helpful. If he or she agrees but thinks it is too soon for Medicare to cover the services, then the person can investigate how to pay for the services that are needed.

Palliative and Hospice Care

What Happens If Someone under Hospice Care Lives Longer than Six Months?

If the doctor continues to certify that the person is still close to dying, Medicare can continue to pay for hospice services. It is also possible to leave hospice care for a while and then later return if the health-care provider still believes that the patient has less than six months to live.[1]

MYTHS ABOUT PALLIATIVE AND HOSPICE CARE

Do you know the differences between palliative and hospice care? Although these two types of care are similar, they also differ in many ways (see Table 51.1).[2]

Table 51.1. Myths and Facts about Palliative and Hospice Care

Palliative Care		Hospice Care	
This is specialized medical care for people living with a serious illness.		This focuses on the care, comfort, and quality of life (QOL) of a person with a serious illness who is approaching the end-of-life.	
Myth: When I begin palliative care, I can no longer receive treatment for my disease.	**Fact:** Palliative care can be provided along with curative treatment.	**Myth:** In hospice care, I cannot receive any treatments.	**Fact:** People may receive medications to help manage symptoms but not treatments to help cure their illness.
Myth: I can no longer see my primary doctor when I start palliative care.	**Fact:** Palliative care teams work with primary doctors.	**Myth:** Hospice care is only provided in a hospital or hospice facility.	**Fact:** It can be provided at home, in a hospital or nursing home, or in a separate hospice center.

---

[1] National Institute on Aging (NIA), "What Are Palliative Care and Hospice Care?" National Institutes of Health (NIH), May 14, 2021. Available online. URL: www.nia.nih.gov/health/what-are-palliative-care-and-hospice-care. Accessed February 16, 2024.

[2] National Institute on Aging (NIA), "Four Myths about Palliative and Hospice Care," National Institutes of Health (NIH), April 28, 2023. Available online. URL: www.nia.nih.gov/health/infographics/four-myths-about-palliative-and-hospice-care. Accessed February 16, 2024.

Part 7 | Legal, Financial, and Insurance Aspects of Disease Management

Chapter 52 | The Americans with Disabilities Act

The Americans with Disabilities Act (ADA) is a federal civil rights law that prohibits discrimination against people with disabilities in everyday activities. The ADA prohibits discrimination on the basis of disability just as other civil rights laws prohibit discrimination on the basis of race, color, sex, national origin, age, and religion. The ADA guarantees that people with disabilities have the same opportunities as everyone else to enjoy employment opportunities, purchase goods and services, and participate in state and local government programs.

WHO IS CONSIDERED A PERSON WITH DISABILITY?
A person with a disability is someone who:
- has a physical or mental impairment that substantially limits one or more major life activities
- has a history or record of such an impairment (such as cancer that is in remission)
- is perceived by others as having such an impairment (such as a person who has scars from a severe burn)

If a person falls into any of these categories, the ADA protects them. Because the ADA is a law, and not a benefit program, you do not need to apply for coverage.

What Does "Substantially Limits" Mean?
The term "substantially limits" is interpreted broadly and is not meant to be a demanding standard. But not every condition will

meet this standard. An example of a condition that is not substantially limiting is a mild allergy to pollen.

What Does "Major Life Activities" Mean?
Major life activities are the kind of activities that you do every day, including your body's own internal processes. There are many major life activities. Some examples include:
- actions such as eating, sleeping, speaking, and breathing
- movements such as walking, standing, lifting, and bending
- cognitive functions such as thinking and concentrating
- sensory functions such as seeing and hearing
- tasks such as working, reading, learning, and communicating
- the operation of major bodily functions, such as circulation and reproduction, and individual organs

Examples of Disabilities
There is a wide variety of disabilities, and the ADA regulations do not list all of them. Some disabilities are visible, and some are not. Some examples of disabilities include:
- cancer
- diabetes
- posttraumatic stress disorder (PTSD)
- human immunodeficiency virus (HIV)
- autism
- cerebral palsy (CP)
- deafness or hearing loss
- blindness or low vision
- epilepsy
- mobility disabilities such as those requiring the use of a wheelchair, walker, or cane
- intellectual disabilities

The Americans with Disabilities Act

- major depressive disorder (MDD)
- traumatic brain injury (TBI)

The ADA covers many other disabilities not listed here.[1]

WHY IS DISABILITY INCLUSION IMPORTANT?

Disability affects approximately 61 million, or nearly one in four (26%), people in the United States living in communities. Disability affects more than 1 billion people worldwide. According to the United Nations Convention on the Rights of Persons with Disabilities (CRPD), people "... with disabilities include those who have long-term physical, mental, intellectual or sensory (such as hearing or vision) impairments which in interaction with various barriers may hinder their full and effective participation in society on an equal basis with others."

People with disabilities experience significant disadvantages when it comes to health:

- Adults with disabilities are three times more likely to have heart disease, stroke, diabetes, or cancer than adults without disabilities.
- Adults with disabilities are more likely than adults without disabilities to be current smokers.
- Women with disabilities are less likely than women without disabilities to have received a breast cancer x-ray test (mammogram) during the past two years.

Although disability is associated with health conditions (such as arthritis, mental, or emotional conditions) or events (such as injuries), the functioning, health, independence, and engagement in society of people with disabilities can vary depending on several factors:

- severity of the underlying impairment
- social, political, and cultural influences and expectations

---

[1] ADA.gov, "Introduction to the Americans with Disabilities Act," U.S. Department of Justice (DOJ), June 17, 2021. Available online. URL: www.ada.gov/topics/intro-to-ada. Accessed March 5, 2024.

- aspects of natural and built surroundings
- availability of assistive technology and devices
- family and community support and engagement

Disability inclusion means understanding the relationship between the way people function and how they participate in society and making sure everybody has the same opportunities to participate in every aspect of life to the best of their abilities and desires.[2]

WHAT DOES THE AMERICANS WITH DISABILITIES ACT DO?

The ADA prohibits discrimination on the basis of disability in employment, state and local government, public accommodations, commercial facilities, transportation, and telecommunications. It also applies to the U.S. Congress.

To be protected by the ADA, one must have a disability or have a relationship or association with an individual with a disability. An individual with a disability is defined by the ADA as a person who has a physical or mental impairment that substantially limits one or more major life activities, a person who has a history or record of such an impairment, or a person who is perceived by others as having such an impairment. The ADA does not specifically name all of the impairments that are covered.

Americans with Disabilities Act Title I: Employment

Title I requires employers with 15 or more employees to provide qualified individuals with disabilities an equal opportunity to benefit from the full range of employment-related opportunities available to others. For example, it prohibits discrimination in recruitment, hiring, promotions, training, pay, social activities, and other privileges of employment. It restricts questions that can be asked about an applicant's disability before a job offer is made, and it requires that employers make reasonable accommodations to the known

---

[2] National Center on Birth Defects and Developmental Disabilities (NCBDDD), "Disability Inclusion," Centers for Disease Control and Prevention (CDC), September 16, 2020. Available online. URL: www.cdc.gov/ncbddd/disabilityandhealth/disability-inclusion.html. Accessed March 5, 2024.

physical or mental limitations of otherwise qualified individuals with disabilities, unless it results in undue hardship. Religious entities with 15 or more employees are covered under Title I.

Title I complaints must be filed with the U.S. Equal Employment Opportunity Commission (EEOC) within 180 days of the date of discrimination or 300 days if the charge is filed with a designated state or local fair employment practice agency. Individuals may file a lawsuit in federal court only after they receive a "right-to-sue" letter from the EEOC.

Charges of employment discrimination on the basis of disability may be filed at any EEOC field office. Field offices are located in 50 cities throughout the United States and are listed in most telephone directories under "U.S. Government." For the appropriate EEOC field office in your geographic area, contact:
- voice: 800-669-4000
- teletypewriter (TTY): 800-669-6820
- videophone (VP): 844-234-5122
- website: www.eeoc.gov

For information on how to accommodate a specific individual with a disability, contact the Job Accommodation Network (JAN) at:
- voice: 800-526-7234
- TTY: 877-781-9403
- website: https://askjan.org

Americans with Disabilities Act Title II: State and Local Government Activities

Title II covers all activities of state and local governments regardless of the government entity's size or receipt of federal funding. Title II requires that state and local governments give people with disabilities an equal opportunity to benefit from all of their programs, services, and activities (e.g., public education, employment, transportation, recreation, health care, social services, courts, voting, and town meetings).

State and local governments are required to follow specific architectural standards in the new construction and alteration of their buildings. They must also relocate programs or otherwise provide access in inaccessible older buildings and communicate effectively with people who have hearing, vision, or speech disabilities. Public entities are not required to take actions that would result in undue financial and administrative burdens. They are required to make reasonable modifications to policies, practices, and procedures where necessary to avoid discrimination, unless they can demonstrate that doing so would fundamentally alter the nature of the service, program, or activity being provided.

Complaints of Title II violations may be filed with the U.S. Department of Justice (DOJ) within 180 days of the date of discrimination. In certain situations, cases may be referred to a mediation program sponsored by the DOJ. The DOJ may bring a lawsuit where it has investigated a matter and has been unable to resolve violations.

Title II may also be enforced through private lawsuits in federal court. It is not necessary to file a complaint with the DOJ or any other federal agency, or to receive a "right-to-sue" letter, before going to court.

Americans with Disabilities Act Title II: Public Transportation

The transportation provisions of Title II cover public transportation services, such as city buses and public rail transit (e.g., subways, commuter rails, Amtrak). Public transportation authorities may not discriminate against people with disabilities in the provision of their services. They must comply with requirements for accessibility in newly purchased vehicles, make good faith efforts to purchase or lease accessible used buses, remanufacture buses in an accessible manner, and, unless it would result in an undue burden, provide paratransit where they operate fixed-route bus or rail systems. Paratransit is a service where individuals who are unable to use the regular transit system independently (because of a physical or mental impairment) are picked up and dropped off at their destinations.

Americans with Disabilities Act Title III: Public Accommodations

Title III covers businesses and nonprofit service providers that are public accommodations, privately operated entities offering certain types of courses and examinations, privately operated transportation, and commercial facilities. Public accommodations are

The Americans with Disabilities Act

private entities who own, lease, lease to, or operate facilities such as restaurants, retail stores, hotels, movie theaters, private schools, convention centers, doctors' offices, homeless shelters, transportation depots, zoos, funeral homes, day care centers, and recreation facilities including sports stadiums and fitness clubs. Transportation services provided by private entities are also covered by Title III.

Public accommodations must comply with basic nondiscrimination requirements that prohibit exclusion, segregation, and unequal treatment. They must also comply with specific requirements related to architectural standards for new and altered buildings; reasonable modifications to policies, practices, and procedures; effective communication with people with hearing, vision, or speech disabilities; and other access requirements. Additionally, public accommodations must remove barriers in existing buildings where it is easy to do so without much difficulty or expense, given the public accommodation's resources.

Courses and examinations related to professional, educational, or trade-related applications, licensing, certifications, or credentialing must be provided in a place and manner accessible to people with disabilities, or alternative accessible arrangements must be offered.

Commercial facilities, such as factories and warehouses, must comply with the ADA's architectural standards for new construction and alterations.

Complaints of Title III violations may be filed with the DOJ. In certain situations, cases may be referred to a mediation program sponsored by the DOJ. The DOJ is authorized to bring a lawsuit where there is a pattern or practice of discrimination in violation of Title III or where an act of discrimination raises an issue of general public importance. Title III may also be enforced through private lawsuits. It is not necessary to file a complaint with the DOJ (or any federal agency), or to receive a "right-to-sue" letter, before going to court.

Americans with Disabilities Act Title IV: Telecommunications Relay Services

Title IV addresses telephone and television access for people with hearing and speech disabilities. It requires common carriers (telephone companies) to establish interstate and intrastate telecommunications relay services (TRSs) 24 hours a day, 7 days a week. TRS enables callers with hearing and speech disabilities who use TTYs (also known as "telecommunications device for the deaf" (TDDs) and callers who use voice telephones to communicate with each other through a third-party communications assistant. The Federal Communications Commission (FCC) has set minimum standards for TRSs. Title IV also requires closed captioning of federally funded public service announcements.[3]

---

[3] ADA.gov, "Guide to Disability Rights Laws," U.S. Department of Justice (DOJ), February 28, 2020. Available online. URL: www.ada.gov/resources/disability-rights-guide. Accessed March 5, 2024.

Chapter 53 | The Family and Medical Leave Act

WHAT IS THE FAMILY AND MEDICAL LEAVE ACT?
The Family and Medical Leave Act (FMLA) provides eligible employees of covered employers with job-protected leave for qualifying family and medical reasons and requires continuation of their group health benefits under the same conditions as if they had not taken leave. FMLA leave may be unpaid or used at the same time as employer-provided paid leave. Employees must be restored to the same or virtually identical position when they return to work after FMLA leave.

Eligible Employees
Employees are eligible if they work for a covered employer for at least 12 months, have at least 1,250 hours of service with the employer during the 12 months before their FMLA leave starts, and work at a location where the employer has at least 50 employees within 75 miles.

Covered Employers
Covered employers under the FMLA include:
- private-sector employers who employ 50 or more employees in 20 or more workweeks in either the current calendar year or the previous calendar year
- public agencies (including federal, state, and local government employers, regardless of the number of employees)

- local educational agencies (including public school boards, public elementary and secondary schools, and private elementary and secondary schools, regardless of the number of employees)

The FMLA protects leave for:
- the birth of a child or placement of a child with the employee for adoption or foster care
- the care for a child, spouse, or parent who has a serious health condition
- a serious health condition that makes the employee unable to work
- reasons related to a family member's service in the military, including the following:
  - **Qualifying exigency leave.** This leave is applicable for certain reasons related to a family member's foreign deployment.
  - **Military caregiver leave.** This leave is applicable when a family member is a current service member or recent veteran with a serious injury or illness.

USING FAMILY AND MEDICAL LEAVE ACT LEAVE

Eligible employees may take:
- up to 12 workweeks of leave in a 12-month period for any FMLA leave reason except military caregiver leave
- up to 26 workweeks of military caregiver leave during a single 12-month period

Intermittent or Reduced Schedule Leave

Employees have the right to take FMLA leave all at once or in separate blocks of time when medically necessary or by reducing the time they work each day or week. Intermittent or reduced schedule leave is also available for military family leave reasons. However, employees may use FMLA leave intermittently or on a reduced leave schedule for bonding with a newborn or newly placed child only if they and their employer agree.

The Family and Medical Leave Act

Paid Leave
The FMLA is job-protected, unpaid leave. Employees may use employer-provided paid leave at the same time that they take FMLA leave if the reason they are using FMLA leave is covered by the employer's paid leave policy. An employer may also require an employee to use their paid leave during FMLA leave.

Requesting Family and Medical Leave Act Leave
Employees do not have to specifically ask for FMLA leave but do need to provide enough information, so the employer is aware the leave may be covered by the FMLA. Employees must provide notice to their employer as soon as possible and practical that they will need to use FMLA leave. For example, if an employee knows that they have a procedure for a serious medical condition scheduled in three weeks, the employee needs to provide notice to the employer as soon as the procedure is scheduled. Employers may ask for information from the heath-care provider before approving FMLA leave and must allow 15 calendar days to provide the information. In some circumstances, such as when the employee's health-care provider is not able to complete the certification information timely, employees must be allowed additional time.

FAMILY AND MEDICAL LEAVE ACT LEAVE BENEFITS AND PROTECTIONS
Job Protection
Employees who use FMLA leave have the right to go back to work at their same job or to an equivalent job that has the same pay, benefits, and other terms and conditions of employment at the end of their FMLA leave. Violations of an employee's FMLA rights may include changing the number of shifts assigned to the employee, moving the employee to a location outside their normal commuting area, or denying the employee a bonus for which they qualified before their FMLA leave.

An employer cannot threaten, discriminate against, punish, suspend, or fire an employee because they requested or used FMLA leave. Violations of an employee's FMLA rights may include actions such as writing up the employee for missing work when using FMLA leave, denying a promotion because the employee has used FMLA leave, or assessing negative attendance points for FMLA leave use.

Group Health Plan Benefits
Employers are required to continue group health insurance coverage for an employee on FMLA leave under the same terms and conditions as if the employee had not taken leave. For example, if family member coverage is provided to an employee, it must be maintained during the employee's FMLA leave.

SPECIAL FAMILY AND MEDICAL LEAVE ACT RULES FOR SOME WORKERS
- **Teachers.** Special rules apply to employees of elementary schools, secondary schools, and school boards. Generally, these rules apply when an employee needs intermittent leave or leave near the end of a school term.
- **Airline flight crew employees.** These employees have special hours of service eligibility requirements.

FAMILY AND MEDICAL LEAVE ACT ELIGIBILITY FOR SERVICE MEMBERS UNDER THE UNIFORMED SERVICES EMPLOYMENT AND REEMPLOYMENT RIGHTS ACT
Returning service members are entitled to receive all rights and benefits of employment that they would have obtained if they had been continuously employed. Any period of absence from work due to the service covered by the Uniformed Services Employment and Reemployment Rights Act (USERRA) counts toward an employee's months and hours of service requirements for FMLA leave eligibility.

ADDITIONAL PROTECTIONS
State Laws
Some states have their own family and medical leave laws. Nothing in the FMLA prevents employees from receiving protections under

other laws. Workers have the right to benefit from all the laws that apply.

Protection from Retaliation

The FMLA is a federal worker protection law. Employers are prohibited from interfering with, restraining, or denying the exercise of (or the attempt to exercise) any FMLA right. Any violations of the FMLA or the FMLA regulations constitute interfering with, restraining, or denying the exercise of rights provided by the FMLA.

Enforcement

The Wage and Hour Division (WHD) is responsible for administering and enforcing the FMLA for most employees. If you believe that your rights under the FMLA have been violated, you may file a complaint with the WHD or file a private lawsuit against your employer in court. State employees may be subject to certain limitations in pursuit of direct lawsuits regarding leave for their own serious health conditions. Most federal and certain congressional employees are also covered by the law but are subject to the jurisdiction of the U.S. Office of Personnel Management (OPM) or Congress.[1]

---

[1] "Fact Sheet #28: The Family and Medical Leave Act," U.S. Department of Labor (DOL), February 2023. Available online. URL: www.dol.gov/agencies/whd/fact-sheets/28-fmla. Accessed February 16, 2024.

Chapter 54 | Advance Directives

During an emergency or at the end-of-life, you may face questions about your loved one's medical treatment and not be able to answer them. You may assume your loved ones know what you would want, but that is not always true. In one study, people guessed nearly one out of three end-of-life decisions for their loved one incorrectly.

Research shows that you are more likely to get the care you want if you have conversations about your future medical treatment and put a plan in place. It may also help your loved ones grieve more easily and feel less burden, guilt, and depression.

WHAT IS ADVANCE CARE PLANNING?
Advance care planning involves discussing and preparing for future decisions about your medical care if you become seriously ill or unable to communicate your wishes. Having meaningful conversations with your loved ones is the most important part of advance care planning. Many people also choose to put their preferences in writing by completing legal documents called "advance directives."

WHAT ARE ADVANCE DIRECTIVES?
Advance directives are legal documents that provide instructions for medical care and only go into effect if you cannot communicate your own wishes.

The following are the two most common advance directives for health care:
- **Living will.** This is a legal document that tells doctors how you want to be treated if you cannot make your own decisions about emergency treatment. In a living will, you can say which common medical treatments or care you would want, which ones you would want to avoid, and under which conditions each of your choices applies.
- **Durable power of attorney (POA) for health care.** This is a legal document that names your health-care proxy, a person who can make health-care decisions for you if you are unable to communicate these yourself. Your proxy, also known as a "representative," "surrogate," or "agent," should be familiar with your values and wishes. A proxy can be chosen in addition to or instead of a living will. Having a health-care proxy helps you plan for situations that cannot be foreseen, such as a serious car accident or stroke.

Think of your advance directives as living documents that you review at least once each year and update if a major life event occurs, such as retirement, moving out of state, or a significant change in your health.

WHO NEEDS AN ADVANCE CARE PLAN?

Advance care planning is not just for people who are very old or ill. At any age, a medical crisis could leave you unable to communicate your own health-care decisions. Planning now for your future health care can help ensure you get the medical care you want and that someone you trust will be there to make decisions for you.

WHAT HAPPENS IF YOU DO NOT HAVE AN ADVANCE DIRECTIVE?

If you do not have an advance directive and you are unable to make decisions on your own, the laws of the state where you live

Advance Directives

will determine who may make medical decisions on your behalf. This is typically your spouse, your parents if they are available, or your children if they are adults. If you are unmarried and have not named your partner as your proxy, it is possible they could be excluded from decision-making. If you have no family members, some states allow a close friend who is familiar with your values to help, or they may assign a physician to represent your best interests. To find out the laws in your state, contact your state legal aid office or state bar association.

WILL AN ADVANCE DIRECTIVE GUARANTEE YOUR WISHES ARE FOLLOWED?

An advance directive is legally recognized but not legally binding. This means that your health-care provider and proxy will do their best to respect your advance directives, but there may be circumstances in which they cannot follow your wishes exactly. For example, you may be in a complex medical situation where it is unclear what you would want. This is another key reason why having conversations about your preferences is so important. Talking with your loved ones ahead of time may help them better navigate unanticipated issues.

There is the possibility that a health-care provider refuses to follow your advance directives. This might happen if the decision goes against:
- the health-care provider's conscience
- the health-care institution's policy
- the accepted health-care standards

In these situations, the health-care provider must inform your health-care proxy immediately and consider transferring your care to another provider.

OTHER ADVANCE CARE PLANNING FORMS AND ORDERS

You might want to prepare documents to express your wishes about a single medical issue or something else not already covered in your advance directives, such as an emergency. For these types

of situations, you can talk with a doctor about establishing the following orders:
- **Do-not-resuscitate (DNR) order**. A DNR order becomes part of your medical chart to inform medical staff in a hospital or nursing facility that you do not want cardiopulmonary resuscitation (CPR) or other life-support measures to be attempted if your heartbeat and breathing stop. Sometimes this document is referred to as a "do-not-attempt-resuscitation (DNAR) order" or an "allow natural death (AND) order." Even though a living will might state that CPR is not wanted, it is helpful to have a DNR order as part of your medical file if you go to a hospital. Posting a DNR order next to your hospital bed might avoid confusion in an emergency. Without a DNR order, medical staff will attempt every effort to restore your breathing and the normal rhythm of your heart.
- **Do-not-intubate (DNI) order**. A similar document, a DNI order informs medical staff in a hospital or nursing facility that you do not want to be on a ventilator.
- **Do-not-hospitalize (DNH) order**. A DNH order indicates to long-term care providers, such as nursing home staff, that you prefer not to be sent to a hospital for treatment at the end-of-life.
- **Out-of-hospital DNR order**. An out-of-hospital DNR order alerts emergency medical personnel to your wishes regarding measures to restore your heartbeat or breathing if you are not in a hospital.
- **Physician orders for life-sustaining treatment (POLST) and medical orders for life-sustaining treatment (MOLST) forms**. These forms provide guidance about your medical care that health-care professionals can act on immediately in an emergency. They serve as a medical order in addition to your advance directive. Typically, you create a POLST or MOLST form when you are near the end-of-life

Advance Directives

or critically ill and understand the specific decisions that might need to be made on your behalf. These forms may also be called "portable medical orders" or "physician orders for scope of treatment" (POST). Check with your state department of health to find out if these forms are available where you live.

You may also want to document your wishes about organ and tissue donation and brain donation. As well, learning about care options such as palliative care and hospice care can help you plan ahead.

HOW CAN YOU GET STARTED WITH ADVANCE CARE PLANNING?

To get started with advance care planning, consider the following steps:

- **Reflect on your values and wishes.** This can help you think through what matters most at the end-of-life and guide your decisions about future care and medical treatment.
- **Talk with your doctor about advance directives.** Advance care planning is covered by Medicare as part of your annual wellness visit. If you have private health insurance, check with your insurance provider. Talking to a health-care provider can help you learn about your current health and the kinds of decisions that are likely to come up. For example, you might ask about the decisions you may face if your high blood pressure (HBP) leads to a stroke.
- **Choose someone you trust to make medical decisions for you.** Whether it is a family member, a loved one, or your lawyer, it is important to choose someone you trust as your health-care proxy. Once you have decided, discuss your values and preferences with them. If you are not ready to discuss specific treatments or care decisions yet, try talking about your general preferences. You can also try other ways to share your

wishes, such as writing a letter or watching a video on the topic together.
- **Complete your advance directive forms.** To make your care and treatment decisions official, you can complete a living will. Similarly, once you decide on your health-care proxy, you can make it official by completing a durable POA for health care.
- **Share your forms with your health-care proxy, doctors, and loved ones.** After you have completed your advance directives, make copies and store them in a safe place. Give copies to your health-care proxy, health-care providers, and lawyer. Some states have registries that can store your advance directive for quick access by health-care providers and your proxy.
- **Keep the conversation going.** Continue to talk about your wishes and update your forms at least once each year or after major life changes. If you update your forms, file and keep your previous versions. Note the date the older copy was replaced by a new one. If you use a registry, make sure the latest version is on record.

Everyone approaches the process differently. Remember to be flexible and take it one step at a time. For example, try simply talking with your loved ones about what you appreciate and enjoy most about life. Your values, treatment preferences, and even the people you involve in your plan may change over time. The most important part is to start the conversation.

HOW TO FIND ADVANCE DIRECTIVE FORMS

You can establish your advance directives for little or no cost. Many states have their own forms that you can access and complete for free. The following are some ways you might find free advance directive forms in your state:
- Contact your State Attorney General's Office.
- Contact your local Area Agency on Aging (AAA; https://eldercare.acl.gov/Public/About/Aging_Network/AAA.aspx). You can find your area agency

Advance Directives

> phone number by visiting the Eldercare Locator (https://eldercare.acl.gov/Public/Index.aspx) or by calling 800-677-1116.
- Download your state's form online from one of these national organizations: the American Association of Retired Persons (AARP), the American Bar Association (ABA), or the National Hospice and Palliative Care Organization (NHPCO).
- If you are a veteran, contact your local Veterans Affairs (VA) office (www.va.gov/contact-us/#contact-your-local-va-facility). The VA office offers an advance directive specifically for veterans.

Some people spend a lot of time in more than one state. If that is your situation, consider preparing advance directives using the form for each state and keep a copy in each place, too.

There are also organizations that enable you to create, download, and print your forms online, but they may charge fees. Before you pay, remember there are several ways to get your forms for free. The following are some free online resources:
- **PREPARE for Your Care.** This is an interactive online program that was funded in part by the National Institute on Aging (NIA; https://prepareforyourcare.org). It is available in English and Spanish.
- **The Conversation Project.** A series of online conversation guides and advance care documents available in English, Spanish, and Chinese. The Conversation Project is a public engagement initiative led by the Institute for Healthcare Improvement (IHI; https://theconversationproject.org).

If you use forms from a website, check to make sure they are legally recognized in your state. You should also make sure the website is secure and will protect your personal information. Read the website's privacy policy and check that the website link begins with "https" (make sure it has an "s") and that it has a small lock icon next to its web address.

Some people also choose to carry a card (e.g., from the American Hospital Association (AHA)) in their wallet, indicating they have an advance directive and where it is kept.[1]

---

[1] National Institute on Aging (NIA), "Advance Care Planning: Advance Directives for Health Care," National Institutes of Health (NIH), October 31, 2022. Available online. URL: www.nia.nih.gov/health/advance-care-planning-advance-directives-health-care. Accessed February 16, 2024.

Chapter 55 | Legal and Financial Planning for People with Chronic Disease

Many people are unprepared to deal with the legal and financial consequences of a serious illness such as Alzheimer disease (AD) or related dementia. Legal and medical experts encourage people recently diagnosed with a serious illness—particularly one that is expected to cause declining mental and physical health—to examine and update their financial and health-care arrangements as soon as possible. Basic legal and financial documents, such as a will, a living trust, and advance directives, are available to ensure that the person's late-stage or end-of-life health-care and financial decisions are carried out.

A complication of diseases such as AD and related dementias is that the person may lack or gradually lose the ability to think clearly. This change affects his or her ability to make decisions and participate in legal and financial planning.

People with early-stage AD or related dementia can often understand many aspects and consequences of legal decision-making. However, legal and medical experts say that many forms of planning can help the person and his or her family address current issues and plan for the next steps, even if the person is diagnosed with late-stage dementia.

There are good reasons to retain a lawyer when preparing advance planning documents. For example, a lawyer can help interpret different state laws and suggest ways to ensure that the person's and family's wishes are carried out.

It is important to understand that laws vary by state, and changes in a person's situation—for example, a divorce, relocation, or death in the family—can influence how documents are prepared and maintained. Life changes may also mean a document needs to be revised to remain valid.

LEGAL, FINANCIAL, AND HEALTH-CARE PLANNING DOCUMENTS

Families beginning the legal planning process should discuss their approach, what they want to happen, and which legal documents they will need. Depending on the family situation and the applicable state laws, a lawyer may introduce a variety of documents to assist in this process, including documents that communicate:
- health-care wishes of someone who can no longer make health-care decisions
- financial management and estate plan wishes of someone who can no longer make financial decisions

ADVANCE HEALTH-CARE DIRECTIVES FOR PEOPLE WITH DEMENTIA

Advance directives for health care are documents that communicate a person's health-care wishes (see Table 55.1). Advance directives go into effect after the person no longer can make decisions on their own. In most cases, these documents must be prepared while the person is legally able to execute them. Health-care directives may include the following:
- **Durable power of attorney (POA).** A durable POA for health care designates a person, sometimes called an "agent" or "proxy," to make health-care decisions when the person with dementia can no longer do so.
- **Living will.** This records a person's wishes for medical treatment near the end-of-life or if the person is permanently unconscious and cannot make decisions about emergency treatment.
- **Do-not-resuscitate (DNR) order.** This instructs health-care professionals not to perform

Legal and Financial Planning for People with Chronic Disease

cardiopulmonary resuscitation (CPR) if a person's heart stops or if he or she stops breathing. A DNR order is signed by a doctor and put in a person's medical chart.

In addition to these, there may be other documents for specific health-care procedures including organ and tissue donation, dialysis, brain donation, and blood transfusions.

Table 55.1. Overview of Medical Documents

Medical Document	How It Is Used
Durable power of attorney (POA) for health care	This document gives a designated person the authority to make health-care decisions on behalf of the person with dementia.
Living will	This document describes and instructs how and when the person wants different types of end-of-life health care.
Do-not-resuscitate (DNR) order	This document instructs health-care professionals not to perform cardiopulmonary resuscitation (CPR) in case of stopped heart or stopped breathing.

ADVANCE DIRECTIVES FOR FINANCIAL AND ESTATE MANAGEMENT

Advance directives for financial and estate management must be created while the person with AD or related dementia has "legal capacity" to make decisions on their own, meaning they can still understand the decisions and what they might mean (see Table 55.2). These directives may include the following:

- **Durable POA for finances**. This document names someone to make financial decisions when the person with AD or a related dementia no longer can. It can help avoid court actions that may take away control of financial affairs.
- **Will**. This document indicates how a person's assets and estate will be distributed upon their death. It can also specify:
  - arrangements for care of minors or pets
  - gifts
  - trusts to manage the estate
  - funeral and/or burial arrangements

Medical and legal experts say that the person newly diagnosed with AD or related dementia and his or her family should create or update a will as soon as possible after diagnosis.

- **Living trust.** This document trust addresses the management of money and property while a person is still living. The trust provides instructions about the person's estate and appoints someone, called the "trustee," to hold titles to property and money on the person's behalf. Using the instructions in the living trust, the trustee can pay bills or make other financial and property decisions when the person with dementia can no longer manage his or her affairs. A living trust can:
  - cover a wide range of property (including cars, homes, jewelry, bonds, cash, etc.)
  - provide a detailed plan for property transfer or sale
  - avoid the expense and delay of probate (in which the courts establish the validity of a will)
  - state how property and funds should be distributed when the last beneficiary dies

Table 55.2. Overview of Legal and Financial Documents

Legal/Financial Document	How It Is Used
Durable power of attorney (POA) for health care	This document gives a designated person the authority to make legal and financial decisions on behalf of the person with Alzheimer disease (AD) or related dementia.
Living will	This document indicates how a person's assets and estate will be distributed among beneficiaries after his or her death.
Do-not-resuscitate (DNR) order	This document gives a designated person (trustee) the authority to hold and distribute property and money for the person with AD or related dementia.

WHERE CAN YOU GET HELP WITH LEGAL AND FINANCIAL PLANNING?

- **Health-care providers.** These professionals cannot act as legal or financial advisers, but they can encourage

planning discussions between patients and their families. Doctors can also guide patients, families, the care team, attorneys, and judges regarding the patient's ability to make decisions. Discussing advance care planning decisions with a doctor is free through Medicare during the annual wellness visit. Private health insurance may also cover these discussions.
- **Elder law attorney.** This lawyer helps older adults and their families interpret state laws, plan how wishes will be carried out, understand financial options, and learn how to preserve financial assets. It is a good idea to ask about a lawyer's fees before making an appointment. The National Academy of Elder Law Attorneys (NAELA) and the American Bar Association (ABA) can help families find qualified attorneys. Also, a local bar association can help identify free legal aid options.
- **Geriatric care managers.** They are trained social workers or nurses who can help people with dementia and their families.

ADVANCE PLANNING ADVICE FOR PEOPLE WITH DEMENTIA
- **Start discussions early.** The rate of decline differs for each person with dementia, and his or her ability to be involved in planning will decline over time. People in the early stages of the disease may be able to understand the issues, but they may also be defensive, frustrated, and/or emotionally unable to deal with difficult questions. The person may even be in denial or not ready to face their diagnosis. This is normal. Be patient and seek outside help from a lawyer or geriatric care manager, if needed. Remember that not all people are diagnosed at an early stage. Decision-making may already be difficult by the time the person with dementia is diagnosed.
- **Gather important papers.** When an emergency arises or when the person with dementia can no longer manage their own affairs, family members or a proxy will need access to important papers, such as a living will or

financial documents. To make sure the wishes of the person with dementia are followed, put important papers in a secure place and provide copies to family members or another trusted person. A lawyer can keep a set of the papers as well.
- **Review plans over time.** Changes in personal situations—such as a divorce, relocation, or death in the family—and in state laws can affect how legal documents are prepared and maintained. Review plans regularly and update documents as needed.
- **Reduce anxiety about funeral and burial arrangements.** Advance planning for the funeral and burial can provide a sense of peace and reduce anxiety for the person with dementia as well as his or her family.

LEGAL AND FINANCIAL PLANNING RESOURCES FOR LOW-INCOME FAMILIES

Families who cannot afford a lawyer can still plan for the future. Samples of basic health planning documents are available online. Area Agency on Aging (AAA) officials may provide legal advice or help. Other possible sources of legal assistance and referrals include state legal aid offices, state bar associations, local nonprofit agencies, foundations, and social service agencies.[1]

---

[1] National Institute on Aging (NIA), "Legal and Financial Planning for People Living with Dementia," National Institutes of Health (NIH), October 2020. Available online. URL: https://order.nia.nih.gov/sites/default/files/2021-01/legal-financial-planning-dementia-factsheet.pdf. Accessed March 5, 2024.

Chapter 56 | Health-Care Benefit Laws

HEALTH INSURANCE PORTABILITY AND ACCOUNTABILITY ACT
The Health Insurance Portability and Accountability Act (HIPAA) offers protections for millions of American workers that improve portability and continuity of health insurance coverage.

The HIPAA protects workers and their families by:
- providing additional opportunities to enroll in group health plan coverage when they lose other health coverage, get married, or add a new dependent
- prohibiting discrimination in enrollment and in premiums charged to employees and their dependents, based on any health factors
- preserving the states' role in regulating health insurance, including the states' authority to provide greater protections than those available under federal law

Special Enrollment Rights
Special enrollment allows individuals who previously declined health coverage to enroll for coverage outside a plan's open enrollment period. There are two types of special enrollment:
- **Loss of eligibility for other coverage**. Employees and dependents who decline coverage due to other health coverage and then lose eligibility or employer contributions have special enrollment rights. For example, an employee who turns down health benefits for himself/herself and his/her family because the

family already has coverage through his/her spouse's plan can request special enrollment for his/her family in his/her own company's plan.
- **Certain life events**. Employees, spouses, and new dependents are permitted to special enroll because of marriage, birth, adoption, or placement for adoption.

For both types, the employee must request enrollment within 30 days of the loss of coverage or life event triggering the special enrollment.

Nondiscrimination Prohibitions

Employees and their family members cannot be denied eligibility or benefits based on certain health factors. They also cannot be charged more than similarly situated individuals based on any health factors. Health factors include medical conditions, claims experience, and genetic information.

The HIPAA and the Affordable Care Act (ACA) also provide protections from impermissible discrimination based on a health factor in wellness programs related to group health plan coverage (such as those that encourage employees to work out, stop smoking, or meet certain health standards such as a target cholesterol level).

Preserving the States' Role

If a health plan provides benefits through an insurance company or health maintenance organization (HMO; an insured plan), the HIPAA may be complemented by state laws that offer additional protections. For example, states may increase the number of days parents have to enroll newborns, adopted children, and children placed for adoption or require additional special enrollment circumstances.

Preexisting Condition Exclusions

The ACA prohibits plans from imposing preexisting condition exclusions for plan years beginning on or after January 1, 2014. For

Health-Care Benefit Laws

prior years, the HIPAA limited these exclusions and required plans to offset preexisting condition exclusion periods if the individual had prior health coverage.[1]

CONSOLIDATED OMNIBUS BUDGET RECONCILIATION ACT CONTINUATION COVERAGE

Throughout a career, workers will face multiple life events, job changes, or even job losses. The continuation coverage provisions of the Consolidated Omnibus Budget Reconciliation Act (COBRA) help workers and their families keep their group health coverage during times of voluntary or involuntary job loss, reduction in the hours worked, transition between jobs, and in certain other cases.

- The COBRA generally requires that group health plans offer employees and their families the opportunity for a temporary extension of health coverage (called "continuation coverage") in certain instances where coverage under the plan would otherwise end.
- The law generally applies to all group health plans maintained by employers (private sector and state/local government) that have at least 20 employees on more than 50 percent of its typical business days in the previous calendar year. Both full- and part-time employees are counted to determine whether a plan is subject to the COBRA. The law does not apply to plans sponsored by the federal government or by churches and certain church-related organizations.
- Several events that can cause workers and their family members to lose group health coverage may result in the right to COBRA coverage. These include:
  - termination of the covered employee's employment for any reason other than gross misconduct
  - reduction in the covered employee's hours of employment

---

[1] "Health Insurance Portability and Accountability Act (HIPAA)," U.S. Department of Labor (DOL), March 23, 2019. Available online. URL: www.dol.gov/sites/dolgov/files/EBSA/about-ebsa/our-activities/resource-center/fact-sheets/hipaa.pdf. Accessed March 4, 2024.

- covered employee becomes entitled to Medicare
- divorce or legal separation of the spouse from the covered employee
- death of the covered employee
- loss of dependent child status under the plan rules
- Under the COBRA, the employee or family member may qualify to keep their group health plan benefits for a set period of time, depending on the reason for losing the health coverage. Table 56.1 represents some basic information on periods of continuation coverage.
- However, the COBRA also provides that your continuation coverage may be cut short in certain cases.

Table 56.1. Consolidated Omnibus Budget Reconciliation Act Continuation Coverage

Qualifying Event	Qualified Beneficiaries	Maximum Period of Continuation Coverage
Termination (for reasons other than gross misconduct) or reduction in hours of employment	Employee, spouse, and dependent child	18 months (In certain circumstances, qualified beneficiaries may become entitled to a disability extension of an additional 11 months or an extension of an additional 18 months due to the occurrence of a second qualifying event.)
Employee enrollment in Medicare	Spouse and dependent child	36 months (The actual period of continuation coverage may vary depending on factors such as whether the Medicare entitlement occurred prior to or after the end of the covered employee's employment or reduction in hours.)
Divorce or legal separation	Spouse and dependent child	36 months
Death of the employee	Spouse and dependent child	36 months
Loss of "dependent child" status under the plan	Dependent child	36 months

Health-Care Benefit Laws

Notification Requirements
- A general notice must be furnished to covered employees and spouses, within the first 90 days of coverage under the plan, informing them of their rights under the COBRA and describing provisions of the law. COBRA information is also required to be contained in the plan's Summary Plan Description (SPD).
- Under the COBRA, the covered employee or a family member has the responsibility to inform the plan administrator of a divorce, legal separation, disability, or a child losing dependent status under the plan.
- Employers have a responsibility to notify the plan administrator of the employee's death, termination of employment or reduction in hours, Medicare entitlement, or bankruptcy of a private-sector employer.
- When the plan administrator is notified that a qualifying event has happened (by the covered employee or family member or by the employer), it must in turn notify each qualified beneficiary of the right to choose continuation coverage.
- The COBRA allows at least 60 days from the date the election notice is provided to inform the plan administrator that the qualified beneficiary wants to elect continuation coverage.

Premium Payments
- Qualified individuals may be required to pay the entire premium for coverage up to 102 percent of the cost to the plan. Premiums may be higher for persons exercising the disability extension provisions of the COBRA. Failure to make timely payments may result in loss of coverage.
- Premiums may be increased by the plan; however, premiums generally must be set in advance of each 12-month premium cycle.[2]

---

[2] "COBRA Continuation Coverage," U.S. Department of Labor (DOL), November 2016. Available online. URL: www.dol.gov/sites/dolgov/files/EBSA/about-ebsa/our-activities/resource-center/fact-sheets/cobra.pdf. Accessed March 4, 2024.

Chapter 57 | Medicaid and Hill-Burton Free and Reduced-Cost Health Care

Chapter Contents
Section 57.1—Medicaid..559
Section 57.2—Hill-Burton Free and Reduced-Cost
 Health Care..562

Section 57.1 | Medicaid

Good health is important to everyone. If you cannot afford to pay for medical care right now, Medicaid can make it possible for you to get the care that you need so that you can get healthy and stay healthy.

Medicaid is available only to certain low-income individuals and families who fit into an eligibility group that is recognized by federal and state law. Medicaid does not give money directly to you; instead, it sends payments directly to your health-care providers. Depending on your state's rules, you may also be asked to pay a small part of the cost (a co-payment) for some medical services. In general, you should apply for Medicaid if you have limited income and resources and match one of the following descriptions.

PREGNANT WOMEN

Apply for Medicaid if you think you are pregnant. You may be eligible if you are married or single. If you are on Medicaid when your child is born, both you and your child will be covered.

CHILDREN AND TEENAGERS

Apply for Medicaid if you are the parent or guardian of a child who is 18 years old or younger and your family's income is limited or if your child is sick enough to need nursing home care but could stay home with good quality care at home. If you are a teenager living on your own, the state may allow you to apply for Medicaid on your own behalf or allow any adult to apply for you. Many states also cover children up to the age of 21.

PEOPLE WHO ARE AGED, BLIND, AND/OR DISABLED

Apply if you are 65 years of age or older, blind, or disabled and have limited income and resources. Apply if you are terminally ill and want to receive hospice services. Apply if you are elderly, blind, or disabled; live in a nursing home, and have limited income and resources. Apply if you are elderly, blind, or disabled and need nursing home care but can stay at home with special community care services. Apply if you are eligible for Medicare and have limited income and resources.

OTHER SITUATIONS

Apply if you are losing welfare coverage and need health coverage. Apply if you are a family with children under the age of 18 and have limited income and resources. (You do not need to be receiving a welfare check to qualify.)

Medicaid is a state-administered program, and each state sets its own guidelines regarding eligibility and services.[1]

MANDATORY AND OPTIONAL MEDICAID BENEFITS

Following are the mandatory and optional Medicaid state plan benefits and the relevant section of the Social Security Act (SSA) and applicable coverage regulation(s) under which each benefit is authorized. States are required to provide all mandatory benefits under federal law. States may provide optional benefits if they choose to add them through the state plan process.

Mandatory Benefits
- transportation to medical care
- inpatient hospital services
- outpatient hospital services
- rural health clinic services
- federally qualified health center services
- laboratory and x-ray services
- nursing facility services
- early and periodic screening, diagnostic, and treatment (EPSDT) services

---

[1] "What Is the Medicaid Program?" U.S. Department of Health and Human Services (HHS), February 12, 2014. Available online. URL: www.hhs.gov/answers/medicare-and-medicaid/what-is-the-medicaid-program/index.html. Accessed March 5, 2024.

Medicaid and Hill-Burton Free and Reduced-Cost Health Care

- family planning services
- tobacco cessation counseling for pregnant women
- physician services
- home health services
- nurse midwife services
- certified pediatric and family nurse practitioner services
- freestanding birth center services when licensed or otherwise recognized by the state
- medication-assisted treatment (MAT)
- routine patient costs of items and services for beneficiaries enrolled in qualifying clinical trials

Optional Benefits
- other licensed practitioner services
- private duty nursing services
- clinic services
- dental services
- physical therapy
- occupational therapy
- speech, hearing, and language disorder services
- prescription drugs
- dentures
- prosthetics
- eyeglasses
- other diagnostic, screening, preventive, and rehabilitative services
- services for individuals aged 65 or older in an institution for mental disease (IMD)
- services in an intermediate care facility for individuals with intellectual disability
- inpatient psychiatric services for individuals under the age of 21
- hospice
- case management
- services related to tuberculosis (TB)
- respiratory care for ventilator-dependent individuals
- personal care

- primary care case management
- primary and secondary medical strategies, treatment, and services for individuals with sickle cell disease (SCD)
- state plan home- and community-based services
- self-directed personal assistance services
- Community First Choice (CFC) Option
- Alternative Benefit Plan (ABP)*
- health homes for enrollees with chronic conditions
- other services approved by the Secretary**

* *The ABP is mandatory for the Medicaid expansion population.*
** *This includes services furnished in a religious nonmedical healthcare institution, emergency hospital services by a non-Medicare-certified hospital, and critical access hospital (CAH).*[2]

Section 57.2 | Hill-Burton Free and Reduced-Cost Health Care

In 1946, Congress passed a law that gave hospitals, nursing homes, and other health facilities grants and loans for construction and modernization. In return, they agreed to provide a reasonable volume of services to people unable to pay and to make their services available to all persons residing in the facility's area.

The program stopped providing funds in 1997, but about 127 health-care facilities nationwide are still obligated to provide free or reduced-cost care. Since 1980, more than $6 billion in uncompensated services have been provided to eligible patients through Hill-Burton.[3]

---

[2] "Mandatory & Optional Medicaid Benefits," Centers for Medicare & Medicaid Services (CMS), April 10, 2023. Available online. URL: www.medicaid.gov/medicaid/benefits/mandatory-optional-medicaid-benefits/index.html. Accessed March 5, 2024.

[3] "Hill-Burton Free and Reduced-Cost Health Care," Health Resources and Services Administration (HRSA), September 2023. Available online. URL: www.hrsa.gov/get-health-care/affordable/hill-burton. Accessed March 5, 2024.

FREQUENTLY ASKED QUESTIONS ABOUT HILL-BURTON FREE AND REDUCED-COST HEALTH CARE
What Services Does the Hill-Burton Program Cover?
Each facility chooses which services it will provide at no or reduced cost. The covered services are specified in a notice which is published by the facility and also in a notice provided to all persons seeking services in the facility. Services fully covered by a third-party insurance or a government program (e.g., Medicare and Medicaid) are not eligible for Hill-Burton coverage. However, Hill-Burton may cover services not covered by the government programs.

Can I Receive Hill-Burton Assistance to Cover My Medicare Deductible and Coinsurance Amounts or Medicaid Co-pay and Spend-Down Amounts?
Medicare deductible and coinsurance amounts are not eligible under the program. However, Medicaid co-payment amounts are eligible, except in a long-term care facility. In addition, Medicaid spend-down amounts (the liability a patient must incur before being eligible for Medicaid) are eligible in all Hill-Burton facilities.

Where Can I Get Hill-Burton Free or Reduced-Cost Care?
Hill-Burton-obligated facilities must provide a certain amount of free or reduced-cost health care each year. Obligated facilities may be hospitals, nursing homes, clinics, or other types of healthcare facilities. See the Hill-Burton-obligated facilities list (www.hrsa.gov/get-health-care/affordable/hill-burton/facilities) to find a Hill-Burton-obligated facility in your state. You may apply for free or reduced-cost care before or after they are provided at the Admissions Office, Business Office, or Patient Accounts Office at the obligated facility.

Who Can Receive Free or Reduced-Cost Care through the Hill-Burton Program?
Eligibility for Hill-Burton free or reduced-cost care is based on a person's family size and income. Income is calculated based on

your actual income for the last 12 months or your last 3 month's income times four, whichever is less. You may qualify if your income falls within the U.S. Department of Health and Human Services (HHS) poverty guidelines (www.federalregister.gov/documents/2021/02/01/2021-01969/annual-update-of-the-hhs-poverty-guidelines) or, at some facilities, if your income is as much as twice (or triple for nursing home services) the poverty guidelines.

What Does "Income" Include?

Gross income (before taxes), interest/dividends earned, and child support payments are examples of income. Assets, food stamps, gifts, loans, or onetime insurance payments are examples of items not included as income when considering eligibility. For self-employed people, income is determined after deductions for business expenses.

When Can I Apply for Hill-Burton Assistance?

You may apply for Hill-Burton assistance at any time, before or after you receive care. You may even apply after a bill has been sent to a collection agency. If a hospital obtains a court judgment before you applied for Hill-Burton assistance, the solution must be worked out within the judicial system. However, if you applied for Hill-Burton assistance before a judgment was rendered and were found eligible, you will receive Hill-Burton assistance even if a judgment was rendered while you were waiting for a response to your application.

Must I Be a U.S. Citizen for Hill-Burton Eligibility?

No, however, to determine your Hill-Burton eligibility, you must have lived in the United States for at least three months.

Can I Apply for Hill-Burton Assistance on Behalf of an Uninsured Relative or Friend?

Yes, you can apply for Hill-Burton assistance on behalf of any patient for whom you can provide the information required to establish eligibility (i.e., you must be able to provide information regarding the patient's family size and income).

Medicaid and Hill-Burton Free and Reduced-Cost Health Care

Do I Have to Wait until I Am Sick before I Can Apply for Hill-Burton Assistance?

Hill-Burton is not health insurance. To apply for Hill-Burton assistance, you must have already received services or know that you will require a specific service in the near future.

What Are Some Reasons I Could Be Denied Hill-Burton Care?

The facility may deny your request if:
- for nonnursing homes, your income is more than the current poverty guidelines or more than twice the guidelines, if specified in the facility's allocation plan
- for nursing home services, your income is more than the poverty guidelines or double or triple the guidelines, if specified in the facility's allocation plan
- the facility has given out its required amount of free care as specified in its allocation plan
- the services you requested or received are not covered in the facility's allocation plan
- the services you requested or received are to be paid by Medicare/Medicaid, insurance, or other financial assistance program
- the facility asks you to first apply for Medicaid/Medicare or a financial assistance program and you do not cooperate
- you do not give the facility requested proof of your income, such as a pay stub

What Can I Do If I Have a Complaint against a Hill-Burton Facility?

If you feel you were unfairly denied free care or reduced-cost care, a complaint must be filed in writing to the Central Office. You must include:
- the name and address of the person making the complaint

- the name and location of the facility
- a statement of the actions that the complainant considers to violate the requirements of the Hill-Burton program

What Other Service Obligation Does a Hill-Burton Facility Have?

Under the community service assurance, Hill-Burton facilities are responsible for providing emergency treatment and for treating all persons residing in the service area, regardless of race, color, national origin, creed, or Medicare or Medicaid status. This assurance is in effect for the life of the facility. If you feel you were unfairly denied services or discriminated against, you should contact the Office for Civil Rights (OCR) at 800-368-1019.

How Do I Apply for Free Care?

You should contact the Admissions, Business, or Patient Accounts Office at a Hill-Burton-obligated facility to find out if you qualify for assistance and whether or not a facility provides the specific services needed.

How Can I Find Out Which Facilities in My Area Are Hill-Burton Facilities?

Check Hill-Burton-obligated facilities list (www.hrsa.gov/get-health-care/affordable/hill-burton/facilities) for a facility in your state. Be aware that although a facility may be listed, you still need to call the facility to be certain that it still has funds available and that the service you desire would be covered.[4]

---

[4] "Hill-Burton Free and Reduced-Cost Health Care—Frequently Asked Questions," Health Resources and Services Administration (HRSA), October 2023. Available online. URL: www.hrsa.gov/get-health-care/affordable/hill-burton/faq/get-care-faq. Accessed March 5, 2024.

Chapter 58 | Paying for Complementary and Integrative Health Approaches

Most adults and children in the United States use complementary health approaches, and the most commonly used approach is natural products (dietary supplements other than vitamins and minerals). Fish oil is the natural product most often used by adults and children. As for mind and body practices, adults and children most often turn to chiropractic or osteopathic manipulation, yoga, meditation, and massage therapy. People seem to be willing to pay "out of pocket" (not through insurance) for certain complementary health approaches.

INSURANCE COVERAGE OF COMPLEMENTARY HEALTH APPROACHES

Many Americans use complementary health approaches, but the type of health insurance they have affects their decisions to use these practices. In a study, researchers analyzed 2012 National Health Interview Survey (NHIS) data on acupuncture, chiropractic, and massage and compared that with data from 2002. While use rates for all three approaches rose, the increase was much more pronounced among those who did not have health insurance. For those who had health insurance, coverage for these three approaches were more likely to be partial than full.

If you want to try a complementary or integrative approach and do not know if your health insurance will cover it, you should contact your health insurance provider to find out.

Some questions to ask your insurance provider are as follows:
- Is this complementary or integrative approach covered for my health condition?
- Does it need to be:
  - preauthorized or preapproved?
  - ordered by a prescription?
- Do I need a referral?
- Does coverage require seeing a practitioner in the network?
- Do I have coverage if I go out-of-network?
- Are there any limits and requirements, for example, on the number of visits or the amount you will pay?
- How much do I have to pay out of pocket?

Keep records of all contacts you have with your insurance company, including notes on calls and copies of bills, claims, and letters. This may help if you have a claim dispute.

If you are choosing a new health insurance plan, ask the insurance provider about coverage of complementary or integrative health approaches. You should find out if you need a special "rider" or supplement to the standard plan for these approaches to be covered. You should also find out if the insurer offers a discount program in which plan members pay for fees and products out of pocket but at a lower rate.

Sources of Information on Insurers

Your state insurance department may be able to help you determine which insurance companies cover specific complementary or integrative health approaches. The USA.gov provides contact information for state and local consumer agencies, including insurance regulators.

Professional associations for complementary health specialties may monitor insurance coverage and reimbursement in their field. You can ask a reference librarian for help or search for them on the Internet.

Paying for Complementary and Integrative Health Approaches

ASKING PRACTITIONERS ABOUT PAYMENT

If you are planning to see a complementary or integrative practitioner, it is important to understand about payment. Here are some questions to ask:

- **Costs**. What does the first appointment cost? What do follow-up appointments cost? Is there a sliding scale based on income? How many appointments am I likely to need? Are there other costs (e.g., tests, equipment, supplements)?
- **Insurance**. Do you accept my insurance plan? What has been your experience with my plan's coverage for people with my condition? Do I file the claims, or do you take care of that?

FEDERAL HEALTH BENEFIT PROGRAMS

The federal government helps with some health expenses of people who are eligible for federal health benefit programs, such as programs for veterans, people aged 65 and older (Medicare), and people who cannot afford health care (Medicaid, funded jointly with the states).

Information on health benefits for veterans is available from the U.S. Department of Veterans Affairs (VA). Information on Medicare and Medicaid is available from the Centers for Medicare & Medicaid Services (CMS). A handbook, *Medicare & You* (www.medicare.gov/medicare-and-you/medicare-and-you.html), explains what services Medicare covers.

Two other Internet resources—Benefits.gov (www.benefits.gov) and the Health and Insurance page (www.opm.gov/healthcare-insurance/healthcare/plan-information/plans) on the U.S. Office of Personnel Management (OPM) website—explain federal health benefit programs. Benefits.gov has a Benefit Finder that can help you learn more about qualifying for programs.[1]

---

[1] "Paying for Complementary and Integrative Health Approaches," National Center for Complementary and Integrative Health (NCCIH), June 2016. Available online. URL: www.nccih.nih.gov/health/paying-for-complementary-and-integrative-health-approaches. Accessed March 4, 2024.

Chapter 59 | Medicare's Preventive Services

An easy and important way to stay healthy is to get disease prevention and early detection services. They can help you find health problems early, when treatment works best. Talk with your doctor or health-care provider to find out what tests or other services you may need and how often you should get them to stay healthy. If you have Medicare Part B, you get many preventive services at no cost to you.

WHAT YOU WILL PAY
If you have Medicare Part B, you will pay nothing for many preventive services if you get them from a qualified doctor or other health-care provider who accepts assignments. Assignment is an agreement by your doctor, provider, or supplier to be paid directly by Medicare, to accept the payment amount Medicare approves for the service, and not to bill you for any more than the Medicare deductible and coinsurance. If you have a Medicare health plan, some plans may not charge deductibles, co-payments, or coinsurance for certain in-network, Medicare-covered preventive services. Contact your plan or benefits administrator directly to learn more about your costs.

PREVENTIVE SERVICES THAT COME UNDER MEDICARE COVERAGE
Abdominal Aortic Aneurysm Screenings
This is a onetime screening ultrasound for people at risk. If you have a family history of abdominal aortic aneurysms (AAAs) or

you are a man aged 65–75 and have smoked at least 100 cigarettes in your lifetime, you are considered at risk.

Alcohol Misuse Screening and Counseling
Medicare covers one alcohol misuse screening per year for adults (including pregnant women) to identify those who misuse alcohol but are not alcohol dependent. If you screen positive, you can get up to four brief face-to-face counseling sessions per year (if you are competent and alert during counseling). Your primary care doctor or other primary care provider must give you the counseling in a primary care setting (such as a doctor's office).

Bone Mass Measurement
These tests help see if you are at risk for broken bones. Medicare covers these tests once every 24 months (more often if medically necessary) for certain people at risk for osteoporosis.

Cardiovascular Behavioral Therapy
Medicare will cover one visit per year with your primary care doctor or other primary care provider to help lower your risk for cardiovascular disease. During this visit, your doctor may discuss aspirin use (if appropriate), check your blood pressure, and give you tips to make sure you are eating well.

Cardiovascular Disease Screenings
These screenings test your cholesterol, lipid, and triglyceride levels to find out if you are at risk for a heart attack or stroke. Medicare covers a cardiovascular disease screening once every five years.

Cervical and Vaginal Cancer Screenings
Medicare covers Pap tests and pelvic exams to check for cervical and vaginal cancers. All women with Medicare can get these tests and exams once every 24 months, and women at high risk can get them once every 12 months. Medicare also covers human

papillomavirus (HPV) tests (when given with a Pap test) once every five years if they are 30–65 years old without HPV symptoms.

Colorectal Cancer Screenings

These tests help find colorectal cancer early, when treatment works best. If you are 45 years or older or are at high risk for colorectal cancer, Medicare covers one or more of these screening tests: fecal occult blood test (FOBT), blood-based biomarker test, flexible sigmoidoscopy, screening colonoscopy, barium enema, and multitarget stool deoxyribonucleic acid (DNA) test (such as Cologuard™). How often Medicare pays for these tests depends on the test and your level of risk for colorectal cancer. You and your doctor decide which test is best for you.

Counseling to Prevent Tobacco Use and Tobacco-Caused Disease

Medicare covers smoking and tobacco-use cessation counseling for people who use tobacco. You can get up to eight counseling sessions in a 12-month period if you use tobacco.

Depression Screening

Medicare covers one depression screening per year for all people with Medicare. You must get the screening in a primary care setting (such as a doctor's office) where you can get follow-up treatment and referrals, if needed.

Diabetes Screenings

Medicare covers blood screening tests to check for diabetes or prediabetes. You can get these tests if you are considered at risk for diabetes, if you are obese, or if you have high blood pressure (HBP), a history of abnormal cholesterol and triglyceride levels (dyslipidemia), or a history of high blood sugar. Medicare also covers these tests if you meet two or more of these criteria: 65 years or older, overweight, family history of diabetes (parents, brothers, and sisters), a history of gestational diabetes (diabetes during pregnancy), or you delivered a baby weighing more than nine pounds. Based on your test results, you may be eligible for up to two screenings each year.

Diabetes Self-Management Training
This training teaches you how to cope with and manage your diabetes. Your training may include tips for eating healthy, being active, monitoring blood sugar, taking medication, and reducing risks. Medicare covers this training if you have diabetes and you get a written order from your doctor or other health-care provider.

Flu Shots
These shots help prevent influenza or flu virus. Medicare covers these shots once per flu season.

Glaucoma Tests
These tests help check for the eye disease glaucoma. Medicare covers these tests once every 12 months for people at high risk for glaucoma.

Hepatitis B Shots
This series of shots helps protect people from getting hepatitis B. Medicare covers these shots for people at medium or high risk for hepatitis B.

Hepatitis B Virus Infection Screenings
Medicare covers hepatitis B virus (HBV) infection screenings for people at high risk for HBV infection and pregnant women. Medicare will only cover these screenings if a primary care provider orders them. Medicare covers HBV infection screenings yearly for those with continued high risk who do not get a hepatitis B vaccination. Medicare also covers these screenings for pregnant women at the first prenatal visit for each pregnancy, at the time of delivery for those with new or continued risk factors, and at the first prenatal visit for future pregnancies (even if you previously got the hepatitis B shot or had negative HBV screening results).

Hepatitis C Screening Tests
Medicare covers a onetime hepatitis C screening test for people born between 1945 and 1965. Medicare also covers yearly screenings for certain people at high risk, including those who use or have used illicit injection drugs or had a blood transfusion before 1992.

Human Immunodeficiency Virus Screenings
Medicare covers human immunodeficiency virus (HIV) screenings if you ask for one and you are either 15–65 years old and not at risk or younger than 15 years or older than 65 years and at increased risk. Medicare covers this test once every 12 months or up to three times during a pregnancy.

Lung Cancer Screenings
Medicare covers lung cancer screenings with low-dose computed tomography (CT) scans once per year if you meet all of these updated conditions: you are 50–77 years old, do not have signs or symptoms of lung cancer (asymptomatic), are a current smoker or have quit smoking within the last 15 years, have a tobacco smoking history of at least 20 "pack years" (an average of one pack (20 cigarettes) per day for 20 years), and have an order from your doctor. Before your first lung cancer screening, you will need to schedule an appointment with your doctor to discuss the benefits and risks and decide if a screening is right for you.

Mammograms (Breast Cancer Screenings)
Medicare covers mammograms once every 12 months for women aged 40 and older. Medicare also covers one baseline mammogram for women between the ages 35 and 39.

Medicare Diabetes Prevention Program
If you have prediabetes and meet other criteria, Medicare covers a once-per-lifetime proven health behavior change program to help you prevent type 2 diabetes. The program begins with weekly core

sessions offered in a group setting over a six-month period. After the core sessions, you will get six monthly follow-up sessions to help you maintain healthy habits.

Medical Nutrition Therapy Services
Medicare may cover medical nutrition therapy and certain related services if you have diabetes or kidney disease or if you have had a kidney transplant in the last 36 months. A doctor must refer you for the service(s).

Obesity Behavioral Therapy
If you have a body mass index (BMI) of 30 or more, Medicare covers behavioral therapy sessions to help you lose weight. Medicare covers this counseling if your primary care doctor or other primary care provider gives the counseling in a primary care setting (such as a doctor's office), where they can coordinate your personalized prevention plan with your other care.

Pneumococcal Shots
Medicare covers pneumococcal shots (or vaccines) to help prevent pneumococcal infections (such as certain types of pneumonia). You can get up to three doses of the pneumococcal vaccine, depending on certain criteria. Talk with your doctor or other health-care provider to find out which vaccine you should get.

Preventive Visits
- **Onetime "Welcome to Medicare" preventive visit.** Medicare covers a review of your medical and social history related to your health and education and counseling about preventive services (such as screenings, shots, and referrals for other care you may need). Medicare covers this visit within the first 12 months that you have Medicare Part B.
- **Yearly "Wellness" visit.** If you have had Part B for longer than 12 months, you can get a yearly "Wellness" visit to

develop or update your personalized plan to help prevent disease and disability, based on your current health and risk factors. Medicare covers this visit once every 12 months. The yearly "Wellness" visit is not a physical exam.

Prostate Cancer Screenings

These screenings check for prostate cancer. Medicare covers a digital rectal exam and a prostate-specific antigen (PSA) blood test once every 12 months for men over the age of 50 (starting the day after your 50th birthday).

Sexually Transmitted Infections Screenings and Counseling

Medicare covers sexually transmitted infection (STI) screenings for chlamydia, gonorrhea, syphilis, and hepatitis B. Medicare covers these screenings for pregnant women and for certain people who are at increased risk for an STI. Your primary care doctor or other primary care provider must order the screening or refer you for behavioral counseling. Medicare covers these screenings once every 12 months or at certain times during pregnancy. Medicare also covers up to two behavioral counseling sessions each year. Medicare will only cover counseling sessions with a Medicare-eligible primary care provider in a primary care setting (such as a doctor's office). Medicare will not cover counseling as a preventive service in an inpatient setting (such as a skilled nursing facility).[1]

---

[1] "Staying Healthy—Medicare's Preventive Services," Centers for Medicare & Medicaid Services (CMS), March 2023. Available online. URL: www.medicare.gov/Pubs/pdf/11100-Staying-Healthy.pdf. Accessed March 6, 2024.

Chapter 60 | Medicare Coverage of Home Health Care

Many health-care treatments that were once offered only in a hospital or a doctor's office can now be done in your home. Home health care is usually less expensive, more convenient, and as effective as care you get in a hospital or skilled nursing facility. In general, the goal of home health care is to give treatment for an illness or injury. Where possible, home health care may help you recover, regain your independence, and become more self-sufficient. Home health care may also help you maintain your current condition or level of function or slow decline.

Medicare pays for you to get health-care services in your home if you meet certain eligibility criteria and the services are considered reasonable and necessary for the treatment of your illness or injury.

WHO IS ELIGIBLE FOR HOME HEALTH CARE?
If you have Medicare, you can use your home health benefits if:
- you are under the care of a doctor or other health-care provider (including a nurse practitioner, clinical nurse specialist, and physician assistant) and you are getting services as part of a care plan that your doctor or allowed provider establishes and reviews regularly
- your doctor or allowed provider certifies that you need one or more of the following:
  - intermittent skilled nursing care (other than drawing blood)

- physical therapy
- speech-language pathology services
- continued occupational therapy
- home health aide services
- the home health agency caring for you is Medicare-certified
- your doctor or allowed provider certifies that you are homebound. To be homebound means to have the following conditions:
  - You have trouble leaving your home without help (such as using a cane, wheelchair, walker, or crutches; special transportation; or help from another person) because of an illness or injury, or leaving your home is not recommended because of your condition.
  - You are normally unable to leave your home, but if you do, it requires a major effort.
  - You may leave home for medical treatment or short, infrequent absences for nonmedical reasons, such as an occasional trip to the barber, a walk around the block, or attendance at a family reunion, funeral, graduation, or other infrequent or unique event. You can still get home health care if you attend adult day care or religious services.
- your doctor or allowed provider documents that they have had a face-to-face encounter with you (such as an appointment with your primary care doctor) within the required time frames and that the encounter was related to the reason you need home health care

WHO IS NOT ELIGIBLE FOR HOME HEALTH CARE?

If you need more than intermittent skilled nursing care, you do not qualify for home health services. Medicare defines "intermittent" as skilled nursing care that is needed:
- fewer than seven days each week
- daily for less than eight hours each day for up to 21 days (Medicare may extend the three-week limit in exceptional circumstances.)

Medicare Coverage of Home Health Care

If you are expected to need full-time skilled nursing care over an extended period, you will not usually qualify for home health benefits.

HOW DOES MEDICARE PAY FOR HOME HEALTH CARE?

Medicare pays for covered home health services you get during a 30-day period of care. You can have more than one 30-day period of care. Payment for each 30-day period is based on your condition and care needs.

Getting treatment from a home health agency that is Medicare-certified can lower your out-of-pocket costs. A Medicare-certified home health agency agrees to:
- be paid by Medicare
- accept only the amount Medicare approves for their services

Medicare's home health benefit only pays for services you get from the home health agency. Other medical services and equipment are generally still covered as part of your other Medicare benefits.

It is important to note that before your home health care begins, the home health agency should tell you how much of your bill Medicare will pay. The agency should also tell you if Medicare does not cover any of the items or services they give you and how much you will have to pay for them. They should explain it to you both verbally and in writing.

WHAT IS COVERED IN HOME HEALTH CARE?

If you are eligible for home health care, Medicare covers these services if they are reasonable and necessary for the treatment of your illness or injury. Medicare covers skilled nursing and therapy services when your doctor or allowed provider determines that the care you need requires the specialized judgment, knowledge, and skills of a nurse or therapist.

Skilled Nursing Care

Medicare covers skilled nursing care when the services you need are as follows:
- Require the skills of a nurse.
- Are reasonable and necessary for the treatment of your illness or injury.
- Are given on a part-time or intermittent basis. (Medicare will not cover a visit if you are only having blood drawn.) "Part time" or "intermittent" means you may be able to get home health aide and skilled nursing services (combined) any number of days per week as long as the services are given:
  - fewer than eight hours each day
  - 28 or fewer hours each week (or up to 35 hours a week in some limited situations)

You can get skilled nursing services from a registered nurse or a licensed practical nurse. If you get services from a licensed practical nurse, a registered nurse will supervise your care. Home health nurses give direct care and teach you and your caregivers about your care. They also manage, observe, and evaluate your care.

Examples of skilled nursing care include giving certain intravenous (IV) drugs, certain injections, or tube feedings; changing dressings; and teaching about prescription drugs or diabetes care. Any service that you could get safely and effectively from a nonmedical person (including yourself) without the supervision of a nurse is not skilled nursing care.

Physical Therapy, Occupational Therapy, and Speech-Language Pathology Services

Your therapy services are considered reasonable and necessary in the home setting if:
- they are a specific, safe, and effective treatment for your condition
- they are complex enough that you can only get them safely and effectively from a qualified therapist (or under the supervision of a qualified therapist)

- your condition requires one of these:
  - therapy to restore or improve functions affected by your illness or injury
  - a skilled therapist or therapist assistant to safely and effectively perform therapy to help you maintain your current condition or prevent your condition from getting worse
- the amount, frequency, and duration of the services are reasonable

Home Health Aide Services

Medicare will pay for part-time or intermittent home health aide services (such as personal care) if you need them to maintain your health or treat your illness or injury and if they are offered by your home health provider. However, Medicare does not cover home health aide services unless you are also getting skilled care. Skilled care includes:
- skilled nursing care
- physical therapy
- speech-language pathology services
- continuing occupational therapy, if you no longer need any of the previously mentioned skilled care

Medical Social Services

Medicare covers these services when a doctor or allowed provider orders them to help you with social and emotional concerns that may interfere with your treatment or how quickly you recover. This might include counseling or help finding resources in your community. However, Medicare does not cover medical social services unless you are also getting skilled care as mentioned earlier.

Medical Supplies

Medicare covers supplies (such as wound dressings) when your doctor or allowed provider orders them as part of your care.

Medicare pays for durable medical equipment (DME) separately from your home health care. The equipment must meet certain criteria, and your doctor or allowed provider must order it. Medicare usually pays 80 percent of the Medicare-approved amount for certain medical equipment, such as a wheelchair or walker. If your home health agency does not supply DME directly, the home health agency staff will usually arrange for a supplier to bring you the items.

The home health agency must perform an initial assessment of all your care needs and must communicate those needs to the doctor or allowed provider responsible for your plan of care. After that, the home health agency must routinely assess your needs. The home health agency is responsible for meeting all of your medical, nursing, rehabilitative, social, and discharge planning needs, as noted in your home health plan of care.

WHAT IS NOT COVERED IN HOME HEALTH CARE?

Medicare does not pay for:
- 24-hour care at home
- meals delivered to your home
- services such as shopping, cleaning, and laundry
- custodial or personal care such as bathing, dressing, and using the bathroom (when this is the only care you need)

Talk to your doctor (or allowed provider) or the home health agency if you have questions about whether certain services are covered. You can also call 800-MEDICARE (800-633-4227). Teletypewriter (TTY) users can call 877-486-2048.

WHAT YOU PAY FOR IN HOME HEALTH CARE

You may have to pay for:
- services and supplies that Medicare never pays for, such as routine foot care
- services and supplies that Medicare usually pays for but will not pay for in this instance, when you have agreed to pay for them (The home health agency must give

Medicare Coverage of Home Health Care

you a notice called the "Advance Beneficiary Notice of Noncoverage" (ABN) in these situations.)
- 20 percent of the Medicare-approved amount for Medicare-covered medical equipment, such as wheelchairs, walkers, and oxygen equipment[1]

---

[1] "Medicare & Home Health Care," Centers for Medicare & Medicaid Services (CMS), August 2023. Available online. URL: www.medicare.gov/Pubs/pdf/10969-Medicare-and-Home-Health-Care.pdf. Accessed March 6, 2024.

Chapter 61 | **Health Savings Account: Eligible Plans**

One way to manage your health-care expenses is to enroll in a plan eligible for Health Savings Account (HSA) also called a "High Deductible Health Plan" (HDHP) and open an HSA, a type of savings account that lets you set aside money on a pretax basis to pay for qualified medical expenses (such as some dental, drug, and vision expenses).

HOW CAN HEALTH SAVINGS ACCOUNT-ELIGIBLE PLANS LOWER YOUR COSTS?

- If you enroll in an HSA-eligible plan, you may pay a lower monthly premium but have a higher deductible (meaning you pay for more of your health-care items and services before the insurance plan pays).
- If you combine your HSA-eligible plan with an HSA, you can pay that deductible, plus other qualified medical expenses, such as co-payments, coinsurance, and more, using money you set aside in your tax-free HSA.
  - Therefore, if you have an HSA-eligible plan and do not need many health-care items and services, you may benefit from the lower monthly premium.
  - If you need more care, you will save by using the tax-free money in your HSA to pay for it.
- Your HSA balance rolls over year to year, so you can build up reserves to pay for health-care items and services you need later.

WHAT IS CONSIDERED A HEALTH SAVINGS ACCOUNT-ELIGIBLE PLAN?

Under the tax law, HSA-eligible plans must set a minimum deductible and a limit, or maximum, on out-of-pocket costs for both individuals and families.

- The minimum deductible is the amount you pay for health-care items and services per year before your plan starts to pay.
- The maximum out-of-pocket costs are the most you would have to pay per year if you need more health-care items and services.

HSA-eligible plan deductibles are often significantly higher than the minimums and can be as high as the maximum out-of-pocket costs.

HOW DO HEALTH SAVINGS ACCOUNT-ELIGIBLE PLANS WORK?

You can contribute to an HSA only if you have an HSA-eligible plan (see Table 61.1).

Table 61.1. Important Facts about Health Savings Account-Eligible Plans

Benefits of Health Savings Account-Eligible Plans	But Also Think About
Plans eligible for Health Savings Account (HSA) may have lower monthly premiums.	Your deductible—the costs you pay before the plan—is often higher.
You can deduct the amount you deposit in an HSA from the income you pay federal income tax on.	If you have money in your HSA when you turn 65, you can spend it on anything you want—but if you are not spending it for a qualified medical expense, it will be taxed as income at your then current tax rate. You must stop contributing to your HSA when you enroll in any part of Medicare. But you may withdraw money from your HSA at any time to help pay for qualified medical expenses that Medicare or Medicare Supplement Insurance (Medigap) does not cover.

Health Savings Account: Eligible Plans

Table 61.1. Continued

Benefits of Health Savings Account-Eligible Plans	But Also Think About
You can use HSA funds to pay for deductibles, co-payments, coinsurance, and other qualified medical expenses. Withdrawals to pay eligible medical expenses are tax-free.	
Unspent HSA funds roll over from year to year, allowing you to build tax-free savings to pay for medical care later. HSAs may earn interest, which is not subject to taxes.	
HSA-eligible plans are available in most areas and may be available as qualified health plans at the Bronze, Silver, or Gold levels on HealthCare.gov. HSA-eligible plans may also be available for enrollment directly through health insurance companies and may be offered by your employer.	HSA-eligible plans may not be available in your area. You will find out when you compare plans on HealthCare.gov or when you contact an agent, broker, or insurance company.
An HSA-eligible plan may provide certain preventive care benefits without a deductible or with a deductible less than the minimum annual deductible.	

FINDING AND USING HEALTH SAVINGS ACCOUNT-ELIGIBLE PLANS

There are yearly limits for deposits into an HSA. Amounts are adjusted yearly for inflation. When you compare plans on HealthCare.gov (www.healthcare.gov), you can filter to see HSA-eligible plans by selecting "Add filters" on the top left and checking "Eligible for an HSA."

SETTING UP HEALTH SAVINGS ACCOUNTS

After you enroll in an HSA-eligible plan, you will need to open an HSA separately to get started.

How to Find a Health Savings Account Financial Institution
- Research HSA providers online.
- Check with your health insurance company to see if they partner with HSA financial institutions.
- Ask your bank if they offer an HSA option that meets your needs.

What to Think about When Choosing a Health Savings Account
- Some HSAs have fees associated with them, such as a charge for opening or closing the account and monthly maintenance fees.
- Banking options, services, and features, such as debit cards and online banking, may differ by HSA provider.
- How you will make your pretax dollar deposits into your HSA may also vary.

Get more information on HSA-eligible plans including both the minimum and maximum yearly deductible, from the Internal Revenue Service (IRS; www.irs.gov/government-entities/federal-state-local-governments/where-can-i-learn-more-about-health-savings-accounts-hsa-and-health-reimbursement-arrangements-hra).[1]

---

[1] "What Are HSA-Eligible Plans?" Centers for Medicare & Medicaid Services (CMS), September 29, 2014. Available online. URL: www.healthcare.gov/high-deductible-health-plan. Accessed March 6, 2024.

Chapter 62 | Medical Discount Plans: Service or Scam?

Wading through your health insurance options and plans can be complex, overwhelming, and confusing. Dishonest companies and scammers know this and use it to their advantage. Instead of getting the health insurance coverage you and your family need, you could end up with a so-called health plan that covers few if any medical expenses are there. And it could leave you on the hook for major medical bills.

FIVE SIGNS OF A HEALTH INSURANCE SCAM

Medicare and health insurance scams are common. Scammers are always looking for new ways to steal your money and your personal information, but they use familiar techniques. Here are five signs you are dealing with a health insurance scam:

- **Scammers say they are from the government and need money or your personal information.**
  Government agencies do not call people out of the blue to ask them for money or personal information. No one from the government will ask you to verify your Social Security, bank account, or credit card number, and they will not ask you to wire money or pay by gift card or cryptocurrency. If you have a question about Medicare

or the Health Insurance Marketplace®, contact the government directly:
- **Medicare.** Visit www.medicare.gov or call 800-MEDICARE (800-633-4227).
- **Health Insurance Marketplace®.** Visit www.healthcare.gov or call 800-318-2596.
- **Scammers say you need to pay a fee for a new Medicare card or you will lose your Medicare coverage.** But you never need to pay for a new card. And Medicare will never call out of the blue to say you will lose coverage. Those are scams.
- **Scammers try to sell you a fake medical discount plan.** Medical discount plans charge you a monthly fee for discounts on specific medical services or products from a list of participating providers. They are not a substitute for health insurance. While some medical discount plans provide legitimate discounts, others take people's money and offer very little in return. Therefore, if you are considering one, check out every claim the plan makes, including whether your doctor participates in the plan. And be sure to get the details of the discount plan in writing before you sign up.
- **Scammers want your sensitive personal information in exchange for a price quote.** The official government site of the Affordable Care Act (ACA) is www.healthcare.gov. It lets you compare prices on health insurance plans, check your eligibility for health-care subsidies, and begin enrollment. But HealthCare.gov will only ask for your monthly income and your age to give you a price quote. Never enter personal financial information such as your Social Security, bank account, or credit card number to get a quote for health insurance. You will be setting yourself up for robocalls or much worse—identity theft.
- **Scammers want you to pay for help with the Health Insurance Marketplace.** The people who offer legitimate help with the Health Insurance

Medical Discount Plans: Service or Scam?

Marketplace—sometimes called "navigators" or "assisters"—are not allowed to charge you and will not ask you for personal or financial information.

WHAT TO DO BEFORE YOU SIGN UP FOR HEALTH INSURANCE
While we have mentioned things to avoid, there are several steps you can take before signing up for health insurance. Here are a few to keep in mind:
- **Visit a trusted source such as HealthCare.gov to compare plans, coverage, and prices**. HealthCare.gov and state marketplaces are the only places where you are guaranteed to get comprehensive, ACA-compliant coverage.
- **Research any company offering health coverage**. Search online for the name of the company and the words "complaint," "scam," or "fraud." Read reviews and see what others have to say.
- **Check to see if the plan is really health insurance**. All companies selling health insurance must be licensed by your state insurance commissioner. If they do not have a license, what they are selling is not insurance. Check with your state insurance commissioner's office (https://content.naic.org/state-insurance-departments) to find out.
- **Do not accept vague answers**. If a salesperson does not give you specific details about the coverage (e.g., deductibles, co-pays, and finding in-network providers), that is a red flag. So is not clearly answering your questions. A legitimate plan representative should be able to answer your questions without having to pass you on to another source such as a brochure or website.
- **Insist on seeing a statement of benefits or a complete copy of the policy you are considering**. Make sure anything the salesperson told you about coverage is written in the statement of benefits.
- **If a salesperson says the plan is through a major insurer, check with that company**. Some scammers

use fake logos and marketing materials to make themselves look legit. If an unfamiliar company says it sells plans through a major insurer, check with the company to make sure it is true.

MEDICARE SCAMS

People on Medicare—and those who are not—are regularly targeted for scams. You might have gotten a call saying something like "Hello, this is Medicare calling. Your coverage is about to be canceled." Every year during open enrollment season (and plenty of other times too), scammers pretending to be from the government call to steal your money and your personal information. Here is what to do:

- **Hang up**. If someone calls, claiming to be affiliated with Medicare, asking for your Social Security number (SSN) or bank account information to get a new card or new benefits, that is a scam.
- **Never give personal information to a caller claiming to be affiliated with Medicare**. You cannot trust your caller identification (ID). Scammers can make these calls look like they are coming from the government even when they are not. Before you give out any personal information, make your own call to 800-MEDICARE to check it out.
- **Report the call**. Report these impersonators at 800-MEDICARE and https://reportfraud.ftc.gov.

Another scam is related to Medicare Part D, which is an optional prescription drug insurance program for people on Medicare. You pay a monthly premium to an insurance carrier for your Part D plan. In return, you use the insurance carrier's network of pharmacies to buy your prescription medications. To protect people, the law is very specific about how Medicare prescription drug plan providers conduct themselves.

- **Medicare Part D plan representatives may enroll you on the phone only if you call them**. To be on the safe side, call Medicare first to check out any provider you may be tempted to contact. The number

to call is 800-MEDICARE (800-633-4227), and the teletypewriter (TTY) number is 877-486-2048. The Medicare phone line is open 24 hours a day. The government does not recommend any particular prescription drug plan—it simply verifies that a provider is legitimate.
- **Anyone who contacts you about Medicare Part D without you seeking them out first is likely a scammer.** Do not share your information and do not pay them.
- **Do not feel pressure to decide on a Medicare prescription drug plan.** You have from October 15 to December 7 of every year to decide on a plan for the following year. That is plenty of time to consider legitimate offers. Enrolling is not mandatory. Whether you sign up for Medicare Part D or not, it will have no effect on your other benefits from Medicare (Parts A and B) or from Social Security.
- **Medicare Part D providers may come to your home only if you have invited them.** Do not talk to anyone who comes to your door with unsolicited offers of drug coverage. The law says prescription drug benefit companies cannot visit your home unless you have given them permission.

MEDICAL DISCOUNT PLANS AND SCAMS

Medical discount plans, also known as "discount health-care programs," often say they will save you money on products and services your insurance may not cover—such as dental, vision, hearing, or chiropractic services. With a medical discount plan, you generally pay a monthly fee for discounts on specific services or products from a list of participating providers.

While there are medical discount plans that give legitimate discounts, others take people's money and offer very little in return. Dishonest marketers sometimes make it sound like they are selling health insurance or lie about what their plans really offer. When you are in the midst of an emergency, the last thing you want to find out is that you will have to cover most, or all, of the bills if what you have is not really health insurance.

So how can you tell if a medical discount plan is legitimate?

- **Confirm the details.** If you are interested in a discount plan—knowing they are not a substitute for health insurance—check whether the doctors you consult participate. Call your providers, as well as others on the plan's list, before you enroll or pay any fees. Some dishonest plan promoters may tell you that particular local doctors participate when they do not, or they might send you outdated lists. So do your own research.
- **Avoid "up to" discounts.** Scammers might claim you will get "discounts of up to 70 percent," for example. But savings with discount plans typically are a lot less than promised. When you add up a discount plan's monthly premiums and enrollment fees, it might amount to no "discount" at all.
- **Check with your state.** Many states require medical discount programs to be licensed or registered. Ask your state insurance commissioner's office if the medical discount program you are considering is licensed. And, if someone is claiming that a medical discount program is health insurance, check it out with that state insurance commissioner's office. Medical discount plans are not insurance, and they are not a substitute for health insurance.
- **Do not sign up on the spot.** Legitimate plans should be willing to send you written information and give you the chance to check out their claims before you enroll. Pressure to sign up quickly or threats of missing out on a "special deal" are your opportunities to say, "no, thanks." Take the time to check out offers and get the details in writing before you sign up.
- **Never give your financial information to someone who calls you unexpectedly.** Identity thieves use pitches for medical discount plans and insurance to get your personal information.

Medical Discount Plans: Service or Scam?

REPORT SCAMS

If you think you have spotted a scam, tell your friends and family about it, so they can protect themselves and then report it to the Federal Trade Commission (FTC). People who know about scams are much more likely to be able to avoid them. Your reports help the FTC and our law enforcement partners build cases and stop scammers.

Report health insurance and medical discount scams to the FTC at https://reportfraud.ftc.gov and your state attorney general.

Report Medicare scams at www.medicare.gov or 800-633-4227.[1]

---

[1] "Spot Health Insurance Scams," Federal Trade Commission (FTC), May 2021. Available online. URL: https://consumer.ftc.gov/articles/spot-health-insurance-scams. Accessed March 6, 2024.

Chapter 63 | Low-Cost or Free Health Insurance for Children

If your children need health coverage, they may be eligible for the Children's Health Insurance Program (CHIP).

The CHIP provides low-cost health coverage to children in families that earn too much money to qualify for Medicaid. In some states, the CHIP covers pregnant women. Each state offers CHIP coverage and works closely with its state Medicaid program.

SEE IF YOUR CHILDREN QUALIFY

Each state program has its own rules about who qualifies for the CHIP. You can apply right now, any time of year, and find out if you qualify. If you apply for Medicaid coverage to your state agency, you will also find out if your children qualify for the CHIP. If they qualify, you will not have to buy an insurance plan to cover them.

There are two ways to apply for the CHIP:
- Call 800-318-2596 (toll-free teletypewriter (TTY): 855-889-4325).
- Fill out an application through the Health Insurance Marketplace. If it looks like anyone in your household qualifies for Medicaid or CHIP, the Centers for Medicare & Medicaid Services (CMS) will send your information to your state agency. They will contact you

about enrollment. When you submit your Marketplace application, you will also find out if you qualify for an individual insurance plan with savings based on your income instead.

What Does the Children's Health Insurance Program Cover?

The CHIP benefits are different in each state. But all states provide comprehensive coverage, including:
- routine checkups
- immunizations
- doctor visits
- prescriptions
- dental and vision care
- inpatient and outpatient hospital care
- laboratory and x-ray services
- emergency services

What Does the Children's Health Insurance Program Cost?

Routine well-child doctor and dental visits are free under the CHIP. But there may be co-payments for other services. Some states charge a monthly premium for CHIP coverage. The costs are different in each state, but you will not have to pay more than 5 percent of your family's income for the year.[1]

---

[1] "The Children's Health Insurance Program (CHIP)," Centers for Medicare & Medicaid Services (CMS), September 21, 2011. Available online. URL: www.healthcare.gov/medicaid-chip/childrens-health-insurance-program. Accessed March 4, 2024.

Chapter 64 | Things to Know before You Pick a Health Insurance Plan

Choosing a health insurance plan can be complicated. Knowing just a few things before you compare plans can make it simpler.

THE HEALTH PLAN CATEGORIES

Plans in the Marketplace are presented in four health plan categories: Bronze, Silver, Gold, and Platinum. Catastrophic plans are also available to some people. Health plan categories are based on how you and your plan split the costs of your health care (see Table 64.1). They have nothing to do with the quality of care.

Bronze
- lowest monthly premium
- highest costs when you need care

Bronze plan deductibles—the amount of medical costs you pay yourself before your insurance plan starts to pay—can be thousands of dollars a year.

It is a good choice if you want a low-cost way to protect yourself from worst-case medical scenarios, such as serious sickness or injury. Your monthly premium will be low, but you will have to pay for most routine care yourself.

Table 64.1. Insurance Plan Costs Split

Plan Category	The Insurance Company Pays	You Pay
Bronze	60%	40%
Silver	70%	30%
Gold	80%	20%
Platinum	90%	10%

Note: These are estimated averages for a typical population. Your costs will vary.

Silver
- moderate monthly premium
- moderate costs when you need care

Silver deductibles—the costs you pay yourself before your plan pays anything—are usually lower than those of Bronze plans.

It is a good choice if you qualify for extra savings—or, if not, if you are willing to pay a slightly higher monthly premium than Bronze to have more of your routine care covered.

GETTING EXTRA SAVINGS WITH A SILVER PLAN
- **If you qualify for cost-sharing reductions (CSRs).** You must pick a Silver plan to get the extra savings. You can save hundreds or even thousands of dollars per year if you go to the doctor a lot. Silver plans may also be available if you are eligible for a premium tax credit and can enroll through a Special Enrollment Period (SEP) based on estimated household income.
- **If you are enrolled in a Silver plan and lose your CSRs.** You will qualify for an SEP. If you want to change plans, you can enroll in a Bronze, Silver, or Gold plan that meets your needs and fits your budget.

Gold
- high monthly premium
- low costs when you need care

Things to Know before You Pick a Health Insurance Plan

Deductibles—the amount of medical costs you pay yourself before your plan pays—are usually low.

This is a good choice if you are willing to pay more each month to have more costs covered when you get medical treatment. If you use a lot of care, a Gold plan could be a good value.

Platinum
- highest monthly premium
- lowest costs when you get care

Deductibles are very low, meaning your plan starts paying its share earlier than for other categories of plans.

This is a good choice if you usually use a lot of care and are willing to pay a high monthly premium, knowing nearly all other costs will be covered.

Plans in all categories provide free preventive care, and some offer selected free or discounted services before you meet your deductible.

No matter which health plan category you choose, you can save a lot of money on your monthly premium based on your income. When you fill out a Marketplace insurance application, you will find out if you qualify for these savings.

CATASTROPHIC HEALTH PLANS

Catastrophic health insurance plans have low monthly premiums and very high deductibles. They may be an affordable way to protect yourself from worst-case scenarios, such as getting seriously sick or injured. But you pay most routine medical expenses yourself.

Who Can Buy a Catastrophic Plan?
- people under the age of 30
- people aged 30 or older with a hardship exemption or affordability exemption (based on Marketplace or job-based insurance being unaffordable)

If you qualify to buy a catastrophic plan, you will see them displayed when you compare plans in the Marketplace.

How Much Do Catastrophic Plans Cost?
- Monthly premiums are usually low, but you cannot use a premium tax credit to reduce your cost. If you qualify for a premium tax credit based on your income, a Bronze or Silver plan is likely to be a better value. Be sure to compare.
- Deductibles—the amount you have to pay yourself for most services before the plan starts to pay anything—are very high.
- After you spend the deductible amount, your insurance company pays for all covered services, with no co-payment or coinsurance.

What Do Catastrophic Plans Cover?
- Catastrophic plans cover the same essential health benefits as other Marketplace plans.
- Like other plans, catastrophic plans cover certain preventive services at no cost.
- They also cover at least three primary care visits per year before you have met your deductible.

YOUR TOTAL COSTS FOR HEALTH CARE
When choosing a plan, it is a good idea to think about your total health-care costs (including the premium, deductible, and co-payment/coinsurance amounts), the health and drug services you will use, the health plan category that works best for you, and plans with easy pricing.

Think about a Plan's Deductible and Co-pays, Not Just the Premium
In addition to a plan's monthly premium, the out-of-pocket costs you pay when you use services have a big effect on your total health-care spending.

Your total costs for the year include the following in your plan:
- **Monthly premium times 12 months.** The amount you pay to your insurance company each month to have health insurance.

Things to Know before You Pick a Health Insurance Plan

- **Deductible.** How much you have to spend for covered health services before your insurance company pays anything (except free preventive services).
- **Co-payments and coinsurance.** Payments you make to your health-care provider each time you get care, such as $20 for a doctor visit or 30 percent of hospital charges.
- **Out-of-pocket maximum.** The most you have to spend for covered services in a year. After you reach this amount, the insurance company pays 100 percent for covered services.

Estimate the Health and Drug Services You Will Use
Think about the health services and prescription drugs your household usually gets. Then, estimate the services you are likely to use in the year ahead. Get estimated total yearly costs when you preview plans and prices at www.healthcare.gov/see-plans/#/.
- Enter some basic information (such as Zone Improvement Plan (ZIP) code, household size, and income) when asked. Then, select "View plans."
- Select "Add yearly cost" on any of the plans listed.
- Pick the level of care you expect to use this year—low, medium, or high use.
- Select "Save and continue" to get your estimated total yearly costs for each plan listed.

It is important to note that your actual expenses will vary, but the estimate is useful for comparing plans' total effect on your household budget.

Consider Plans with Easy Pricing
Marketplace plans marked easy pricing include some benefits before you reach the deductible. As soon as coverage starts, you will pay only a co-payment for:
- doctor and specialist visits, including mental health
- urgent care

- physical, speech, and occupational therapy
- generic and most preferred drugs

And this may help you compare easy pricing plans because they have the same out-of-pocket costs within their health plan category, such as:
- deductibles
- out-of-pocket maximums
- co-payments/coinsurance

Compare only plans with easy pricing when you shop for coverage.
- When viewing plans, select "Add filters."
- Pick a health plan category (Bronze, Silver, Gold, or Platinum). Then, select with easy pricing.

Once you apply this filter, only plans with easy pricing will appear for the category you picked.

HEALTH INSURANCE PLAN AND NETWORK TYPES

There are different types of Marketplace health insurance plans designed to meet different needs. Some types of plans restrict your provider choices or encourage you to get care from the plan's network of doctors, hospitals, pharmacies, and other medical service providers. Others pay a greater share of costs for providers outside the plan's network.

Types of Marketplace Plans

Depending on how many plans are offered in your area, you may find plans of all or any of these types at each metal level—Bronze, Silver, Gold, and Platinum.

The following are some examples of plan types you will find in the Marketplace:
- **Exclusive provider organization (EPO).** A managed care plan where services are covered only if you use doctors, specialists, or hospitals in the plan's network (except in an emergency).

Things to Know before You Pick a Health Insurance Plan

- **Health maintenance organization (HMO)**. A type of health insurance plan that usually limits coverage to care from doctors who work for or contract with the HMO. It generally will not cover out-of-network care except in an emergency. An HMO may require you to live or work in its service area to be eligible for coverage. HMOs often provide integrated care and focus on prevention and wellness.
- **Point of service (POS)**. A type of plan where you pay less if you use doctors, hospitals, and other health-care providers that belong to the plan's network. POS plans require you to get a referral from your primary care doctor in order to see a specialist.
- **Preferred provider organization (PPO)**. A type of health plan where you pay less if you use providers in the plan's network. You can use doctors, hospitals, and providers outside of the network without a referral for an additional cost.[1]

---

[1] "3 Things to Know before You Pick a Health Insurance Plan," Centers for Medicare & Medicaid Services (CMS), October 3, 2014. Available online. URL: www.healthcare.gov/choose-a-plan/comparing-plans. Accessed March 5, 2024.

Chapter 65 | Filing a Claim for Your Health or Disability Benefits

If you participate in a health plan or a plan that provides disability benefits, you will want to know how to file a claim for your benefits. The steps outlined here describe some of your plan's obligations and briefly explain the procedures and timelines for filing a health or disability benefits claim.

Before you file, however, be aware of the Employee Retirement Income Security Act (ERISA) of 1974, a federal law that protects your health and disability benefits and sets standards for those who administer your plan. Among other things, the law and rules issued by the U.S. Department of Labor (DOL) include requirements for the processing of benefit claims, the timeline for a decision when you file a claim, and your rights when a claim is denied.

The Affordable Care Act (ACA) includes additional requirements for claims processing for group health plans that are nongrandfathered. A nongrandfathered health plan is a plan that was established, or that has made certain significant changes, after March 23, 2010.

REVIEWING INFORMATION FROM YOUR PLAN

A key document related to your plan is the Summary Plan Description (SPD). The SPD is the brochure you receive when you are first covered by your employer's plan. It provides a detailed overview of the plan—how it works, what benefits it provides, and how to file a claim for benefits. It also describes your rights as well as your responsibilities under the ERISA and your plan. You can also find answers to many of your questions in the Summary of Benefits and Coverage (SBC), a short, easy-to-understand summary of the benefits available under your plan and detailed information on the out-of-pocket costs for coverage. For some single-employer collectively bargained plans, you should also check claim filing, grievance, and appeal procedures of the collective bargaining agreement (CBA) as they may apply to claims for health and disability benefits.

Before you apply for health or disability benefits, review the SPD to make sure you meet the plan's requirements and understand the procedures for filing a claim. Sometimes claims procedures are contained in a separate booklet that is handed out with your SPD. If you do not have a copy of your plan's SPD or claims procedures, make a written request for one or both to your plan's administrator. Your plan administrator is required to provide you with a copy.

FILING A CLAIM

An important first step is to check your SPD and the SBC to make sure you meet your plan's requirements to receive benefits. Your plan might say, for example, that a waiting period must pass before you can enroll and receive benefits or that a dependent is not covered after a certain age. Also, be aware of what your plan requires to file a claim. The SPD or claims procedure booklet must include information on where to file, what to file, and whom to contact if you have questions about your plan, such as the process for providing a required preapproval for health benefits. Plans generally cannot charge any filing fees or costs for filing claims and appeals.

If, for any reason, that information is not in the SPD or claims procedure booklet, write your plan administrator, your employer's human resource department (or the office that normally handles claims), or your employer to notify them that you have a claim. Keep a copy of the letter for your records. You may also want to send the letter by certified mail, return receipt requested, so you will have a record that the letter was received and by whom.

If it is not you but an authorized representative who is filing the claim, that person should refer to the SPD and follow your plan's

Filing a Claim for Your Health or Disability Benefits

claims procedure. Your plan may require you to complete a form to name the representative. If it is an emergency situation, the treating physician can automatically become your authorized representative without you having to complete a form.

When a claim is filed, be sure to keep a copy for your records.

TYPES OF CLAIMS
All health and disability benefit claims must be decided within a specific time limit, depending on the type of claim filed.
- **Group health claims.** These are divided into three types: urgent care, preservice, and postservice claims, with the type of claim determining how quickly a decision must be made. The plan must decide what type of claim it is except when a physician determines that the urgent care is needed.
  - **Urgent care claims.** These are a special kind of preservice claim that requires a quicker decision because your health would be threatened if the plan took the normal time permitted to decide a preservice claim. If a physician with knowledge of your medical condition tells the plan that a preservice claim is urgent, the plan must treat it as an urgent care claim.
  - **Preservice claims.** These are requests for approval that the plan requires you to obtain before you get medical care, such as preauthorization or a decision on whether a treatment or procedure is medically necessary.
  - **Postservice claims.** These are all other claims for benefits under your group health plan, including claims after medical services have been provided, such as requests for reimbursement or payment of the costs of the services provided. Most claims for group health benefits are postservice claims.
- **Disability claims.** These are requests for benefits where the plan must make a determination of disability to decide the claim.

WAITING FOR A DECISION ON YOUR CLAIM

As noted, the ERISA sets specific periods of time for plans to evaluate your claim and inform you of the decision. The time limits are counted in calendar days, so weekends and holidays are included. These limits do not govern when the benefits must be paid or provided. If you are entitled to benefits, check your SPD for how and when benefits are paid. Plans are required to pay or provide benefits within a reasonable time after a claim is approved.

- **Urgent care claims.** These must be decided as soon as possible, taking into account the medical needs of the patient, but no later than 72 hours after the plan receives the claim. The plan must tell you within 24 hours if more information is needed; you will have no less than 48 hours to respond. Then, the plan must decide the claim within 48 hours after the missing information is supplied or the time to supply it has elapsed. The plan cannot extend the time to make the initial decision without your consent. The plan must give you notice that your claim has been granted or denied before the end of the time allotted for the decision. The plan can notify you orally of the benefit determination so long as a written notification is furnished to you no later than three days after the oral notification.
- **Preservice claims.** These must be decided within a reasonable period of time appropriate to the medical circumstances, but no later than 15 days after the plan has received the claim. The plan may extend the time period up to an additional 15 days if, for reasons beyond the plan's control, the decision cannot be made within the first 15 days. The plan administrator must notify you prior to the expiration of the first 15-day period, explaining the reason for the delay, requesting any additional information, and advising you when the plan expects to make the decision. If more information is requested, you have at least 45 days to supply it. The plan then must decide the claim no later than 15 days

Filing a Claim for Your Health or Disability Benefits

after you supply the additional information or after the period of time allowed to supply it ends, whichever comes first. If the plan wants more time, the plan needs your consent. The plan must give you written notice that your claim has been granted or denied before the end of the time allotted for the decision.
- **Postservice health claims**. These must be decided within a reasonable period of time, but not later than 30 days after the plan has received the claim. If, because of reasons beyond the plan's control, more time is needed to review your request, the plan may extend the time period up to an additional 15 days. However, the plan administrator has to let you know before the end of the first 30-day period, explaining the reason for the delay, requesting any additional information needed, and advising you when a final decision is expected. If more information is requested, you have at least 45 days to supply it. The claim then must be decided no later than 15 days after you supply the additional information or the period of time given by the plan to do so ends, whichever comes first. The plan needs your consent if it wants more time after its first extension. The plan must give you notice that your claim has been denied in whole or in part (paying less than 100 percent of the claim) before the end of the time allotted for the decision.
- **Disability claims**. These must be decided within a reasonable period of time, but not later than 45 days after the plan has received the claim. If, because of reasons beyond the plan's control, more time is needed to review your request, the plan can extend the time frame up to 30 days. The plan must tell you prior to the end of the first 45-day period that additional time is needed, explaining why, any unresolved issues and additional information needed, and when the plan expects to render a final decision. If more information is requested during either extension period, you will

have at least 45 days to supply it. The claim then must be decided no later than 30 days after you supply the additional information or the period of time given by the plan to do so ends, whichever comes first. The plan administrator may extend the time period for up to another 30 days as long as it notifies you before the first extension expires. For any additional extensions, the plan needs your consent. The plan must give you notice whether your claim has been denied before the end of the time allotted for the decision.

If your claim is denied, the plan administrator must send you a notice, either in writing or electronically, with a detailed explanation of why your claim was denied and a description of the appeal process. In addition, the plan must include the plan rules, guidelines, or exclusions (such as medical necessity or experimental treatment exclusions) used in the decision or provide you with instructions on how you can request a copy of these documents from the plan. The notice may also include a specific request for you to provide the plan with additional information in case you wish to appeal your denial.

APPEALING A DENIED CLAIM

Claims are denied for various reasons. Perhaps you are not eligible for benefits. Perhaps the services you received are not covered by your plan. Or perhaps the plan simply needs more information about your claim. Whatever the reason, you have at least 180 days to file an appeal (check your SPD or claims procedure to see if your plan provides a longer period).

Use the information in your claim denial notice in preparing your appeal. You should also be aware that the plan must provide claimants, on request and free of charge, copies of documents, records, and other information relevant to the claim for benefits. The plan also must identify, at your request, any medical or vocational expert whose advice was obtained by the plan. Be sure to include in your appeal all information related to your claim, particularly any additional information or evidence that you want the

Filing a Claim for Your Health or Disability Benefits

plan to consider, and get it to the person specified in the denial notice before the end of the 180-day period.

REVIEWING AN APPEAL

On appeal, your claim must be reviewed by someone new who looks at all of the information submitted and consults with qualified medical professionals if a medical judgment is involved. This reviewer cannot be the same person or a subordinate of the person who made the initial decision, and the reviewer must give no consideration to that decision.

Plans have specific periods of time within which to review your appeal, depending on the type of claim.

- **Urgent care claims.** These must be reviewed as soon as possible, taking into account the medical needs of the patient, but not later than 72 hours after the plan receives your request to review a denied claim.
- **Preservice claims.** These must be reviewed within a reasonable period of time appropriate to the medical circumstances, but not later than 30 days after the plan receives your request to review a denied claim.
- **Postservice claims.** These must be reviewed within a reasonable period of time, but not later than 60 days after the plan receives your request to review a denied claim. If a group health plan needs more time, the plan must get your consent. If you do not agree to more time, the plan must complete the review within the permitted time limit.
- **Disability claims.** These must be reviewed within a reasonable period of time, but not later than 45 days after the plan receives your request to review a denied claim. If the plan determines special circumstances exist and an extension is needed, the plan may take up to an additional 45 days to decide the appeal. However, before taking the extension, the plan must notify you in writing during the first 45-day period explaining the special circumstances and the date by which the plan expects to make the decision.

There are two exceptions to these time limits. In general, single-employer collectively bargained plans may use a collectively bargained grievance process for their claims appeal procedure if it has provisions on filing, determination, and review of benefit claims. Multiemployer collectively bargained plans are given special time frames to allow them to schedule reviews on appeal of postservice claims and disability claims for the regular quarterly meetings of their boards of trustees. If you are a participant in one of those plans and you have questions about your plan's procedures, you can consult your plan's SPD and CBA or contact the DOL's Employee Benefits Security Administration (EBSA).

Plans can require you to go through two levels of review of a denied health or disability claim to finish the plan's claims process. If two levels of review are required, the maximum time for each review generally is half of the time limit permitted for one review. For example, in the case of a group health plan with one appeal level, as noted previously, the review of a preservice claim must be completed within a reasonable period of time appropriate to the medical circumstances but no later than 30 days after the plan gets your appeal. If the plan requires two appeals, each review must be completed within 15 days for preservice claims. If your claim on appeal is still denied after the first review, the plan has to allow you a reasonable period of time (but not a full 180 days) to file for the second review.

Once the final decision on your claim is made, the plan must send you a written explanation of the decision. The notice must be in plain language that can be understood by participants in the plan. It must include all the specific reasons for the denial of your claim on appeal, refer you to the plan provisions on which the decision is based, tell you if the plan has any additional voluntary levels of appeal, explain your right to receive documents that are relevant to your benefit claim free of charge, and describe your rights to seek judicial review of the plan's decision.

IF YOUR APPEAL IS DENIED

If the plan's final decision denies your claim, you may want to seek legal advice regarding your rights to bring an action in court

Filing a Claim for Your Health or Disability Benefits

to challenge the denial. Normally, you must complete your plan's claim process before filing an action in court to challenge the denial of a claim for benefits. However, if you believe your plan failed to establish or follow a claims procedure consistent with the DOL's rules, you may want to seek legal advice regarding your right to ask a court to review your benefit claim without waiting for a decision from the plan. You may also want to contact the nearest EBSA office about your rights if you believe the plan failed to follow any of the ERISA's requirements in handling your benefit claim.

If your appeal is denied and you are in a nongrandfathered health plan, you also have the right to external review of the decision. To find out if your plan is not grandfathered, check the documents from your plan describing the plan's benefits. If your plan is grandfathered, it must be disclosed. If there is no disclosure in your plan's documents, your plan likely is not grandfathered.

ADDITIONAL PROTECTIONS IF YOUR PLAN IS NOT GRANDFATHERED UNDER THE AFFORDABLE CARE ACT

Nongrandfathered health plans, or insurers to those plans, must provide additional internal claims and appeal rights and a process for external review of benefit claim denials. Internal claims and appeals are your health claims or appeals of denials reviewed by your plan. These rights also apply to rescissions (retroactive cancellations) of coverage.

The additional internal claims and appeal protections include:
- providing you with new or additional evidence or rationale and the opportunity to respond to it, before a final decision is made on the claim
- ensuring that claims and appeals are adjudicated in an independent and impartial manner
- providing details on the claim involved, the reason for denial (including the denial code and meaning), the internal and external appeals processes that are available, and information on consumer assistance, in all claims denial notices

- providing, on request, diagnosis and treatment codes (and their meanings) for any denied claim
- providing notices in a culturally and linguistically appropriate manner
- allowing you to begin the external review process if the plan fails to follow the internal claims requirements (unless the plan's violation is minimal)
- allowing you to resubmit an internal claim if a request for an immediate external review is rejected

Nongrandfathered plans must also provide a process for an external review of claims denials by an independent party. The external review process used depends on whether the plan is self-funded or provides benefits through an insurance company. The notice of the denial of your claim from your plan will describe the external review process and your rights.[1]

---

[1] "Filing a Claim for Your Health or Disability Benefits," U.S. Department of Labor (DOL), September 2015. Available online. URL: www.dol.gov/sites/dolgov/files/legacy-files/ebsa/about-ebsa/our-activities/resource-center/publications/filing-a-claim-for-your-health-or-disability-benefits.pdf. Accessed March 4, 2024.

Part 8 | Additional Help and Information

Chapter 66 | Glossary of Disease Management Terms

activities of daily living (ADLs): The tasks of everyday life. These activities include eating, dressing, getting in or out of a bed or chair, taking a bath or shower, doing the shopping, doing housework, and using a telephone.

advance directive: A legal document that states the treatment or care a person wishes to receive or not receive if he or she becomes unable to make medical decisions (e.g., due to being unconscious or in a coma).

Alzheimer disease (AD): A progressive and fatal disease in which nerve cells in the brain degenerate and brain matter shrinks, resulting in impaired thinking, behavior, and memory.

analyte: The part of the sample that the test is designed to find or measure. For example, a home pregnancy test measures human chorionic gonadotropin (hCG) in urine. The analyte is hCG.

anesthesia: A combination of medications administered to a patient to block pain and other sensations, at times rendering the patient unconscious, so that medical or surgical procedures can be performed; anesthesia can be general, regional, or local.

antibiotic: A drug used to treat infections caused by bacteria and other microorganisms.

anxiety: Feelings of fear, dread, and uneasiness that may occur as a reaction to stress. A person with anxiety may sweat, feel restless and tense, and have a rapid heartbeat.

This glossary contains terms excerpted from documents produced by several sources deemed reliable.

appeal: A special kind of complaint you make if you disagree with a decision to deny a request for health-care services or payment for services you already received. You may also make a complaint if you disagree with a decision to stop services that you are receiving. For example, you may ask for an appeal if Medicare does not pay for an item or service you think you should be able to get. There is a specific process that your Medicare health plan or the original Medicare plan must use when you ask for an appeal.

approved amount: The fee Medicare sets for a covered medical service. This is the amount a doctor or supplier is paid by you and Medicare for a service or supply. It may be less than the actual amount charged by a doctor or supplier. The approved amount is sometimes called the "approved charge."

assistive device: A tool that helps a person with a disability to do a certain task. Examples are a cane, wheelchair, scooter, walker, hearing aid, or special bed.

assistive technology: Any device or technology that helps a disabled person. Examples are special grips for holding utensils and computer screen monitors to help a person with low vision read more easily.

blood transfusion: The administration of blood or blood products into a blood vessel.

cancer: A term for diseases in which abnormal cells divide without control. Cancer cells can invade nearby tissues and can spread to other parts of the body through the blood and lymph systems.

caregiver: Anyone who helps care for an elderly individual or person with a disability who lives at home.

durable power of attorney (POA): A type of POA. A POA is a legal document that gives one person (such as a relative, lawyer, or friend) the authority to make legal, medical, or financial decisions for another person.

genome: An organism's complete set of deoxyribonucleic acid (DNA), including all of its genes. Each genome contains all of the information needed to build and maintain that organism.

home health agency: An organization that provides home care services, such as skilled nursing care, physical therapy, occupational therapy, speech therapy, and care by home health aides.

hospice: A program that provides special care for people who are near the end-of-life and for their families, either at home, in freestanding facilities, or within hospitals.

Glossary of Disease Management Terms

insured plan: A plan that provides benefits through an insurance company or health maintenance organization (HMO). Check your summary plan description (SPD) to see if your plan is insured.

living will: A type of legal advance directive in which a person describes specific treatment guidelines that are to be followed by health-care providers if he or she becomes terminally ill and cannot communicate.

Medicaid: A joint federal and state program that helps with medical costs for some people with limited income and resources. Medicaid programs vary from state to state, but most health-care costs are covered if you qualify for both Medicare and Medicaid.

Medicare health plan: Generally, a plan offered by a private company that contracts with Medicare to provide Part A and Part B benefits to people with Medicare who enroll in the plan. Medicare health plans include all Medicare Advantage plans, Medicare cost plans, and demonstration/pilot programs. Program of All-Inclusive Care for the Elderly (PACE) organizations are special types of Medicare health plans. PACE plans can be offered by public or private entities and provide Part D and other benefits in addition to Part A and Part B benefits.

mental health: A person's overall psychological and emotional condition. Good mental health is a state of well-being in which a person is able to cope with everyday events, think clearly, be responsible, meet challenges, and have good relationships with others.

neurology: A medical specialty concerned with the study of the structures, functions, and diseases of the nervous system.

nursing home: A place that gives care to people who have physical or mental disabilities and need help with ADLs (such as taking a bath, getting dressed, and going to the bathroom) but do not need to be in the hospital.

nutrition: The clinical practice concerned with nutrients and other substances contained in food and their action, interaction, and balance in relation to health and disease.

obstetrics/gynecology: The medical-surgical specialty concerned with the management and care of women during pregnancy, parturition, and puerperium; the physiology and disorders primarily of the female genital tract; and female endocrinology and reproductive physiology.

occupational therapist: A health professional trained to help people who are ill or disabled learn to manage their daily activities.

occupational therapy: Services given to help you return to usual activities (such as bathing, preparing meals, and housekeeping) after illness.

palliative care: Care given to improve the quality of life (QOL) of patients who have a serious or life-threatening disease. The goal of palliative care is to prevent or treat as early as possible the symptoms of the disease, side effects caused by treatment of the disease, and psychological, social, and spiritual problems related to the disease or its treatment. It is also called "comfort care," "supportive care," and "symptom management."

pharmacology: A clinical specialty concerned with the effectiveness and safety of drugs in humans.

physical examination: An exam of the body to check for general signs of disease.

physical therapist: A health professional who teaches exercises and physical activities that help condition muscles and restore strength and movement.

psychological: Having to do with how the mind works and how thoughts and feelings affect behavior.

psychologist: A specialist who can talk with patients and their families about emotional and personal matters and can help them make decisions.

radiology: The specialty concerned with the use of x-ray and other forms of radiant energy in the diagnosis and treatment of disease.

rehabilitation: A process to restore mental or physical abilities lost to injury or disease in order to function in a normal or near-normal way.

screening test: An initial or preliminary test. Screening tests do not tell you if you definitely have a disease or condition. Rather, positive results indicate that you may need additional tests or a doctor's evaluation to see if you have a particular disease or condition.

skilled nursing care: A level of care that includes services that can only be performed safely and correctly by a licensed nurse (either a registered nurse or a licensed practical nurse).

social service: A community resource that helps people in need. Services may include help getting to and from medical appointments, home delivery of medication and meals, in-home nursing care, help paying medical costs not covered by insurance, loaning medical equipment, and housekeeping help.

social worker: A professional trained to talk with people and their families about emotional or physical needs and to find them support services.

Glossary of Disease Management Terms

special enrollment: An opportunity for certain individuals to enroll in a group health plan, regardless of the plan's regular enrollment dates.

speech-language pathology: A clinical profession concerned with the study of speech/language and swallowing disorders and their diagnosis.

summary plan description: A document outlining your plan, usually provided when you enroll in the plan.

support group: A group of people with similar diseases who meet to discuss how better to cope with their disease and treatment.

supportive care: Care given to improve the QOL of patients who have a serious or life-threatening disease.

surgery: A medical specialty concerned with manual or operative procedures used in the diagnosis and treatment of diseases, injuries, or deformities.

tube feeding: A type of enteral nutrition (nutrition that is delivered into the digestive system in a liquid form). For tube feeding, a small tube may be placed through the nose into the stomach or the small intestine.

waiting period: The time that must pass before coverage can become effective under the terms of a group health plan.

x-ray: A type of high-energy radiation. In low doses, x-rays are used to diagnose diseases by making pictures of the inside of the body.

yoga: An ancient system of practices used to balance the mind and body through exercise, meditation (focusing thoughts), and control of breathing and emotions.

Chapter 67 | Resources for Information about Disease Management

GOVERNMENT ORGANIZATIONS

Administration on Aging (AoA)
330 C St., S.W.
Washington, DC 20201
Toll-Free: 800-677-1116
Phone: 202-401-4634
Website: https://acl.gov/about-acl/administration-aging

Agency for Healthcare Research and Quality (AHRQ)
5600 Fishers Ln., 7th Fl.
Rockville, MD 20857
Phone: 301-427-1364
Website: www.ahrq.gov

Centers for Disease Control and Prevention (CDC)
1600 Clifton Rd.
Atlanta, GA 30329-4027
Toll-Free: 800-CDC-INFO
(800-232-4636)
Toll-Free TTY: 888-232-6348
Website: www.cdc.gov

Centers for Medicare & Medicaid Services (CMS)
7500 Security Blvd.
Baltimore, MD 21244
Toll-Free: 877-267-2323
Phone: 410-786-3000
TTY: 410-786-0727
Toll-Free TTY: 866-226-1819
Website: www.cms.gov

Resources in this chapter were compiled from several sources deemed reliable; all contact information was verified and updated in June 2024.

Eunice Kennedy Shriver **National Institute of Child Health and Human Development (NICHD)**
P.O. Box 3006
Rockville, MD 20847
Toll-Free: 800-370-2943
Phone: 301-496-5133
Toll-Free Fax: 866-760-5947
Website: www.nichd.nih.gov
Email: NICHDInformation
ResourceCenter@mail.nih.gov

Federal Trade Commission (FTC)
600 Pennsylvania Ave., N.W.
Washington, DC 20580
Phone: 202-326-2222
Website: www.ftc.gov

Genetic and Rare Diseases Information Center (GARD)
P.O. Box 8126
Gaithersburg, MD 20898-8126
Toll-Free: 888-205-2311
Website: https://rarediseases.info.nih.gov

Health Resources and Services Administration (HRSA)
5600 Fishers Ln.
Rockville, MD 20857
Toll-Free: 877-464-4772
Phone: 301-443-3376
Toll-Free TTY: 877-897-9910
Website: www.hrsa.gov
Email: press@hrsa.gov

InsureKidsNow.gov
7500 Security Blvd.
Baltimore, MD 21244
Toll-Free: 877-KIDS-NOW (877-543-7669)
Website: www.insurekidsnow.gov

MedlinePlus
8600 Rockville Pike
Bethesda, MD 20894
Toll-Free: 888-346-3656
Phone: 301-594-5983
Website: https://medlineplus.gov

National Cancer Institute (NCI)
9609 Medical Center Dr.
Rockville, MD 20850
Toll-Free: 800-4-CANCER (800-422-6237)
Website: www.cancer.gov
Email: NCIinfo@nih.gov

National Center for Complementary and Integrative Health (NCCIH)
9000 Rockville Pike
Bethesda, MD 20892
Toll-Free: 888-644-6226
Toll-Free TTY: 866-464-3615
Website: www.nccih.nih.gov
Email: info@nccih.nih.gov

National Health Information Center (NHIC)
1101 Wootton Pkwy., Ste. 420
Rockville, MD 20852
Website: www.health.gov/nhic

Resources for Information about Disease Management

National Heart, Lung, and Blood Institute (NHLBI)
31 Center Dr.
Bldg. 31
Bethesda, MD 20892
Toll-Free: 877-645-2448
Website: www.nhlbi.nih.gov
Email: nhlbiinfo@nhlbi.nih.gov

National Human Genome Research Institute (NHGRI)
31 Center Dr., MSC 2152, 9000 Rockville Pike
Bldg. 31, Rm. 4B09
Bethesda, MD 20892-2152
Phone: 301-402-0911
Fax: 301-402-2218
Website: www.genome.gov
Email: nhgripressoffice@mail.nih.gov

National Institute of Arthritis and Musculoskeletal and Skin Diseases (NIAMS)
1 AMS Cir.
Bethesda, MD 20892-3675
Toll-Free: 877-22-NIAMS (877-226-4267)
Phone: 301-495-4484
Fax: 301-718-6366
Website: www.niams.nih.gov
Email: niamsinfo@mail.nih.gov

National Institute of Diabetes and Digestive and Kidney Diseases (NIDDK)
9000 Rockville Pike
Bethesda, MD 20892
Toll-Free: 800-860-8747
Website: www.niddk.nih.gov/health-information/diabetes
Email: healthinfo@niddk.nih.gov

National Institute of General Medical Sciences (NIGMS)
45 Center Dr. MSC 6200
Bethesda, MD 20892-6200
Phone: 301-496-7301
Website: www.nigms.nih.gov

National Institute on Aging (NIA)
P.O. Box 8057
Gaithersburg, MD 20898
Toll-Free: 800-222-2225
Toll-Free TTY: 800-222-4225
Website: www.nia.nih.gov
Email: niaic@nia.nih.gov

National Institutes of Health (NIH)
9000 Rockville Pike
Bethesda, MD 20892
Phone: 301-496-4000
TTY: 301-402-9612
Website: www.nih.gov
Email: olib@od.nih.gov

Office of Dietary Supplements (ODS)
6705 Rockledge Dr.
Rm. 730, MSC 7991
Bethesda, MD 20817
Phone: 301-435-2920
Fax: 301-480-1845
Website: https://ods.od.nih.gov
Email: ods@nih.gov

U.S. Department of Health and Human Services (HHS)
200 Independence Ave., S.W.
Hubert H. Humphrey Bldg.
Washington, DC 20201
Toll-Free: 877-696-6775
Website: www.hhs.gov

U.S. Department of Labor (DOL)
200 Constitution Ave., N.W.
Washington, DC 20210
Toll-Free: 866-4-USA-DOL
(866-487-2365)
Website: www.dol.gov

U.S. Equal Employment Opportunity Commission (EEOC)
131 M St., N.E.
Washington, DC 20507
Toll-Free: 800-669-4000
Toll-Free TTY: 800-669-6820
Website: www.eeoc.gov
Email: info@eeoc.gov

U.S. Food and Drug Administration (FDA)
10903 New Hampshire Ave.
Silver Spring, MD 20993-0002
Toll-Free: 888-INFO-FDA
(888-463-6332)
Website: www.fda.gov

National Library of Medicine (NLM)
8600 Rockville Pike
Bethesda, MD 20894
Toll-Free: 888-FIND-NLM
(888-346-3656)
Phone: 301-594-5983
Website: www.nlm.nih.gov
Email: NLMCommunications@nih.gov

PRIVATE ORGANIZATIONS

Alzheimer's Association®
225 N. Michigan Ave.
17th Fl.
Chicago, IL 60601
Toll-Free: 800-272-3900
Website: www.alz.org

American Academy of Family Physicians (AAFP)
11400 Tomahawk Creek Pkwy.
Leawood, KS 66211-2680
Toll-Free: 800-274-2237
Phone: 913-906-6000
Fax: 913-906-6075
Website: www.aafp.org
Email: aafp@aafp.org

American Cancer Society (ACS)
270 Peachtree St., N.W., Ste. 1300
Atlanta, GA 30303
Toll-Free: 800-ACS-2345
(800-227-2345)
Website: www.cancer.org

Resources for Information about Disease Management

American Health Information Management Association (AHIMA)
35 W. Wacker Dr.
16th Fl.
Chicago, IL 60601
Toll-Free: 800-335-5535
Phone: 312-233-1100
Fax: 312-278-0272
Website: www.ahima.org
Email: info@ahima.org

American Heart Association (AHA)
7272 Greenville Ave.
Dallas, TX 75231
Toll-Free: 800-AHA-USA-1 (800-242-8721)
Phone: 214-570-5943
Website: www.heart.org

American Lung Association (ALA)
55 W. Wacker Dr., Ste. 1150
Chicago, IL 60601
Toll-Free: 800-LUNGUSA (800-586-4872)
Website: www.lung.org
Email: info@lung.org

American Medical Association (AMA)
330 N. Wabash Ave., Ste. 39300
AMA Plz.
Chicago, IL 60611-5885
Toll-Free: 800-262-3211
Phone: 312-464-4782
Website: www.ama-assn.org
Email: msc@ama-assn.org

America's Health Insurance Plans (AHIP)
601 Pennsylvania Ave., N.W.
Ste. 500
South Bldg.
Washington, DC 20004
Phone: 202-778-3200
Fax: 202-331-7487
Website: www.ahip.org
Email: info@ahip.org

Association of Maternal and Child Health Programs (AMCHP)
1825 K St., N.W., Ste. 250
Washington, DC 20006
Phone: 202-775-0436
Fax: 202-478-5120
Website: www.amchp.org
Email: info@amchp.org

Caregiver Action Network (CAN)
1150 Connecticut Ave., N.W., Ste. 501
Washington, DC 20036-3904
Toll-Free: 855-227-3640
Phone: 202-454-3970
Website: www.caregiveraction.org
Email: info@caregiveraction.org

Cleveland Clinic
9500 Euclid Ave.
Cleveland, OH 44195
Toll-Free: 800-223-2273
Phone: 216-444-2200
Website: https://my.clevelandclinic.org

Coalition Against Insurance Fraud (CAIF)
1012 14th St., N.W., Ste. 610
Washington, DC 20005
Phone: 202-393-7330
Website: www.insurancefraud.org
Email: coalition@insuranceFraud.org

Families USA
1225 New York Ave., N.W., Ste. 800
Washington, DC 20005
Phone: 202-628-3030
Fax: 202-347-2417
Website: www.familiesusa.org
Email: info@familiesusa.org

Family Voices
561 Virginia Rd., Ste. 300
Bldg. 4
Concord, MA 01742
Toll-Free: 888-835-5669
Phone: 781-674-7224
Website: https://familyvoices.org

HealthCare Choices NY, Inc.
6209 16th Ave.
Brooklyn, NY 11204
Phone: 718-234-0073
Toll-Free TTY: 800-662-1220
Website: www.healthcarechoicesny.org
Email: info@healthcarechoicesny.org

Insurance Information Institute (III)
110 William St.
New York, NY 10038
Phone: 212-346-5500
Website: www.iii.org
Email: info@iii.org

Kaiser Family Foundation (KFF)
185 Berry St., Ste. 2000
San Francisco, CA 94107
Phone: 650-854-9400
Fax: 650-854-4800
Website: www.kff.org

National Association of Insurance Commissioners (NAIC)
1100 Walnut St., Ste. 1500
Kansas City, MO 64106-2197
Phone: 816-842-3600
Website: www.naic.org
Email: help@naic.org

National Health Care Anti-Fraud Association (NHCAA)
1220 L St., N.W., Ste. 815
Washington, DC 20005
Phone: 202-659-5955
Fax: 202-785-6764
Website: www.nhcaa.org
Email: nhcaa@nhcaa.org

National Patient Advocate Foundation (NPAF)
1100 H St., N.W., Ste. 710
Washington, DC 20005
Phone: 202-347-8009
Website: www.npaf.org

Resources for Information about Disease Management

National Rehabilitation Information Center (NARIC)
8400 Corporate Dr., Ste. 500
Landover, MD 20785
Toll-Free: 800-346-2742
Phone: 301-459-5900
TTY: 301-459-5984
Fax: 301-459-4263
Website: www.naric.com
Email: naricinfo@heitechservices.com

Pan American Health Organization (PAHO)
525 23rd St., N.W.
Washington, DC 20037
Phone: 202-974-3000
Fax: 202-974-3663
Website: www.paho.org

INDEX

INDEX

INDEX

Page numbers followed by "n" refer to citation information; by "t" indicate tables; and by "f" indicate figures.

A

AAA *see* abdominal aortic aneurysm
abdominal aortic aneurysm (AAA)
    Medicare 571
    screening tests 48
ACA *see* Affordable Care Act
ACE inhibitors *see* angiotensin-converting enzyme inhibitors
acquired immunodeficiency syndrome (AIDS)
    assistive devices 499
    drugs 369
    health-care scams 309
    white blood cells (WBCs) 157
acute myeloid leukemia (AML), chronic diseases 15
acute respiratory infections (ARIs), tobacco use 14
AD *see* Alzheimer disease
ADA *see* adenosine deaminase
ADA.gov
    publications
        Americans with Disabilities Act (ADA) 525n
        disability rights laws 530n
Addison disease, medications 324
adenocarcinoma, infectious diseases 446
adenosine deaminase (ADA), severe combined immunodeficiency (SCID) 162
Administration on Aging (AoA), contact information 627
adverse drug reactions, overview 403–406
AED *see* automated external defibrillator
aerobic
    fibromyalgia 112
    managing stress 440
    physical inactivity 19
    spinal stenosis 120
Affordable Care Act (ACA)
    disability claims 617
    health information 432
    health insurance scam 592
    medications 360
    nondiscrimination prohibitions 552
Agency for Healthcare Research and Quality (AHRQ)
    contact information 627
    publications
        ambulatory care safety 227n
        health care 188
        health-care quality 218n
        medical errors 308n
        seeking out information 196n
        stay healthy 48n, 50n
        steps after diagnosis 70n
        talking with your doctor 179n, 197n

Agency for Healthcare Research and
    Quality (AHRQ)
    publications, *continued*
        wrong-site, wrong-procedure,
            wrong-patient errors
            (WSPEs) 258n
AI *see* artificial intelligence
AIDS *see* acquired immunodeficiency
    syndrome
airborne transmission
    disease transmission 4
    preventing infection 484
allergy
    benign prostatic
        hyperplasia (BPH) 128
    mental impairment 524
    prescription drug
        advertisements 366
allow natural death (AND) order,
    advance care planning 540
ALS *see* amyotrophic lateral sclerosis
Alzheimer's Association®, contact
    information 630
Alzheimer disease (AD)
    artificial intelligence (AI) 506
    chronic diseases 10, 545
    chronic medical conditions 488
    described 133
    genetic testing 56
ambulatory care, overview 224–227
American Academy of Family
    Physicians (AAFP), contact
    information 630
American Cancer Society (ACS),
    contact information 630
American Health
    Information Management
    Association (AHIMA), contact
    information 631
American Heart Association (AHA),
    contact information 631
American Lung Association (ALA),
    contact information 631

American Medical
    Association (AMA), contact
    information 631
America's Health Insurance
    Plans (AHIP), contact
    information 631
aminosalicylates, ulcerative colitis 108
AML *see* acute myeloid leukemia
amputation
    chronic diseases 16
    diabetes 30
    health-care quality 214
    see also assistive devices
amyotrophic lateral sclerosis (ALS),
    described 134
anabolic steroids, medications 326
analgesics
    Bell palsy 136
    medications 322
anesthesia
    cardiovascular diseases 91
    hospital emergencies 241
    kidney stone 126
    overview 249–251
angiotensin receptor blockers (ARBs),
    cardiovascular diseases 93
angiotensin-converting enzyme (ACE)
    inhibitors
    cardiovascular diseases 86
    prescription drugs 323
antacids
    drug interactions 336
    gastrointestinal (GI) diseases 105
    health care 187
    medications 322
antiinflammatory drugs
    disease transmission 6
    gastrointestinal (GI)
        diseases 100
antianxiety drugs,
    medication 322
antiarrhythmics, prescription
    drugs 322
antibacterials, medication 322

Index

antibiotic resistance
  antibiotics 396
  gastrointestinal (GI) diseases 102
antibiotics
  bladder infection 124
  healthy lifestyle 96
  medications 322
  meningococcal vaccine 469
  overview 396–398
  respiratory diseases 75
  surgical site infection (SSI) 248
anticoagulants, anxiolytics 323
anticonvulsants, prescription drugs 323
antidepressants
  medications 323
  pain relievers 424
antidiarrheals, antibiotics 323
antiemetics, medications 323
antifungals
  over-the-counter (OTC) medications 323
  pneumonia 78
  preventing human diseases 6
antihistamines
  drug interactions 407
  medications 323
  over-the-counter (OTC) medications 351
  pain relievers 424
antihypertensives, antidiarrheal preparations 323
antiinflammatories, bronchial tubes 324
antineoplastics, cough suppressants 323
antiphospholipid syndrome (APS), systemic lupus erythematosus (SLE) 164
antipsychotics, medications 323
antipyretics, rheumatoid arthritis (RA) 323

antiretroviral therapy (ART), human immunodeficiency virus (HIV) 157
antivirals
  Bell palsy 136
  over-the-counter (OTC) drugs 324
  pneumonia 78
  preventing human diseases 6
aortic aneurysm
  family health history 35
  men screening tests 48
  screening ultrasound 571
appendicitis, medical insurance 198
appetite
  chronic illnesses 488
  hepatitis A vaccine 465
  prescription drugs 181
APS *see* antiphospholipid syndrome
ARBs *see* angiotensin receptor blockers
ARIs *see* acute respiratory infections
arrhythmias
  cardiovascular diseases 81
  heart disease 35
ART *see* antiretroviral therapy
arthritis
  biosimilars 385
  corticosteroids 324
  fibromyalgia 112
  high blood pressure (HBP) 190
  major depressive disorder (MDD) 525
  nasal spray 468
  over-the-counter (OTC) medications 349
  preventing falls 447
artificial intelligence (AI), overview 504–507
artificial neurons, artificial intelligence (AI) 505
ASD *see* autism spectrum disorder
Aspergillus, preventing infection 484

aspirin
   Bell palsy 136
   caregivers 240
   health care 187
   heart attack 89
   influenza vaccine 467
   Medicare 572
   over-the-counter (OTC)
      medications 351
assistive devices
   described 139
   occupational therapy 161
   rehabilitative technology 495
Association of Maternal and Child
   Health Programs (AMCHP),
   contact information 631
asthma
   artificial intelligence (AI) 506
   chronic diseases 15
   described 74
   drug interactions 334
   electronic health
      (eHealth) literacy 266
   human diseases 3
   influenza vaccine 466
atherosclerosis, heart disease 35
autism spectrum disorder (ASD)
   defined 457
   human-animal interactions 451
automated external
   defibrillator (AED),
   cardiovascular diseases 81

B

bariatric surgery
   defined 88
   surgery and medical
      procedures 106
beta-blockers
   coronary heart disease 86
   improving health-care quality 215
   medication 324

biofeedback, pain management 448
biofilms, preventing
   infection 482
biologics
   biosimilars 385
   ulcerative colitis 109
biomarker
   colorectal cancer screenings 573
   overview 60–65
biomaterials, described 508
biopsy
   biomarker testing 62
   hemochromatosis 32
   surgery 247
biosimilars, overview 385–387
biventricular pacemaker, defined 94
bladder infection, described 123
blood sugar
   ambulatory care 224
   artificial pancreas 499
   chronic diseases 16
   diabetes screenings 573
   healthy eating plan 434
   heart failure 93
   home-use tests 53
   see also diabetes
BMD *see* bone mineral density
BMI *see* body mass index
body mass index (BMI)
   obesity behavioral
      therapy 576
   screening test 47
bone mineral density (BMD),
   osteoporosis 112
breast cancer
   artificial intelligence (AI) 506
   biomarker tests 63
   chronic diseases 18
   major life activities 525
   neurofibromatosis 153
   osteoporosis 116
   pharmacogenomics 330

Index

bronchitis
    chronic diseases 15
    described 75
    severe combined
        immunodeficiency (SCID) 162
bronchodilators
    chronic obstructive pulmonary
        disease (COPD) 77
    medications 324
brown bagging, preventing medical
    errors 305

C

CABG *see* coronary artery bypass
    grafting
CAD *see* coronary artery disease
calcium channel blockers
    coronary heart disease 86
    over-the-counter (OTC) drugs 323
CAM *see* complementary and
    alternative medicine
cancer
    anesthesia 250
    assistive devices 499
    biomarkers 61
    colorectal cancer 29
    defined 15
    fraud scams 310
    healthy eating plan 434
    hepatitis B vaccine 465
    imported drugs 369
    making decisions 191
    prostate problems 127
    traumatic brain injury (TBI) 525
cardiac arrest
    described 81
    healthy lifestyle 95
cardiac resynchronization therapy
    (CRT), heart failure 94
cardiomyopathy
    alcohol use 21

cardiac arrest 84
    family health history 35
cardiopulmonary resuscitation (CPR)
    advance care planning 540
    blood-vascular system 81
cardiovascular disease (CVD)
    alcohol misuse screening 572
    health-care quality 214
    overview 81–98
    reducing health risk 445
    screening tests 50
Caregiver Action Network (CAN),
    contact information 631
catastrophic plans, health insurance
    plan 601
catheters
    caregivers 241
    oxygen therapy 90
    preventing infection 482
    urinary incontinence 130
CBT *see* cognitive behavioral
    therapy
CCM *see* chronic care model
CDIs *see* child development
    inventories
C. diff see Clostridioides difficile
celiac disease
    described 99
    genetic testing 56
Centers for Disease Control and
    Prevention (CDC)
    contact information 627
    publications
        antibiotics 398n
        artificial intelligence (AI) 506n
        before surgery 249n
        benefits of physical
            activity 447n
        coronavirus
            disease 2019 (COVID-19)
            vaccines 473n
        diabetes 166n

Centers for Disease Control and
    Prevention (CDC)
  publications, *continued*
    electronic health (eHealth)
      literacy 265n
    family health history 26n, 37n
    fibromyalgia 112n
    financial stress and positive
      financial behaviors 360n
    handwash 486n
    health literacy 264n
    how infections spread 484n
    immune system 157n
    laboratory quality assurance
      and standardization
      programs 223n
    nutrition 433n
    pharmacogenomics 333n
    systemic lupus
      erythematosus (SLE) 164n
    tackling electronic health
      (eHealth) literacy 265n
Centers for Medicare & Medicaid
    Services (CMS)
  contact information 627
  publications
    Children's Health Insurance
      Program (CHIP) 600n
    choosing a hospital 233n
    e-prescribing 361n
    health insurance plan 607n
    health insurance rights and
      protections 277n
    Health Savings Account (HSA)-
      eligible plans 590n
    home health care 585n
    hospital inpatient or
      outpatient 238n
    Medicaid benefits 562n
    Medicare's preventive
      services 577n
    prescription medications 359n
    second opinion 200n

central nervous system (CNS)
  human diseases 3
  multiple sclerosis (MS) 148
cerebral palsy (CP)
  assistive devices 499
  described 137
  major life activities 524
  screening tests 457
cervical cancer
  children vaccines 461
  health-care quality 215
  women screening test 46
CF *see* cystic fibrosis
CGM *see* continuous glucose monitor
chemotherapy
  antibiotics 397
  biomarker tests 63
  hospice care 518
  neurofibromatosis 153
chickenpox, rotavirus
  vaccines 471
child development inventories (CDIs),
  defined 459
ChildCare.gov
  publication
    children's physical
      health 156n
chlamydia
  lung cancer 48
  prostate cancer screenings 577
cholera, disease transmission 5
cholesterol testing
  health-care quality 215
  home-use tests 53
chronic care model (CCM),
  ambulatory care 224
chronic illness
  medications 359
  mental health 488
  overview 431–452
chronic kidney disease (CKD)
  healthy eating 435
  oxygen therapy 91

Index

chronic obstructive pulmonary
   disease (COPD)
   cigarette smoking 15
   described 76
cirrhosis, hemochromatosis 31
CKD *see* chronic kidney disease
Cleveland Clinic, contact
   information 631
CLIA *see* Clinical Laboratory
   Improvement Amendments of 1988
Clinical Laboratory Improvement
   Amendments of 1988 (CLIA),
   laboratory-developed
   tests (LDTs) 51
clinical trials
   cancer treatments 62
   choosing hospital 231
   making decisions 190
   Medicaid 561
   nervous system diseases 134
closed distribution system, drug safety
   concerns 367
Clostridioides difficile (*C. diff*)
   antibiotics 397
   gastroesophageal reflux (GER) 105
CNS *see* central nervous system
Coalition Against Insurance
   Fraud (CAIF), contact
   information 632
COBRA *see* Consolidated Omnibus
   Budget Reconciliation Act
cognitive behavioral therapy (CBT),
   fibromyalgia 112
collard greens, healthy eating plan 434
colon cancer
   artificial intelligence (AI) 507
   screening test 46
colonoscopy
   anesthesia 250
   colorectal cancer 28
   health-care quality 215
   Medicare 573
   screening test 46

colorectal cancer
   family health history 26
   health-care quality 215
   Medicare 573
   poor nutrition 18
   screening tests 49
   ulcerative colitis 109
coma, pain relievers 425
companion diagnostic test, heart
   disease 62
complementary and alternative
   medicine (CAM),
   overview 201–208
computed tomography (CT)
   human diseases 6
   Medicare 575
   robotic interventions 253
congenital heart defects, family health
   history 35
Consolidated Omnibus Budget
   Reconciliation Act (COBRA),
   health-care laws 553
continuous glucose monitor (CGM),
   artificial pancreas systems 500
control algorithm, artificial
   pancreas 500
COPD *see* chronic obstructive
   pulmonary disease
coronary artery bypass
   grafting (CABG), weight
   management 88
coronary artery disease (CAD)
   cardiac arrest 84
   heart disease 35
coronavirus disease 2019 (COVID-19)
   human diseases 5
   metabolic syndrome 445
   preventive care 511
   rotavirus disease 472
corticosteroids
   defined 108
   multiple sclerosis (MS) 149
   over-the-counter (OTC) drugs 324
   rheumatoid arthritis (RA) 160

643

cost-sharing reductions (CSRs), health insurance plan 602
counterfeit drugs
　imported drugs 367
　unapproved drugs 422
COVID-19 *see* coronavirus disease 2019
CP *see* cerebral palsy
CPR *see* cardiopulmonary resuscitation
Crohn's disease, described 100
CRT *see* cardiac resynchronization therapy
cryptosporidiosis, human disease transmission 5
CSRs *see* cost-sharing reductions
CT *see* computed tomography
CVD *see* cardiovascular disease
cystic fibrosis (CF)
　assistive devices 499
　genetic testing 55
　pharmacogenomics 333
cystoscopy, kidney stone 126
cytotoxins, medications 324

D

DASH eating plan *see* Dietary Approaches to Stop Hypertension eating plan
decongestants, medications 325
defense mechanisms, human diseases 6
dementia
　activities of daily living (ADLs) 10
　Alzheimer disease (AD) 545
　chronic disease conditions 442
　palliative care 516
dengue, human diseases 5
dentures
　caregivers 240
　chronic diseases 40
　Medicaid 561

deoxyribonucleic acid (DNA)
　genetic testing 55
　medical care 163
　Medicare 573
　pharmacogenomics 329
　precision medicine 391
DESI *see* drug efficacy study implementation
DEXA *see* dual-energy x-ray absorptiometry
diabetes
　Americans with Disabilities Act (ADA) 524
　artificial intelligence (AI) 506
　cardiac arrest 84
　chronic illnesses 488
　electronic health (eHealth) literacy 266
　health benefits 451
　health-care quality 214
　health-care scams 309
　heart disease 35
　home health 582
　human diseases 3
　over-the-counter (OTC) medications 351
　see also blood sugar; prediabetes
diarrhea
　antibiotics 398
　children vaccines 465
　gastroesophageal reflux (GER) 105
　human diseases 5
　medication 344
　oral treatments 151
　preventing infection 485
diet
　chronic diseases 18
　coronary heart disease 88
　healthy eating plan 435
　human diseases 3
　Paget disease 117
　Parkinson disease (PD) 155
　personal health record (PHR) 291

Index

Dietary Approaches to Stop
  Hypertension (DASH) eating plan,
  coronary heart disease 85
dietary supplements
  cerebral palsy (CP) 140
  chronic illnesses 490
  complementary and alternative
    medicine (CAM) 202
  coronary heart disease 86
  drug interactions 336, 409
  human diseases 7
  medical errors 305
  over-the-counter (OTC)
    medications 353
Dilaudid, pain relievers 424
diphtheria, nasal sprays 461
diphtheria, tetanus, and
  pertussis (DTaP), children
  vaccine 470
direct-to-consumer genetic testing,
  overview 55–60
disease-modifying antirheumatic
  drugs (DMARDs), rheumatoid
  arthritis (RA) 160
diuretics
  heart failure 93
  medications 323
  prostate problems 128
dizziness
  antibiotics 397
  human papillomavirus (HPV)
    vaccine 466
  pain relievers 425
DMARDs *see* disease-modifying
  antirheumatic drugs
DME *see* durable medical
  equipment
DNA *see* deoxyribonucleic acid
drug breakdown,
  pharmacogenomics 332
drug efficacy study
  implementation (DESI), counterfeit
  drugs 419

Drug Facts label, medication
  errors 413
drug interactions
  Bell palsy 136
  described 334
  overview 407–410
drug receptors,
  pharmacogenomics 329
drug uptake, pharmacogenomics 331
DTaP *see* diphtheria, tetanus, and
  pertussis
dual-energy x-ray
  absorptiometry (DEXA), screening
  test 47
durable medical equipment (DME),
  home health care 583

E

ECMO *see* extracorporeal membrane
  oxygenation
eHealth *see* electronic health
EHRs *see* electronic health records
electric nerve stimulation, pain
  management 449
electronic health (eHealth),
  overview 265–268
electronic health
  records (EHRs)
  electronic health (eHealth)
    literacy 266
  patient portal 292
  precision medicine 390
  see also ambulatory care
emphysema
  chronic obstructive pulmonary
    disease (COPD) 76
  tobacco use 15
end-stage renal disease (ESRD),
  antibiotic resistance 397
endometrium, chronic illness
  management 446

endoscopy, gastroesophageal reflux disease (GERD) 106
EOB *see* explanation of benefits
epilepsy
    depression 488
    nervous system diseases 140
    rehabilitative and assistive technologies 499
    vaccines 463
ESRD *see* end-stage renal disease
Eunice Kennedy Shriver National Institute of Child Health and Human Development (NICHD)
    contact information 628
    publication
        rehabilitative and assistive technology 499n
exercise
    chronic obstructive pulmonary disease (COPD) 77
    coronary heart disease 85
    epilepsy 143
    fibromyalgia 112
    heart valve diseases 96
    human health 7
    motor neuron diseases (MNDs) 148
    osteoporosis 34
    Parkinson disease (PD) 155
    personal health record (PHR) 291
expectorant, defined 325
explanation of benefits (EOB), medical identity theft 313
extracorporeal membrane oxygenation (ECMO), defined 83

F

familial hypercholesterolemia (FH), family health history 36
Families USA, contact information 632
Family and Medical Leave Act (FMLA), overview 531–535
family health history, overview 25–26
Family Voices, contact information 632
FASDs *see* fetal alcohol spectrum disorders
fatigue
    chronic illness 487
    epilepsy 141
    fibromyalgia 112
    hepatitis B vaccine 465
    human diseases 5
    minimally invasive surgery 253
fatty liver disease, alcohol use 21
FD&C Act *see* Federal Food, Drug, and Cosmetic Act
fecal occult blood testing (FOBT)
    cancer screening 215
    Medicare 573
Federal Food, Drug, and Cosmetic Act (FD&C Act), laboratory-developed tests (LDTs) 52
Federal Trade Commission (FTC)
    contact information 628
    publications
        health insurance scams 597n
        medical identity theft 316n
fetal alcohol spectrum disorders (FASDs), alcohol use 22
FH *see* familial hypercholesterolemia
fibromyalgia, described 112
fibrosis, alcohol use 21
flexible spending accounts (FSAs), direct-to-consumer genetic testing 60
flu shot
    Medicare 574
    quality health care 214
FMLA *see* Family and Medical Leave Act
FOBT *see* fecal occult blood testing
food transmission, human diseases 5
foot exam, health-care quality 214
FSAs *see* flexible spending accounts

Index

functional limitation,
  chronic illness 446
fundoplication, gastroesophageal
  reflux disease (GERD) 106

G

gastritis and gastropathy,
  described 102
gastroenteritis, rotavirus 470
gastroesophageal reflux (GER),
  described 104
gastrointestinal (GI) diseases,
  overview 99–110
GBS *see* Guillain-Barré syndrome
gelatin, measles, mumps, and rubella
  (MMR) vaccine 468
generally recognized as safe and
  effective (GRASE), unapproved
  prescription drugs 420
generic drug, overview 375–381
Genetic and Rare Diseases
  Information Center (GARD),
  contact information 628
GER *see* gastroesophageal reflux
German measles, nasal spray 468
germline mutations, biomarker test 64
glaucoma, Medicare 574
glucagon, artificial pancreas
  systems 502
gonorrhea, Medicare 577
GRASE *see* generally recognized as
  safe and effective
Guillain-Barré syndrome (GBS),
  vaccines for children 467

H

HBOT *see* hyperbaric oxygen
  treatment
HBP *see* high blood pressure
HD *see* Huntington disease
HDL *see* high-density lipoprotein

HealthCare Choices NY, Inc., contact
  information 632
health insurance
  chronic diseases 13
  complementary and alternative
    medicine (CAM) 206
  genetic testing 55
  health-care benefit laws 551
  health-care rights and
    responsibilities 277
  hospitalization 239
  medical identity theft 313
  prescription medications 357
  scams 591
Health Insurance Portability and
  Accountability Act (HIPAA)
  described 551
  electronic
    health (eHealth) literacy 267
health literacy
  ambulatory care 225
  overview 261–264
Health Resources and Services
  Administration (HRSA)
  contact information 628
  publications
    Hill-Burton free and reduced-
      cost health care 562n, 566n
Health Savings Account (HSA),
  overview 587–590
HealthIT.gov
  publications
    electronic health
      record (EHR) 266n
    electronic prescribing 361n
    health information rights 281n
    health information
      technology 290n
    patient participation in
      care 267n
    patient portal 292n
    personal health
      record (PHR) 291n, 292n

HealthIT.gov
   publications, *continued*
      protecting privacy and security 288n
heart attack
   adverse drug reactions 403
   artificial intelligence (AI) 504
   chronic illness and depression 487
   coronary heart disease 84
   family health history 35
   health-care fraud scams 309
   healthy eating plan 436
   Medicare 572
   quality health care 214
heart failure
   coronary heart disease 88
   family health history 35
   palliative care 515
   quality health care 214
   vaccines 463
heart valve diseases, described 95
hemoglobin A1C (blood glucose) testing, quality health care 214
hemolytic anemia, systemic lupus erythematosus (SLE) 164
hepatitis
   alcohol use 21
   home-use tests 53
   Medicare 574
   vaccines for children 464
hepatocellular carcinoma, hereditary hemochromatosis 31
hereditary hemochromatosis, described 31
heroin, prescription pain relievers 425
HER2 *see* human epidermal growth factor receptor 2
high blood cholesterol
   chronic diseases 17
   coronary heart disease 85
   family health history 34

high blood pressure (HBP)
   advance care planning 541
   benign prostatic hyperplasia (BPH) 128
   chronic diseases 17
   coronary heart disease 85
   drug interactions 408
   family health history 34
   hospice care 518
   Medicare 237t
   medications 325
   prescription drugs 370
   quality health care 213
   screenings 47
   stress 438
high-density lipoprotein (HDL), chronic diseases 15, 445
HIPAA *see* Health Insurance Portability and Accountability Act
HIV *see* human immunodeficiency virus
HIV.gov
   publication
      human immunodeficiency virus (HIV) treatment 159n
home-use test, overview 52–54
hormone replacement therapy (HRT), medications 325
hormone therapy, osteoporosis 116
hormones
   artificial pancreas systems 502
   medications 324
   osteoporosis 115
hospice care
   advance care planning 541
   overview 517–519
hospital-borne transmission, human diseases 5
HRT *see* hormone replacement therapy
H2 blockers, gastroesophageal reflux disease (GERD) 105

Index

human epidermal growth
   factor receptor 2 (HER2),
   pharmacogenomics 330
human immunodeficiency virus (HIV)
   alcohol use 22
   described 157
   Medicare 575
human papillomavirus (HPV),
   vaccines 461
Huntington disease (HD),
   described 146
hybrid artificial pancreas systems,
   defined 500
hyperbaric oxygen treatment (HBOT),
   cerebral palsy (CP) 140
hyperglycemia, artificial pancreas
   systems 503
hypoglycemia, artificial pancreas
   systems 501
hypothyroidism, depression 488

I

idiopathic thrombocytopenia
   purpura (ITP), systemic lupus
   erythematosus (SLE) 164
ileoanal reservoir surgery, defined 109
ileostomy, defined 109
immune system dysregulation, human
   diseases 4
immunization
   Children's Health Insurance
     Program (CHIP) 600
   electronic health record (EHR) 266
   personal health record (PHR) 292
   quality health care 214
immunosuppressants, ulcerative
   colitis 108
immunosuppressives, defined 325
implantable cardioverter
   defibrillator (ICD)
   defined 83
   heart failure 94

infection
   antibiotics 397
   bronchitis 75
   choosing a hospital 231
   heart valve diseases 96
   human disease transmission 4
   immune system diseases 157
   medical errors 307
   Medicare 574
   medications 323
   prevention at home 481
   screening tests 43
   surgery 247
   urinary system diseases 124
   vaccines 464
infectious diseases
   managing chronic illness 445
   preventive care 511
influenza
   human disease transmission 4
   Medicare 574
   medications 324
   vaccines 461
informed consent
   genetic testing 59
   health-care laws 277
   overview 299–303
   precision medicine 391
injury
   Bell palsy 136
   health insurance plan 601
   heart valve diseases 98
   Medicare 579
   muscle and bone diseases 111
   preventive care 512
   surgery 247
insomnia, prescription pain
   relievers 426
insulin
   ambulatory care 224
   artificial pancreas 499
   biosimilar 385

insulin, *continued*
   medications 325
   nutrition 18
   systemic lupus
      erythematosus (SLE) 165
Insurance Information Institute (III),
   contact information 632
InsureKidsNow.gov, contact
   information 628
intellectual disabilities (IDs)
   Americans with Disabilities Act
      (ADA) 524
   Medicaid 561
   screening test 457
intravenous (IV)
   anesthesia 249
   cardiac arrest 82
   hospitalization 241
   kidney infection 125
intussusception, rotavirus vaccine 471
itchiness, human papillomavirus
   (HPV) vaccine 466

J

Janus kinase (JAK) inhibitors,
   rheumatoid arthritis (RA) 160
joint replacement
   biomaterials 508
   rheumatoid arthritis (RA) 161

K

Kaiser Family Foundation (KFF),
   contact information 632
kidney disease
   chronic diseases 16
   Medicare 576
   over-the-counter (OTC) drugs 351
   quality health care 214
kidney failure
   bladder infection 174
   chronic diseases 10

kidney stones
   described 125
   epilepsy 143
   healthy eating 435
   Paget disease 117

L

laboratory-developed tests (LDTs),
   overview 51–52
laser capture microdissection, Barrett
   esophagus 255
laxatives
   defined 325
   drug interactions 351
lipid, Medicare 572
liquid biopsy, biomarkers 63
lockjaw, vaccines 462
low-density lipoprotein (LDL), familial
   hypercholesterolemia (FH) 37
lung cancer
   Medicare 575
   preventive care 513
   screening tests 47
   tobacco use 15
lung disease
   respiratory system 74
   tobacco use 14
Lyme disease, human disease
   transmission 5
Lynch syndrome, described 29

M

magnetic resonance imaging (MRI)
   diagnosing human diseases 6
   image-guided robotic
      interventions 252
major depressive disorder (MDD),
   Americans with Disabilities
      Act (ADA) 525
malaria, human disease
   transmission 5

Index

mammogram
  family health history 26
  Medicare 575
  screenings tests 45
massage therapy
  complementary and integrative health approaches 567
  defined 449
  human diseases prevention 7
  Parkinson disease (PD) 155
measles
  human disease transmission 5
  vaccines 468
measles, mumps, and rubella (MMR), vaccines for children 461
mechanical heart pump, defined 94
Medicaid
  biosimilars 387
  Children's Health Insurance Program (CHIP) 599
  Health Insurance Portability and Accountability Act (HIPAA) 280
  hospitalization 236
  overview 559–562
  palliative care 516
medical errors
  ambulatory care 225
  prevention 305
medical identity theft, overview 313–316
medical insurance
  hospitalization 235
  second opinion 198
medical orders for life-sustaining treatment (MOLST), advance directives 540
Medicare
  advance care planning 541
  Health Insurance Portability and Accountability Act (HIPAA) 280
  health insurance scams 591
  home health care 579
  hospitalization 231
  medical errors 305
  palliative care 516
  preventive services 571
  second opinion 198
medication-assisted treatment (MAT), Medicaid 561
meditation
  complementary health approaches 567
  coronary heart disease 86
  defined 449
  fibromyalgia 112
  stress 440
MedlinePlus
  contact information 628
  publications
    asthma 75n
    celiac disease 100n
    chronic obstructive pulmonary disease (COPD) 78n
    Crohn's disease 102n
    developmental and behavioral screening tests 460n
    direct-to-consumer genetic testing 60n
    medications 321n
    nondrug pain management 449n
    patient rights 278n
    pneumonia 78n
    precision medicine 391n
    surgery 247n
    tuberculosis (TB) 79n
    urinary incontinence 131n
MedWatch
  adverse drug reactions 404
  generic drugs 381
  medication error 411
  robotically assisted surgery (RAS) 256

meningitis
    infection at home 484
    vaccines 464
meningococcal vaccines, described 468
meridians, managing pain 448
metabolic disruptions, human
    diseases 4
metabolism
    genetic tests 56
    medications 327
    respiratory system 73
methicillin-resistant *Staphylococcus aureus* (MRSA)
    human disease transmission 5
    infection at home 483
microscope, surgery 247
middle ear disease, tobacco use 14
minimally invasive surgery
    defined 122
    image-guided robotic
        interventions 252
misdiagnosis, defined 44
mobile health (mHealth), defined 265
monoamine oxidase inhibitors
    (MAOIs), medications 323
motor neuron diseases (MNDs),
    described 146
multiple sclerosis (MS)
    described 148
    rehabilitative and assistive
        technology 499
muscle relaxants
    cerebral palsy (CP) 139
    defined 326
muscle-strengthening, chronic
    diseases prevention 39, 442
myelopathy, rehabilitative and assistive
    technology 499

N

nasal decongestant, drug
    interactions 334, 408

National Association of Insurance
    Commissioners (NAIC), contact
    information 632
National Cancer Institute (NCI)
    contact information 628
    publications
        biomarker testing 65n
        clinical trials 299n
        Paget disease 118n
National Center for Chronic
    Disease Prevention and Health
    Promotion (NCCDPHP)
    publications
        chronic disease prevention 40n
        chronic diseases 9n, 22n
        health and economic costs 11n
        healthy eating tips 437n
        physical activity 443n
        preventive care 513n
National Center for Complementary
    and Integrative Health (NCCIH)
    contact information 628
    publications
        complementary health
            approach 206n, 208n, 569n
        complementary health
            practitioner 207n
National Center on Birth Defects
    and Developmental Disabilities
    (NCBDDD)
    publication
        disability inclusion 526n
National Health Information Center
    (NHIC), contact information 628
National Healthcare Anti-Fraud
    Association (NHCAA), contact
    information 632
National Heart, Lung, and Blood
    Institute (NHLBI)
    contact information 629
    publications
        bronchitis 76n
        cardiac arrest 84n

Index

National Heart, Lung, and Blood
　Institute (NHLBI)
　publications, *continued*
　　coronary heart disease 89n
　　heart attack 92n
　　heart failure 95n
　　heart valve diseases 98n
National Human Genome Research
　Institute (NHGRI)
　contact information 629
　publication
　　severe combined
　　　immunodeficiency (SCID)
　　　164n
National Institute of Arthritis
　and Musculoskeletal and Skin
　Diseases (NIAMS)
　contact information 629
　publications
　　osteoporosis 117n
　　rheumatoid arthritis (RA) 162n
　　scoliosis 119n
　　spinal stenosis 122n
National Institute of
　Biomedical Imaging and
　Bioengineering (NIBIB)
　publications
　　artificial intelligence (AI) 505n
　　biomaterials 509n
　　image-guided robotic
　　　interventions 255n
　　sensors 508n
National Institute of Diabetes
　and Digestive and Kidney
　Diseases (NIDDK)
　contact information 629
　publications
　　acid reflux 106n
　　artificial pancreas 504n
　　bladder infection 124n
　　gastritis and gastropathy 104n
　　kidney infection
　　　(pyelonephritis) 125n

kidney stones 127n
peptic ulcers 107n
prostate problems 129n
ulcerative colitis 110n
National Institute of Environmental
　Health Sciences (NIEHS)
　publication
　　biomarkers 61n
National Institute of General Medical
　Sciences (NIGMS)
　contact information 629
　publications
　　anesthesia 251n
　　medication in your
　　　body 327n, 329n
National Institute of Mental
　Health (NIMH)
　publication
　　depression 491n
National Institute of Neurological
　Disorders and Stroke (NINDS)
　publications
　　amyotrophic lateral
　　　sclerosis (ALS) 136n
　　Bell palsy 136n
　　cerebral palsy (CP) 140n
　　epilepsy and seizures 145n
　　Huntington disease (HD) 146n
　　motor neuron
　　　diseases (MNDs) 148n
　　multiple sclerosis (MS) 152n
　　neurofibromatosis 154n
National Institute of Nursing
　Research (NINR)
　publication
　　palliative care 479n
National Institute on Aging (NIA)
　contact information 629
　publications
　　advance care planning 544n
　　Alzheimer disease (AD) 134n
　　choosing a doctor 173n
　　doctor's visit 182n, 185n, 186n

653

National Institute on Aging (NIA)
    publications, *continued*
        health information online 298n
        hospitalization 244n
        legal and financial
            planning 550n
        myths about palliative and
            hospice care 519n
        palliative care and hospice
            care 519n
        Parkinson disease (PD) 155n
        talking with your doctor 192n
National Institutes of Health (NIH),
    contact information 629
National Library of Medicine (NLM),
    contact information 630
National Patient Advocate
    Foundation (NPAF), contact
    information 632
National Rehabilitation Information
    Center (NARIC), contact
    information 633
Neisseria meningitidis, vaccines 469
neurofibromatosis, described 152
neurological disorder
    nervous system 134
    palliative care 476
    vaccine 467
neurotransmitters
    anesthesia 251
    Parkinson disease (PD) 154
NIH News in Health
    publications
        artificial intelligence (AI) 507n
        benefits and harms of screening
            tests 45n
        power of pets 452n
nonprescription medications
    complementary health
        approaches 203
    drug interactions 407
    health care 187
    medication usage 347

nonsteroidal antiinflammatory
    drugs (NSAIDs)
        Crohn's disease 100
        peptic ulcer 107
novel small molecule medicines,
    ulcerative colitis 109
Novo Nordisk, counterfeit
    medications 422
nutrition
    celiac disease 100
    children's health 455
    chronic illnesses 13, 433
    chronic obstructive pulmonary
        disease (COPD) 77
    direct-to-consumer genetic
        testing 56
    osteoporosis 113
    preventive care 512
    scoliosis 119
Nutrition Facts labels
    healthy eating plan 436
    preventing medication errors 413

O

obesity
    chronic diseases 10, 40
    coronary heart disease 85
    electronic health record (EHR) 266
    family health history 35
    gastroesophageal reflux
        disease (GERD) 104
    healthy eating 433
Office for Civil Rights (OCR)
    health information rights 280
    Hill-Burton facility 566
    privacy rights 287
Office of Dietary Supplements (ODS),
    contact information 629
Office of Disease Prevention and
    Health Promotion (ODPHP)
    publications
        health care 433n

Index

Office of Disease Prevention and
    Health Promotion (ODPHP)
    publications, *continued*
        health communication
            and health information
            technology 271n
        manage stress 441n
        National Action Plan
            to Improve Health
            Literacy 273n
        preventive care 511n
opioids
    cardiac arrest 82
    excessive alcohol use 22
    misuse of prescription pain
        relievers 424
oral syringe, medication
    errors 413
osteogenesis imperfecta (OI), assistive
    devices 499
osteoporosis
    depression 490
    exercise and physical activity 191
    family health history 26
    Medicare preventive services 572
    preventing chronic diseases 40
    preventive care services 512
    rheumatoid arthritis (RA) 161
    treatment options 112
    women's screening test 47
ovarian cancer, family health
    history 27
over-the-counter (OTC)
    Bell palsy 136
    bronchitis 75
    defined 322
    doctor appointments 335
    drug interactions 408
    gastroesophageal reflux
        disease (GERD) 104
    medical errors 305
    medication errors 413
    medications and children 400

    misuse of prescription pain
        relievers 424
    overview 349–354
    safe medications usage 341
overdiagnosis, screening tests 44
overstimulation, hospital stay 242
overweight
    coronary heart disease 85
    family health history 30
    gastroesophageal reflux
        disease (GERD) 104
    Medicare preventive services 573
    poor nutrition 17
    women's screening test 46
OxyContin, misuse of prescription
    pain relievers 424
oxygen therapy
    bronchitis 76
    cardiac arrest 83
    described 90

P

Paget disease, treatment options 117
pain
    amyotrophic lateral
        sclerosis (ALS) 136
    artificial intelligence (AI) 507
    bladder infection 124
    coronary heart disease 86
    depression 487
    diabetes 16
    doctor's visit 186
    economic costs 10
    fibromyalgia 112
    gastritis and gastropathy 103
    health-care partner 177
    hereditary hemochromatosis 31
    hospice care 518
    human diseases 5
    Medicare 237t
    medications categories 322
    men's screening tests 48

pain, *continued*
   misuse of prescription
     medications 424
   over-the-counter (OTC)
     medications 349
   palliative care 473
   pets 450
   pharmacogenomics 331
   physical activity 447
   preventing chronic diseases 40
   rheumatoid arthritis (RA) 159
   robotic interventions 252
   safe medications usage 341
   surgery 247
   vaccines for children 463
palliative care
   advance care planning 541
   overview 515–516
   seriously ill child 473
Pan American Health
   Organization (PAHO), contact
   information 633
Pap test, Medicare preventive
   services 572
paralysis
   Bell palsy 136
   rehabilitative and assistive
     technology 498
   vaccines for children 463
parathyroid hormone (PTH) analog,
   osteoporosis 116
parathyroid hormone related-protein
   (PTHrP) analog, osteoporosis 116
paratransit, Americans with
   Disabilities Act (ADA) 528
Parkinson disease (PD)
   depression 488
   direct-to-consumer genetic
     testing 56
   palliative care 516
   treatment options 154
pathologists, rehabilitative and
   assistive technology 498

peptic ulcer, treatment options 106
percutaneous coronary
   intervention (PCI)
   described 90
   family health history 35
percutaneous
   nephrolithotomy (PCNL), kidney
   stones 126
personal health record (PHR)
   electronic health (eHealth)
     literacy 265
   health information 431
   overview 291–292
   privacy and security 289
pharmacogenomics
   direct-to-consumer genetic
     testing 56
   overview 329–333
   precision medicine 388
pharmacy-level substitution,
   biosimilars 386
physical activity
   children's health 456
   chronic obstructive pulmonary
     disease (COPD) 77
   coronary heart disease 85
   disease prevention 6
   health and medical apps 297
   overview 442–447
   poor nutrition 17
   preventing chronic diseases 39
   preventive care services 512
   stress 440
   type 1 diabetes 165
physical therapy
   Bell palsy 136
   home health care 580
   Medicaid state plan 561
   motor neuron
     diseases (MNDs) 147
   pain management 449
   rheumatoid arthritis (RA) 159
   scoliosis 119

Index

physician orders for life-sustaining treatment (POLST), advance care planning 540
pills
    human immunodeficiency virus (HIV) 158
    imported drugs 368
    medication errors 414
    over-the-counter (OTC) medications 353
    robotic interventions 255
    tuberculosis (TB) 79
    type 1 diabetes 165
plague, vector transmission 5
pneumonia
    antibiotics 397
    chronic obstructive pulmonary disease (COPD) 77
    hospital-borne transmission 5
    Medicare preventive services 576
    physical activity 445
    severe combined immunodeficiency (SCID) 162
    vaccines for children 464
point of service (POS), defined 607
polysaccharides, vaccines for children 462
posttraumatic stress disorder (PTSD)
    Americans with Disabilities Act (ADA) 524
    rehabilitative and assistive technology 498
    stress 441
power of attorney (POA)
    defined 538
    financial planning 546
pramlintide, artificial pancreas 502
precision medicine, overview 387–391
prediabetes
    economic costs 10
    family health history 30
    Medicare preventive services 573
preferred provider organization (PPO)
    choosing a doctor 170
    choosing a hospital 231
    defined 607
pregnancy
    adverse drug reactions 403
    coronary heart disease 87
    epilepsy and seizures 141
    health-care rights 277
    home-use tests 53
    Medicare preventive services 573
    medications 321
    over-the-counter (OTC) medications 352
    tobacco use 14
    vaccines for children 468
prescription medications
    complementary and alternative medicine (CAM) 208
    gastroesophageal reflux disease (GERD) 104
    health-care professionals 336
    purchasing online 362
    tips for patients 187
preventive care
    health insurance plan 603
    health insurance rights and protections 277
    Health Savings Account (HSA) 589t
    health-care quality 214
    overview 511–513
primary care doctor
    choosing a doctor 171
    health-care professionals 336
    home health care 580
    Marketplace 607
    medical errors 307
    Medicare preventive services 572
    second opinion 200
    type 1 diabetes 165
prostate problems
    drug interactions 351
    treatment options 127

prostate-specific antigen (PSA),
    Medicare preventive services 577
prostatitis, treatment options 127
prosthetics
    Medicaid state plan 561
    rehabilitative and assistive
        technology 495
proton pump inhibitor (PPI), gastritis
    and gastropathy 102
proximal, physical activity 446
psoriasis, depression 488
psychosis, rehabilitative and assistive
    technology 498
psychotherapy
    depression 491
    pain management 449
    stress 441
pulse oximeters, biosensors 508

Q

qi, pain management 448
quality of life (QOL)
    amyotrophic lateral sclerosis
        (ALS) 134
    artificial pancreas 503
    depression 491
    developmental and behavioral
        screening tests 457
    disease prevention 39
    health communication 272
    pain management 448
    palliative care 474, 515
    physical activity 442
    preventive care services 511
    rheumatoid arthritis (RA) 159
    scoliosis 118
    seeking out information 193
    support groups 69

R

radiofrequency ablation (RFA), robotic
    interventions 254

recreation therapy, defined 138
red blood cell (RBC), urinary system
    diseases 123
rehabilitative technology,
    overview 495–499
resilience, children's health 456
respiratory diseases
    overview 73–79
    vaccines for children 468
respiratory droplets, disease
    transmission 4
retinal eye exam, health-care
    quality 214
Reye syndrome, vaccines for
    children 467
rheumatoid arthritis (RA)
    depression 488
    medication categories 323
    osteoporosis 113
    treatment options 159
robotic interventions,
    overview 252–255
robotic prostatectomy, robotic
    interventions 253

S

scoliosis
    neurofibromatosis 153
    treatment options 118
screening tests
    children's development and
        behavior 456
    family health history 25
    health information 431
    health-care quality 215
    Medicare preventive
        services 573
    overview 43–50
    preventive care services 512
second opinion
    health-care quality 212
    overview 197–200

Index

secondhand smoke
  chronic obstructive pulmonary
    disease (COPD) 76
  osteoporosis 114
  preventable chronic diseases 14
seizure
  anticonvulsants 323
  economic costs 10
  neurofibromatosis 153
  overdose 425
  treatment options 140
  vaccines for children 463
selective serotonin reuptake inhibitors (SSRIs), medications 323
self-administered drugs, Medicare 235
semaglutide
  coronary heart disease 88
  counterfeit drugs 422
sepsis
  antibiotics 397
  disease transmission 5
severe combined immunodeficiency (SCID), treatment options 162
sexually transmitted infection (STI)
  alcohol use 22
  disease transmission 4
  Medicare preventive services 577
  screening tests 48
shock wave lithotripsy, kidney stones 126
sickle cell disease (SCD)
  direct-to-consumer genetic testing 56
  Medicaid 562
sigmoidoscopy, health-care quality 215
Sjögren syndrome, systemic lupus erythematosus (SLE) 164
skilled nursing facility (SNF)
  home health care 579
  Medicare 234
  Medicare preventive services 577

skin cancer
  artificial intelligence (AI) 504
  family health history 30
  health-care fraud scams 310
  healthy eating plan 434
smoking
  bronchitis 76
  doctor's appointment 183
  family health history 26
  health-care benefit laws 552
  health-care quality 215
  heart failure 92
  Medicare preventive services 573
  preventable chronic diseases 14
  preventing chronic diseases 39
  preventive care services 512
  screening tests 44
  surgery 248
  urinary incontinence 130
Social Security Act (SSA), Medicaid state plan 560
Social Security number (SSN)
  health information 296
  medical identity theft 313
  Medicare scams 594
soreness
  coronary heart disease 90
  vaccines for children 463
spasms
  bronchodilators 324
  motor neuron diseases (MNDs) 147
  urinary incontinence 130
  vaccines for children 463
spina bifida, rehabilitative and assistive technology 499
spinal cord injuries (SCIs), rehabilitative and assistive technology 499
spinal stenosis, treatment options 119
stability tests, generic drugs 378
standard operating procedures (SOPs), quality assurance (QA) 219

stent
    biomaterials 508
    cardiac arrest 83
    family health history 35
    kidney stones 127
    palliative care 515
steroids
    Bell palsy 136
    chronic obstructive pulmonary
        disease (COPD) 77
    infection prevention 483
    male sex hormones 326
    multiple sclerosis (MS) 149
    ulcerative colitis 108
Streptococcus pneumoniae, vaccines for
    children 469
streptomycin, vaccines for
    children 470
stroke
    advance care planning 538
    biosensors 507
    coronary heart disease 87
    depression 488
    disability inclusion 525
    economic costs 9
    family health history 30
    health-care fraud scams 309
    health-care quality 214
    healthy eating plan 436
    Medicare preventive services 572
    rehabilitative and assistive
        technology 496
    screening tests 47
subcutaneous cardioverter device
    (SCD), cardiac arrest 84
sudden infant death syndrome (SIDS)
    healthy eating plan 433
    tobacco use 14
summary plan description (SPD)
    disability benefits 609
    health-care benefit laws 555
surgery
    antibiotics 397

    artificial intelligence (AI) 506
    Bell palsy 136
    biomarker testing 62
    cardiac arrest 83
    Crohn's disease 100
    decision-making 189
    doctor's visits 178
    family health history 35
    health information privacy
        rights 286
    health-care quality 212
    hospital stay 242
    infection prevention 483
    medical errors 305
    Medicare 234
    overview 245–249
    Paget disease 117
    pain management 449
    prostatitis 128
    rheumatoid arthritis (RA) 159
    second opinion 198
    tobacco use 16
    vaccines for children 471
surgical site infection (SSI),
    surgery 247
surrogate, advance care planning 538
Surveillance, Epidemiology, and End
    Results (SEER) Program
    publications
        cardiovascular system 81n
        digestive system 99n
        muscular system 111n
        nervous system 133n
        respiratory system 73n
        skeletal system 112n
        urinary system 123n
systemic lupus erythematosus (SLE)
    depression 488
    treatment options 164

T

tai chi
    disease prevention 7
    Parkinson disease (PD) 155

Index

tamper-evident packaging (TEP), over-the-counter (OTC) medications 353
targeted temperature management (TTM), cardiac arrest 83
tetanus, vaccines for children 461
Therapeutic Lifestyle Changes (TLC) program, coronary heart disease 85
three-dimensional (3D) near-infrared imaging, robotic interventions 254
thrombolytics, defined 323
thyroid
  depression 488
  drug interactions 351
  medications 325
  osteoporosis 115
  systemic lupus erythematosus (SLE) 164
thyroiditis, systemic lupus erythematosus (SLE) 164
total artificial heart, heart failure 94
toxoids, vaccines for children 461
tranquilizer
  defined 327
  drug interactions 351
transcatheter aortic valve replacement (TAVR), heart valve disease 98
transcranial direct current stimulation (tDCS), rehabilitative and assistive technology 497
transcranial magnetic stimulation (TMS), rehabilitative and assistive technology 496
transcutaneous electrical nerve stimulation (TENS), nondrug pain management 448
transmyocardial laser revascularization (TMR), coronary heart disease 88
trauma, health-care quality 214
traumatic brain injury (TBI)
  Americans with Disabilities Act (ADA) 525
  rehabilitative and assistive technology 499
tricyclics, antidepressants 323
triglyceride
  coronary heart disease 87
  Medicare preventive services 572
  tobacco use 15
tuberculosis (TB)
  disease transmission 5
  infection prevention 484
  Medicaid benefits 561
  treatment options 78
tumor
  biomarker testing 61
  disease classification 3
  heart valve disease 97
  neurofibromatosis 152
  pharmacogenomics 330
  robotic interventions 253
typhoid fever, disease transmission 5

U

ulcerative colitis, treatment options 108
ultrasound
  Medicare preventive services 571
  men's screening test 48
  radiological examinations 6
  robotic interventions 252
ureteroscopy, kidney stones 126
urinary incontinence, treatment options 129
urinary system diseases, overview 123–131
urinary tract infections (UTIs)
  bladder infection 123
  disease transmission 5

U.S. Department of Health and
    Human Services (HHS)
    contact information 630
    publications
        health information 286n
        Health Insurance Portability
            and Accountability Act
            (HIPAA) 285n
        informed consent 303n
        Medicaid program 560n
        privacy, security, and electronic
            health records (EHRs) 268n
U.S. Department of Labor (DOL)
    contact information 630
    publications
        Consolidated Omnibus
            Budget Reconciliation
            Act (COBRA) 555n
        disability benefits 618n
        Family and Medical Leave
            Act (FMLA) 535n
        Health Insurance Portability
            and Accountability
            Act (HIPAA) 553n
U.S. Equal Employment Opportunity
    Commission (EEOC), contact
    information 630
U.S. Food and Drug
    Administration (FDA)
    contact information 630
    publications
        biosimilar and interchangeable
            biologics 387n
        buying medications online 364n
        counterfeit medication 424n
        drug interactions 410n
        general drug categories 327n
        generic drugs 381n
        health fraud scams 311n
        home use tests 53n, 54n
        image-guided robotic
            interventions 256n

laboratory developed tests 52n
managing benefits and risks of
    medications 344n
medical device 504n
medications 339n
medications and
    children 401n
misuse of prescription pain
    relievers 426n
over-the-counter (OTC)
    medications 349n, 354n
prescription drugs 366n
reducing medication
    errors 415n
safety concerns of imported
    drugs 374n
side effects (adverse
    reactions) 406n
taking medications 396n
unapproved drugs 421n
using medications safely 347n
vaccines for children 472n

V

vaccines
    chronic obstructive pulmonary
        disease (COPD) 77
    disease prevention 6
    health information 431
    Medicare preventive services 576
    overview 460–473
    preventive care services 512
    rheumatoid arthritis (RA) 162
    see also antibiotics
vancomycin-resistant
    Enterococcus (VRE), infection
    prevention 483
vector transmission 5
ventilators
    infection prevention 482
    motor neuron
        diseases (MNDs) 148

Index

viral load, human immunodeficiency virus (HIV) 158
vitamins
  celiac disease 99
  complementary and alternative medicine (CAM) 567
  doctor's appointment 180
  healthy eating plan 436
  medical errors 305
  medication categories 327
  medications and children 400
  safe medications usage 341

W

wearable cardioverter device (WCD), cardiac arrest 84
weight management
  coronary heart disease 88
  see also physical activity
wheezing
  antibiotics 398
  vaccines for children 467
  see also asthma
white blood cells (WBCs)
  immune system diseases 157
  multiple sclerosis (MS) 151
  musculoskeletal diseases 111
whole exome sequencing (WES)
  biomarker tests 63
  direct-to-consumer genetic testing 60
whole genome sequencing (WGS), biomarker tests 63
whooping cough, vaccines for children 462
wrong-site surgery, medical errors 257
wrong-site, wrong-procedure, wrong-patient errors (WSPEs), overview 257–258

X

x-linked severe combined immunodeficiency (XSCID), immune disease management 162
x-ray
  Children's Health Insurance Program (CHIP) 600
  disability inclusion 525
  health-care quality 212
  heart attack 90
  human diseases 6
  medical benefits 560
  Medicare 234
  osteoporosis 34
  patient privacy 286
  rheumatoid arthritis (RA) 161
  safe medications usage 346
  women's screening test 47
  see also screening tests

Y

yoga
  complementary and alternative medicine (CAM) 207
  disease prevention 7
  fibromyalgia 112
  insurance coverage 567
  Parkinson disease (PD) 155

Z

Zika, vector transmission 5
zinc, complementary and alternative medicine (CAM) 207